Society and Psychosis

Psychiatry is in the process of rediscovering its roots. It seemed as if the long history of interest in the impact of society on the rates and course of serious mental illness had been forgotten, overtaken by the advances of neuroscience and genetics. However, as our knowledge of physiological and genetic processes improves, it becomes increasingly clear that social conditions and experiences over the life course are crucial to achieving a full understanding. Old controversies are giving way to genuinely integrated models in which social, psychological and biological factors interact over time, culminating in the onset of psychosis. This book reviews these issues from an international perspective, laying the foundations for a new understanding of the psychotic disorders, with profound implications for health policy and clinical practice. It will be of interest to academics, researchers, clinicians and all those who work with people with a serious mental illness.

Craig Morgan is Senior Lecturer at the Institute of Psychiatry, King's College London, UK.

Kwame McKenzie is Professor of Psychiatry at the University of Toronto and the University of Central Lancashire, and Senior Scientist and Clinician at the Centre for Addictions and Mental Health, Toronto, Canada.

Paul Fearon is Senior Lecturer and Head of the Section of Epidemiology and Social Psychiatry at the Institute of Psychiatry, King's College, London, UK.

Society and Psychosis

Craig Morgan

Section of Social and Cultural Psychiatry, Health Service and Population Research Department, Institute of Psychiatry, King's College London, UK

Kwame McKenzie

University of Toronto, Canada; University of Central Lancashire, UK

Paul Fearon

Section of Epidemiology and Social Psychiatry, Department of Psychological Medicine and Psychiatry, Institute of Psychiatry, King's College London, UK

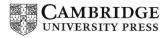
CAMBRIDGE
UNIVERSITY PRESS

CAMBRIDGE
UNIVERSITY PRESS

University Printing House, Cambridge CB2 8BS, United Kingdom

One Liberty Plaza, 20th Floor, New York, NY 10006, USA

477 Williamstown Road, Port Melbourne, VIC 3207, Australia

314-321, 3rd Floor, Plot 3, Splendor Forum, Jasola District Centre, New Delhi - 110025, India

103 Penang Road, #05-06/07, Visioncrest Commercial, Singapore 238467

Cambridge University Press is part of the University of Cambridge.

It furthers the University's mission by disseminating knowledge in the pursuit of education, learning and research at the highest international levels of excellence.

www.cambridge.org
Information on this title: www.cambridge.org/9780521689595

First published 2008

A catalogue record for this publication is available from the British Library

ISBN 978-0-521-68959-5 Paperback

Cambridge University Press has no responsibility for the persistence or
accuracy of URLs for external or third-party internet websites referred to in
this publication, and does not guarantee that any content on such websites is,
or will remain, accurate or appropriate.

....

Every effort has been made in preparing this book to provide accurate and
up-to-date information which is in accord with accepted standards and practice
at the time of publication. Although case histories are drawn from actual cases,
every effort has been made to disguise the identities of the individuals involved.
Nevertheless, the authors, editors and publishers can make no warranties that the
information contained herein is totally free from error, not least because clinical
standards are constantly changing through research and regulation. The authors,
editors and publishers therefore disclaim all liability for direct or consequential
damages resulting from the use of material contained in this book. Readers
are strongly advised to pay careful attention to information provided by the
manufacturer of any drugs or equipment that they plan to use.

Contents

Contributors

Jennifer H. Barnett
Department of Psychiatry
University of Cambridge
Box 189
Addenbrooke's Hospital
Cambridge
UK

Paul Bebbington
Department of Mental Health Sciences
University College London (Bloomsbury Campus)
Wolfson Building
48 Riding House Street
London
UK

Jane Boydell
Section of Epidemiology and Social Psychiatry
Department of Psychiatry and Psychological Medicine
Box 63
Institute of Psychiatry
De Crespigny Park
London
UK

Michaeline Bresnahan
Department of Epidemiology
Mailman School of Public Health
Columbia University
Presbyterian Hospital
722 West 168th Street
New York, NY
USA

Tom Craig
Section of Social and Cultural Psychiatry
Health Service and Population Research Department
Box 33
Institute of Psychiatry
De Crespigny Park
London
UK

Paul Fearon
Section of Epidemiology and Social Psychiatry
Department of Psychological Medicine and Psychiatry
Box 63
Institute of Psychiatry
De Crespigny Park
London
UK

Helen Fisher
Department of Psychiatry and Psychological
Medicine, and Social, Genetic and
Developmental Psychiatry Centre
Box 63
Institute of Psychiatry
De Crespigny Park
London
UK

David Fowler
School of Medicine, Health Policy and
Practice
University of East Anglia
Norwich
UK

Daniel Freeman
Department of Psychology
Box 77
Institute of Psychiatry
De Crespigny Park
London
UK

Philippa Garety
Department of Psychology
Box 77
Institute of Psychiatry
De Crespigny Park
London
UK

Kim Hopper
Nathan Klein Institute for Psychiatric
Research and Mailman School of Public
Health
Colombia University
722 West 168th Street
Sociomedical Sciences #928
New York, NY
USA

Gerard Hutchinson
Psychiatry Unit
Department of Clinical Medical Sciences
University of the West Indies
Mount Hope
Champs Fleurs
Trinidad

Peter B. Jones
Department of Psychiatry
University of Cambridge
Box 189
Addenbrooke's Hospital
Cambridge
UK

Aliya Kassam
Health Service and Population Research
Department
Box 29
Institute of Psychiatry
De Crespigny Park
London
UK

Elizabeth Kuipers
Department of Psychology
Box 77
Institute of Psychiatry
De Crespigny Park
London
UK

Julian Leff
Department of Psychiatry and Psychological
Medicine
Box 63
Institute of Psychiatry
De Crespigny Park
London
UK

Dana March
Department of Epidemiology
Mailman School of Public Health
Columbia University
Presbyterian Hospital
722 West 168th Street
New York, NY
USA

Kwame McKenzie
Centre for Addictions and Mental Health
University of Toronto
455 Spadina Av.
Toronto
Canada

Craig Morgan
Section of Social and Cultural Psychiatry
Health Service and Population Research
Department
Box 33
Institute of Psychiatry
De Crespigny Park
London
UK

Inez Myin-Germeys
Department of Psychiatry and
Neuropsychology
Maastricht University
PO Box 616 (Location DOT10)
6200 MD Maastricht
The Netherlands

Ezra Susser
Department of Epidemiology
Mailman School of Public Health
Columbia University
Presbyterian Hospital
722 West 168th Street
New York, NY
USA

Graham Thornicroft
Health Service and Population Research
Department
Box 29
Institute of Psychiatry
De Crespigny Park
London
UK

Pekka Tienari
Department of Psychiatry
The University of Oulu
PO Box 5000
90014 Oulu
Finland

Jim van Os
Department of Psychiatry and
Neuropsychology
Maastricht University
PO Box 616 (Location DOT10)
6200 MD Maastricht
The Netherlands

Karl-Erik Wahlberg
Department of Psychiatry
The University of Oulu
PO Box 5000
90014 Oulu
Finland

Richard Warner
Department of Psychiatry
University of Colorado at Boulder
233 UCB
Boulder, CO
USA

Acknowledgements

We would like to thank Sonya Levin for early assistance, and Dr Helen Billinge for invaluable help with referencing and proofreading.

Introduction

Craig Morgan, Kwame McKenzie and Paul Fearon

Psychiatry has recently rediscovered its roots. It seemed as if its long history of interest in the impact of society on the rates and course of serious mental illness had been forgotten, overtaken by the inexorable advance of neuroscience and genetics. However, as our knowledge of the physiological and genetic processes linked to psychosis has advanced, it has become increasingly clear that social conditions and experiences over the life course are important in the aetiology of psychosis. Old dichotomies and controversies are giving way to genuinely integrated models, in which social, psychological and biological factors are seen to interact over time, culminating in the onset of psychosis. The influence of society extends beyond onset to shape course and outcome, with important implications for public policy and service delivery. In this context, it is useful to take stock of what is currently known about the links between society and psychosis, limitations to this knowledge, unanswered questions and future research priorities. *Society and Psychosis* aims to do this.

Categories and continua

There have been many attempts to define psychosis. Wing (1978), for example, gave a relatively narrow description: 'A 'psychotic' state is one characterised by delusions or hallucinations, in which the individual is unable to differentiate his grossly abnormal thought processes from external reality and remains unaware of his deficiency.' (pp. 44–5.) Less restrictive definitions include hallucinatory experiences that the sufferer realises are abnormal and, more broadly still, others include disorganised speech and grossly disorganised behaviour (APA, 1994). Psychotic symptoms can occur in a range of disorders identified in the *Diagnostic and Statistical Manual* (APA, 1994) and the *International Classification of Diseases* (WHO, 1992), including schizophrenia spectrum disorders, affective disorders, a range of brief psychotic disorders and grief reactions.

The purposes of classification and diagnosis in psychiatry are the same as in the rest of medicine. That is, diagnosis is intended to communicate information about symptoms, aetiology, prognosis and optimal treatment. In relation to psychotic mental disorders, there have been recurrent questions about whether specific diagnoses, particularly schizophrenia, provide such information reliably. For example, it has long been acknowledged that the outcome of schizophrenia is variable. While the textbook account – that approximately a third recover, a third have an episodic course and a third have a continuous course – may need to be revised as new research emerges, there is, nevertheless, clear heterogeneity in outcome for those diagnosed with schizophrenia (and those with other psychotic disorders) (Menezes *et al.*, 2006). Likewise, responsiveness to antipsychotic medication is not uniform, and there is a sizeable minority of subjects who remain resistant to most common forms of treatment. Furthermore, an increasing body of recent research suggests that large numbers of people in the general population experience psychotic (or psychotic-like) symptoms: 10–15% in some studies (Verdoux and van Os, 2002). As a consequence, the debate has resurfaced on whether psychotic disorders are discrete entities, marked by a clear disjunction from normal experience, or whether they lie on a continuum with normality (van Os *et al.*, 2000). This debate is fuelled by research in cognitive psychology focusing on specific psychotic symptoms, such as hallucinations and delusions, rather than on diagnostic categories (see Chapter 14). The lack of diagnostic specificity of such positive psychotic symptoms is one observation that has led some to argue that it is negative symptoms (e.g., blunted affect, asociality, anhedonia, poor self-care, etc.) that are at the core of schizophrenia. This is also contributing to the renewed debate about the validity and utility of schizophrenia as a diagnostic entity (Bentall, 2003; Lieberman and First, 2007).

This book is concerned with psychosis in a broad sense, and the tension between whether the focus should be on psychotic symptoms, conceived as lying on a continuum with normality, or on discrete diagnosable psychotic disorders will be evident throughout these pages. As this issue remains unresolved, this tension is welcome; research from both perspectives promises to increase understanding and in time will, hopefully, contribute to resolving this debate. This is not simply an academic point. Efforts to understand and treat psychosis will depend to a large degree on accurate conceptualisations, and it may be that our current efforts are hampered by lack of clarity over what the unit of investigation should be: symptoms, such as delusions and hallucinations, or categories, such as schizophrenia and bipolar disorder. This is one of the central issues in psychosis research.

A final point on this is necessary. While this book is concerned with psychosis in a broad sense, as much of the existing research focuses on schizophrenia, this will frequently be used as an example, on the basis that understanding schizophrenia in particular may give us insights into psychosis in general.

Changing views of the epidemiology of schizophrenia

One of the basic tenets of the epidemiology of schizophrenia has been that the incidence is more or less uniform around the world (Crow, 2000). The WHO multi-country studies of the 1970s and 1980s contributed much to establishing this orthodoxy, particularly the finding from the Determinants of Outcomes of Severe Mental Disorders (DOSMeD) study that there were no statistically significant differences between the 12 centres studied in the incidence of narrowly defined schizophrenia (Jablensky et al., 1992). The apparent invariance of schizophrenia has been taken as evidence that the disorder is primarily genetic; the usual variability that would be expected if the occurrence of schizophrenia was influenced by local social environments was simply not evident (Crow, 2000).

In recent years, new research and meta-analyses have challenged the interpretation that schizophrenia, even narrowly defined, has a uniform incidence (Cantor-Graae and Selten, 2005; McGrath et al., 2004). A comprehensive meta-analysis of 100 incidence studies by John McGrath and his colleagues (2004) at the University of Queensland found marked variations in the incidence of psychosis by place and persons. For example, the variation in incidence rates between sites covered in the studies reviewed was more than fivefold. The review further confirmed higher rates in urban centres and in migrant groups, this latter finding being replicated in a more specific review (Cantor-Graae and Selten, 2005). In fact, from the beginning, the interpretation of a uniform incidence did not go unchallenged. A number of commentators pointed out that, although statistically non-significant, there was a twofold difference between the highest and lowest reported incidence rates for narrow schizophrenia in the DOSMeD study, and, for broadly defined schizophrenia, there were marked differences between the various centres (Kleinman, 1991). As McGrath (2007) has commented, it seems that the contours of the epidemiology of schizophrenia are not flat after all.

An uneven epidemiological terrain does not, in itself, point towards a particular aetiology, but it does open the door for investigating causes through the lens of differences in incidence between populations and places.

The aetiology of psychosis

The causes of schizophrenia and other psychoses have been the subject of intense research efforts and frequently acrimonious debates. In the crudest terms, these debates have centred on the question of whether the causes reside in individual biology, intrapsychic conflict or socioenvironmental stress. At various points there have been attempts to bridge these positions within biopsychosocial frameworks (e.g., Engel, 1980). However, it is arguable that, for all the lip service paid to some kind of vague biopsychosocial model of aetiology, at various points one side or other has dominated. In the past 20 years, for example, the dominant view has been that schizophrenia (psychosis) is a genetic brain disease, the onset of which is the product of a neurodevelopmental process (Andreasen, 2000). Social factors, if they have been assigned a role at all, have been relegated to the status of triggers, serving merely to hasten the onset of a largely biologically determined disease. This view, however, is changing.

The proposition that socioenvironmental factors are aetiologically important in psychosis has, in the past, been undermined by two particular problems. First, as schizophrenia and other psychoses are often preceded by a period of functional decline, leading to problems in maintaining social relationships and employment, it is extremely difficult to determine the causal direction of any association between markers of socioeconomic adversity and schizophrenia. Second, the mechanisms by which society impacts on individuals to increase risk of schizophrenia and other psychoses have been poorly specified. The numbers of people who are exposed to adverse social conditions, traumatic life events, and so on, far outstrip the numbers who ever experience serious mental illness. The types of adverse social conditions associated with psychosis are not specific (they are also associated with a range of other disorders), and most people who are exposed do not develop a serious mental illness. If such experiences are relevant to the onset of psychosis, how is it that such a relatively small proportion develops schizophrenia? The chapters in Part II of this book address these questions directly.

There are at least three developments that are contributing to the renewed interest in the role of the social environment in the aetiology of psychosis. First, as already discussed, it is becoming clear that there are notable variations in the incidence of psychosis both between and within countries. The higher incidences in urban centres and in migrant and ethnic minority groups, in the absence of concrete evidence one way or the other, at the very least suggests that there are social factors that occur more commonly in these settings and groups and that merit further study. Second, there has been a series of recent studies that have overcome the problem of direction of causation by using data from large population-based registers and prospective cohorts (Janssen *et al.*, 2004; Pedersen and Mortensen, 2001). These have continued to produce findings that link exposure to negative social experiences and circumstances prior to the development of psychosis and subsequent onset (e.g., Spauwen *et al.*, 2006). Where the extent of exposure, either in terms of frequency or severity, has been measured, some of these studies have found evidence of dose–response relationships, such that the greater the exposure to, say, sexual abuse, the greater the risk of psychosis (e.g., Janssen *et al.*, 2004). Finally, and perhaps most importantly, one consequence of the recent rapid advances in neuroscience and genetics is that we are beginning to understand how social experience along the life course interacts with genotype, and impacts on biological development, to shape adult outcomes. These insights are now being used to produce biological models linking adverse social experiences, including childhood trauma, and adult psychosis (e.g., Spauwen et al., 2006; Teicher et al., 2003). All of the chapters in this book that address aetiology reflect this development; they all propose candidate mechanisms that, at least in theory, could account for the observed associations between the various social exposures and psychosis. Vague notions of susceptibility or diathesis, proposed in the past, are being replaced by concrete evidence-based biological mechanisms linking social experience with brain development and psychosis (Teicher et al., 2003).

Course and outcome of psychosis

In contrast to the controversy that surrounds the possible role of socioenvironmental factors in the aetiology of psychosis, it is generally accepted that the social environment can influence the course and outcome of psychosis. Over 30 years ago, Wing and Brown (1970) showed how living in long-stay institutions contributed to the development of behaviours and symptoms that had been assumed to be intrinsic features of schizophrenia. There is now a considerable body of research showing that critical and hostile (i.e., high expressed emotion) home environments can increase the risk of relapse, particularly in the absence of antipsychotic medication (Kavanagh, 1992). Further, negative social attitudes and responses towards those with psychosis exclude many from opportunities for employment and productive social relationships, opportunities that have been shown to promote recovery (Warner, 2000). The finding from the WHO DOSMeD study, that outcomes are better in developing than in developed countries, is usually interpreted in these terms (Jablensky et al., 1992), i.e., as reflecting the fact that responses to psychosis in the developing world are less stigmatising and sufferers are more readily reintegrated back into family and social groups. This interpretation, however, has never been fully tested and new analyses are beginning to question whether the course and outcome really is more benign in the developing world (Patel et al., 2006).

Research further shows that interventions designed to modify social environments and promote social reintegration can improve course and outcome (Leff and Warner, 2006). The classic example is family intervention to reduce levels of expressed emotion (Kuipers et al., 2002). However, the use of specific targeted social interventions in routine mental health care is sporadic at best, and research on social interventions is swamped by that on psychopharmacology. To a degree, the introduction of novel antipsychotic medication has provided further impetus to psychopharmacological research; whether these deliver the advertised benefits over and above first-generation neuroleptics is questionable (Jones et al., 2006; Lieberman *et al.*, 2005). In contrast, research on psychosocial interventions is slight; again, however, there are signs of change, particularly with an increasing number of studies of cognitive interventions for psychosis (e.g., Kuipers *et al.*, 2006).

Society and psychosis

The primary purpose of this book is to reflect these current trends in the study of society and psychosis, and to contribute to developing an agenda for future research. There have been many swings and trends in psychosis research, as noted above. In Chapter 2, Julian Leff sets the scene by surveying the shifting fashions of psychiatric research. By reflecting on his own involvement in research over the past 30 years, and analysing trends in the publication of psychosocial and biological papers in the *British Journal of Psychiatry* and the *American Journal of Psychiatry*, Leff argues that the wider social, economic and political context often determines what research is funded and published. It is for future analyses to assess the external pressures that are shaping current shifts towards more fully integrated biopsychosocial models of psychosis. The hope is that, with each shift, we move closer to a fuller understanding that allows for more effective interventions.

Theoretical and conceptual foundations

The first part of the book provides a series of orientating chapters. In attempting to understand the relationship between society and psychosis, there is much that can be learned from the social sciences. The historical relationship between psychiatry and the social sciences, however, has been fraught, and scepticism concerning the role of the social environment in the aetiology of psychosis is reflected in continuing scepticism about the value of the social sciences. In Chapter 3, Craig Morgan provides an overview of this often acrimonious relationship and outlines a number of areas in which the social sciences can provide important contributions to current efforts at investigating links between society and psychosis. In Chapter 4, Dana March and her colleagues provide an introduction to conceptualising the social world. To understand how social conditions and experiences impact on individuals, we need conceptual tools that allow us to define and measure what are continual social processes. As research now shows broad associations between relatively crude variables (e.g., urbanicity, migration) and risk of psychosis, there is a need to move on to investigating directly the social processes that potentially underpin these relationships. In this, basic conceptual and theoretical work will be essential.

Perhaps the one area with the greatest potential for clarifying the nature of the relationship between the social environment and risk of psychosis is that of gene–environment interaction. As more research emerges, showing that the impact of a specific environmental factor, such as life events or cannabis consumption, on the risk of psychosis is influenced by genotype, this will become an increasingly important area of study. In Chapter 5, Jennifer Barnett and Peter Jones provide a detailed conceptual and methodological overview of gene–environment interplay in psychosis. The ideas introduced here are picked up and illustrated with specific examples in many of the chapters in the second part of the book. The prominence given to gene–environment interactions in these chapters further emphasises the extent to which the social and biological are being combined in current psychosis research.

Social factors and the onset of psychosis

The social environment can be considered at different stages and at different levels: for example, at the level of the individual, the family or society. The chapters in the second part of the book review specific areas of research, setting out what is currently known, the limitations to what is known and, as appropriate, methodological issues and challenges for future research.

In the first of these, Chapter 6, Jane Boydell and Kwame McKenzie examine ecological-level research, an area gaining increasing attention, partly because of the repeated finding that rates of psychosis are higher in urban centres (van Os, 2004), and partly because of increasing interest in social capital and mental illness (e.g., McKenzie and Harpham, 2006). In Chapters 7 and 8, research on early childhood adversity and intrafamilial factors is reviewed. These are contentious areas. In Chapter 7, Helen Fisher and Tom Craig consider the evidence for a link between forms of childhood trauma, including sexual and physical abuse, and the risk of psychosis. Their review reaches a more tentative conclusion than other recent commentators in this area (Read *et al.*, 2005), pointing to important methodological issues for future research. Fisher and Craig present a preliminary theoretical framework as a guide for subsequent research. In Chapter 8, Pekka Tienari and Karl-Erik Wahlberg examine research on families and psychosis. This is a particularly sensitive topic given the unfortunate history of families, particularly mothers, being blamed for causing schizophrenia. As Tienari and Wahlberg explain, families do not cause psychosis. It may, nonetheless, be that certain forms of communication within families impact on child development in such a way as to increase vulnerability to later emotional and mental disorder, Where there is also a genetic susceptibility, the two may interact to increase risk of psychosis. However, these are not predestined pathways, and individual resources and subsequent positive experiences may be protective. The potential links between early adversity and later adversity is one of the themes of Chapter 9, in which Inez Myin-Germeys and Jim van Os consider research on adult adversity. While reviewing the field in general, Myin-Germeys and van Os also present data from a series of innovative studies assessing the impact of daily hassles on the development and exacerbation of psychotic symptoms. It is apparent from this work that a range of different factors operate over the life course to increase susceptibility to psychosis. The development, or exacerbation, of psychotic symptoms in the vulnerable may be provoked by specific life events or regular daily stresses.

In the final chapter in this part, Chapter 10, Kwame McKenzie and his colleagues focus on migration, ethnicity and psychosis. Within a broad review of this field, they focus in detail on the evidence that the African-Caribbean population in the UK is at greatly increased risk of psychosis and, from this, propose a preliminary sociodevelopmental model of psychosis.

Social factors and outcomes

The third part of the book contains three chapters focusing, broadly, on social responses to psychosis and their effects. In the first, Chapter 11, Richard Warner shows that social interventions can impact positively on the course of psychosis and sufferers' quality of life. In Chapter 12, Graham Thornicroft and his colleagues provide a detailed and wide-ranging review of literature on stigma and psychosis. Schizophrenia remains heavily stigmatised, and sufferers frequently experience discrimination and social exclusion. Such adverse societal responses may worsen outcomes and quality of life for those with schizophrenia. What Chapter 12 makes clear is the need for urgent strategies to tackle stigma and promote social reintegration. In Chapter 13, Kim Hopper reviews the intriguing finding that the outcomes of schizophrenia may be better in developing than developed countries; a finding that, as noted above, has long been considered as evidence that social and cultural contexts are major determinants of course and outcome.

Models and conclusions

In parallel with a resurgence of interest in social factors and psychosis, there has been a rapid development of research from a cognitive psychology perspective, focusing on specific symptoms and examining the role of variables, such as attributions and emotion, in the aetiology of psychosis (e.g., Bentall, 2003). In much of the book, the focus is very much on how social experience interacts with biology to increase the risk of psychosis. A further framework for linking these is a cognitive model of psychosis. In Chapter 14, Paul Bebbington and his colleagues review this expanding field and explain how a cognitive model can provide a further explanatory link between social adversity and psychosis; a framework, moreover, that retains the important role of biology and, arguably, begins to resemble a genuinely biopsychosocial model of psychosis.

In the final chapter, we present a formulation of the state of the art of research into the impact of society on psychosis, and offer thoughts on an agenda for future research. However, distinguishing social from biological research, particularly in relation to aetiology, is increasingly artificial. Studies on the impact of social factors will need to take account of the potential mediating role of a number of biological variables, including genotype and biochemistry. There appears to be an emerging consensus that new research needs to be undertaken with, rather than in isolation from, specialists in the biological and psychological sciences. Integration of different fields and different types of knowledge is the way forward for research into psychosis and is reflected throughout the chapters of *Society and Psychosis*.

Despite the clear importance of investigating social aspects of psychosis and all the work that has been done to date, there is still much more that needs to be done. Scientists always seem to conclude with a call for more research. We argue for a different type of research, using new methodologies and conceptualisations, which will help us to link knowledge of the social world with knowledge of genetics, biology and psychology to increase our understanding of psychosis.

REFERENCES

American Psychiatric Association (1994). *Diagnostic and Statistical Manual of Mental Disorders*, 4th edn. Washington, DC: American Psychiatric Association.

Andreasen, N. (2000). Schizophrenia: the fundamental questions. *Brain Research Reviews*, **31**, 106–12.

Bentall, R. (2003). *Madness Explained: Psychosis and Human Nature*. London: Allen Lane.

Cantor-Graae, E. and Selten, J. P. (2005). Schizophrenia and migration: a meta-analysis and review. *American Journal of Psychiatry*, **162** (1), 12–24.

Crow, T. J. (2000). Schizophrenia as the price that *Homo sapiens* pays for language: a resolution of the central paradox in the origin of the species. *Brain Research Reviews*, **31**, 118–29.

Engel, G. L. (1980). The clinical application of the biopsychosocial model. *American Journal of Psychiatry*, **137**, 535–44.

Jablensky, A., Sartorius, N., Ernberg, G. *et al.* (1992). Schizophrenia: manifestations, incidence and course in different cultures. A World Health Organization ten-country study. *Psychological Medicine. Monograph Supplement*, **20**, 1–97.

Janssen, I., Krabbendam, L., Bak, M. *et al.* (2004). Childhood abuse as a risk factor for psychosis. *Acta Psychiatrica Scandinavica*, **109**, 38–45.

Jones, P. B., Barnes, T. R. E., Davies, L. *et al.* (2006). Randomized controlled trial of the effect on quality of life of second- vs first-generation antipsychotic drugs in schizophrenia: cost utility of the latest antipsychotic drugs in schizophrenia study (CUtLASS 1). *Archives of General Psychiatry*, **63**, 1079–87.

Kavanagh, N. (1992). Recent developments in Expressed Emotion and schizophrenia. *British Journal of Psychiatry*, **160**, 601–20.

Kleinman, A. (1991). *Rethinking Psychiatry: From Cultural Category to Personal Experience*. New York: The Free Press.

Kuipers, E., Leff, J. and Lam, D. (2002). *Family Work for Schizophrenia: A Practical Guide*, 2nd edn. London: Gaskell.

Kuipers, E., Garety, P., Fowler, D. *et al.* (2006). Cognitive, emotional, and social processes in psychosis: refining cognitive behavioural therapy for persistent positive symptoms. *Schizophrenia Bulletin*, **32** (suppl. 1), s24–s31.

Leff, J. and Warner, R. (2006). *Social Inclusion of People with Mental Illness*. Cambridge: Cambridge University Press.

Lieberman, J. A. and First, M. B. (2007). Renaming schizophrenia. *British Medical Journal*, **334**, 108.

Lieberman, J. A., Stroup, T. S., McEvoy, J. P. *et al.* (2005). Effectiveness of antipsychotic drugs in patients with chronic schizophrenia. *New England Journal of Medicine*, **353** (12), 1209–23.

McGrath, J. (2007). The surprisingly rich contours of schizophrenia epidemiology. *Archives of General Psychiatry*, **64**, 14–15.

McGrath, J., Saha, S., Wellham, J. *et al.* (2004). A systematic review of the incidence of schizophrenia: the distribution of rates and the influence of sex, urbanicity, migrant status, and methodology. *BMC Medicine*, **2**, 13.

McKenzie, K. and Harpham, T. (eds) (2006). *Social Capital and Mental Health*. London: Jessica Kingsley.

Menezes, N. M., Arenovich, T. and Zipursky, R. B. (2006). A systematic review of longitudinal outcome studies of first-episode psychosis. *Psychological Medicine*, **36** (10), 1349–62.

Patel, V., Cohen, A., Thara, R. *et al.* (2006). Is the outcome of schizophrenia really better in developing countries? *Revista Brasileira Psiquiatria*, **28** (2), 129–52.

Pedersen, C. and Mortensen, P. (2001). Evidence of a dose-response relationship between urbanicity during upbringing and schizophrenia risk. *Archives of General Psychiatry*, **58**, 1039–46.

Read, J., van Os, J., Morrison, A. P. *et al.* (2005). Childhood trauma, psychosis and schizophrenia: a literature review with theoretical and clinical implications. *Acta Psychiatrica Scandinavica*, **112**, 330–50.

Spauwen, J., Krabbendam, L., Lieb, R. *et al.* (2006). Impact of psychological trauma on the development of psychotic symptoms: relationship with psychosis proneness. *British Journal of Psychiatry*, **188**, 527–33.

Teicher, M. H., Andersen, S. L., Polcari, A. *et al.* (2003). The neurobiological consequences of early stress and childhood maltreatment. *Neuroscience and Behavioral Reviews*, **27**, 33–44.

van Os, J. (2004). Does the urban environment cause psychosis? *British Journal of Psychiatry*, **184**, 287–8.

van Os, J., Hanssen, M., Bijl, R. *et al.* (2000). Strauss (1969) revisited: a psychosis continuum in the general population? *Schizophrenia Research*, **45**, 11–20.

Verdoux, H. and van Os, J. (2002). Psychotic symptoms in non-clinical populations and the continuum of psychosis. *Schizophrenia Research*, **54** (1–2), 59–65.

Warner, R. (2000). *The Environment of Schizophrenia*. London: Routledge.

Wing, J. (1978). *Reasoning about Madness*. Oxford: Oxford University Press.

Wing, J. and Brown, G. (1970). *Institutionalism and Schizophrenia*. London: Cambridge University Press.

World Health Organization (1992). *The ICD-10 Classification of Mental and Behavioural Disorders (International Classification of Diseases)*, 10th edn. Geneva: World Health Organization.

2

Climate change in psychiatry: periodic fluctuations or terminal trend?

Julian Leff

Introduction

The direction of research and practice in all fields of medicine is determined by a multiplicity of pressures, including government policy, public demands, economic factors, technical advances and the intellectual zeitgeist. All of these operate in psychiatry, but in addition the social and psychological elements of psychiatric conditions are so prominent that they apply extra pressure. With a few exceptions, such as Alzheimer's disease and Huntington's chorea, the underlying pathology of psychiatric illnesses remains unknown or at best controversial. This situation nurtures the flourishing of many theories and opinions in the domains of biology, psychology and sociology. Opposing camps have grown up with adherents from psychology and sociology in one camp (humanist) and proponents of biological explanations in the other (reductionist, according to the humanists). Over the past decades there have been regular pleas from integrationists to merge differences between the two camps and develop a holistic biopsychosocial approach (e.g., Engel, 1980). Major barriers to this resolution have been the absence of a unifying language to describe the integrated phenomena, and the scepticism of biologists about the ability of the humanists to adopt a 'hard-nosed' scientific approach to the testing of their theories (see Clare, 1980; Sedgwick, 1982).

As a result of the polarisation of these two camps, there has been a struggle for the ascendancy of one over the other that has continued throughout the last century (Sedgwick, 1982). The theoretical disputes have been closely paralleled by arguments over the clinical practice of psychiatry. The current political emphasis on evidence-based medicine has brought theory and practice closer together, and has sharpened some of the arguments between the two camps. It has been recognised that much of what psychiatric professionals do in their daily practice is without an evidence base (www.cochrane.org/colloquia/abstracts/capetown/capetownPB19.html). We should not feel too dejected about this since the same

Society and Psychosis, ed. Craig Morgan, Kwame McKenzie and Paul Fearon. Published by Cambridge University Press. © Cambridge University Press 2008.

is true for a high proportion of medical, surgical and obstetric practices (www.medlib.iupui.edu/ebm/home.html).

Influences on research output

Innovations in the practice of psychiatry can influence the direction of research. The introduction of psychoanalysis at the opening of the twentieth century, which in time came to dominate the training of US psychiatrists, had a limited impact on training in the UK. Psychoanalysts did not espouse quantitative research, and psychotherapists were equally averse to scientific evaluation until recently. Eric Kandel (2005), one of the three psychiatric Nobel Laureates, abandoned his psycho-analytic training in the 1960s to pursue a research career focused on elucidating the mechanisms of neural signal transduction, studying sea snails and mice. While the introduction of electroconvulsive therapy (ECT) and insulin coma stimulated evaluative research, which supported ECT and made insulin coma obsolete (Ackner et al., 1957; Brandon et al., 1984), there has been no randomised controlled trial (RCT) of leucotomy, which is still in active use in some countries. During a recent visit to Chile, I was told that a neurosurgical unit in one of the psychiatric hospitals in Santiago was performing three leucotomies a week.

Three decades ago, I was a member of a small committee set up by the UK Medical Research Council to design a randomised controlled trial in conjunction with some neurosurgeons. It failed to materialise because the neurosurgeons refused to accept even a waiting list control, on the grounds that their intervention represented the last resort of desperate patients who could brook no further delay. This type of clinical opposition is another force determining what research comes to fruition and eventual publication. Increasingly, ethical committees play a determining role in what research is acceptable and what is rejected. Many studies that were mounted and published in past years would now fall at this hurdle.

The development of specific psychoactive drugs and their introduction into clinical practice from the 1950s onward have created a vast industry of research, which floods the market with papers and has contributed to the multiplication of specialist journals. Innovations in the organisation of psychiatric services have also stimulated an extensive research effort, although not on the same scale as psycho-pharmacology and drug trials. This is partly because of the extensive financial support by the pharmaceutical industry of trials of their products, and partly because of the time it takes to evaluate a complex organisational change. For example, the Team for the Assessment of Psychiatric Services (TAPS) spent 13 years evaluating the policy of UK governments (both left and right) of replacing psychiatric hospitals with community services (Leff et al., 2000). The development of new psychological treatments, such as cognitive behavioural therapy and family interventions for schizophrenia, has also given birth to a growing research literature (e.g., Kuipers *et al.*, 1998; Leff *et al.*, 1985), although, again, this is no rival to the millions of words expended on the value of medication.

In the biological arena, technological advances in brain imaging and in the visualisation of neural processes in the brain have also led to an expansion in specialist journals and in a burgeoning literature. For example, *Biological Psychiatry* was launched in 1976, *Human Brain Mapping* in 1993, *Neuroimage* in 1993 and an e-journal, *Public Library of Science (PLoS) Biology*, in 2005. The completion of the human genome project in 2003 and the refinement of molecular genetics are beginning to have an impact on psychiatric publications, which are certain to grow exponentially over the next decade.

Another major growth area in the psychiatric literature comes from a surprising source: the official classificatory systems for psychiatric diseases. The introduction of the nosological category post-traumatic stress disorder (PTSD) into the US Diagnostic and Statistical Manual, DSM-III, in 1980 and into the WHO International Classification of Diseases has resulted in a huge number of articles on this subject. Certainly, research was conducted on psychological reactions to traumatic events previously, but not on the current scale. Part of the impetus for this in the USA is that the cost of services for an officially recognised diagnostic entity can be reimbursed by the Health Insurance companies.

Policies of the bodies funding research also exert an influence on the type of research conducted. The main government funding body for psychiatric research in the USA is the National Institute of Mental Health. Representatives of the National Alliance for Mental Patients, a non-governmental organisation, sit on the key committee and influence decisions about funding. This organisation is strongly in favour of biological research, and reputedly against any project involving the measurement of relatives' expressed emotion, because of the presumed imputation that families play a part in causing psychiatric illnesses. In the UK, the main government supported funding body is the Medical Research Council, which is genuinely independent of government policies. However, it has policies of its own that determine what types of research applications are likely to be successful. The UK Department of Health has a relatively large research budget and regularly calls for applications in specific areas. These are closely linked to government policy, which influences priorities for research (HMSO, 1995).

The rise of biological research

The net effect of this plethora of influences (see Table 2.1) on the balance between psychosocial and biological research is hard to predict, but prediction should not be attempted without taking into account macro-social changes, which may constitute

Table 2.1 Some influences on the balance between biological and psychosocial research

Introduction of new treatments – biological or psychosocial
Resistance by practitioners to evaluation of their therapies
Increasing control by ethical committees
Technological advances in brain science
Unravelling the human genome and refining molecular genetics
Policies of funding bodies
Incorporation of new disease categories in official systems of classification
Grass-roots ideological movements
Governments of the right or the left

the main overriding factor. Brown (1985) charts the rise and decline of the community mental health movement in the USA, pointing out that cycles of institutional change and reform have been common. The first stirrings of the revolution in psychiatric care were apparent in the UK before World War II, but it was the experiences of military psychiatrists in the war that changed the custodial atmosphere in many psychiatric hospitals in the UK and the USA and initiated an increase in the discharge of patients into the community. This began before the introduction of chlorpromazine into clinical practice in 1955: some British psychiatric hospitals had begun to reduce their beds a few years before this (Leff, 1997).

The shift in the locus of psychiatric care was officially endorsed and facilitated in the USA by the Community Mental Health Centers Acts of 1963 and 1965. These were components of the larger social welfare package of the New Frontier and Great Society programmes of Presidents Kennedy and Johnson. Brown (1985, p. 149) considers that, 'the last era of general optimism was the community mental health period, roughly located in the decade and a half from 1960–1975 ... many of the great promises of this approach were not met. In this failure we can locate the preconditions for the rise of a new biologism, a more strictly biomedical and asocial view of mental health and illness.'

The community mental health movement partly came to grief because of the aspirations and activities of its front-line workers. Many of them were young idealistic people who viewed themselves as agents of social change and came into conflict with local landlords and politicians. They had no chance against vested interests because of their naivety and political inexperience. The movement mainly foundered because in 1973 US President Nixon illegally impounded community mental health centre funds already appropriated by Congress. Brown (1985, p. 166) asserts that, 'such activities were made possible by the rightist government policies of the Nixon period, characterised by domestic espionage, international destabilisation and support of reactionary coups, and disruption of liberal and radical groups involved in antiwar, civil rights and feminist activities.' He predicted that, 'Current rightwards trends in the 1980s could potentiate a renewed interest in a wide range of authoritarian responses, including psychotechnology.' (p. 166.)

In the UK, we have seen regular swings between left-leaning and right-leaning governments, with distinctly different attitudes to social change. One of the most dramatic shifts is attributable to UK Prime Minister Margaret Thatcher, who famously declaimed, 'There is no such thing as society!' (*Women's Own* magazine, 31 October 1987), and insisted on altering the name of the UK's Social Science Research Council by heading it the 'Economic and Social Research Council'. Thatcherite economic policies have not been repudiated, and the great social reforms of the post-war Attlee government are currently being eroded by a Labour government that lurches to the right. It is characterised by belligerence abroad, increased surveillance of the domestic population and restriction of civil rights. The latter includes a proposed amendment to the Mental Health Act, which, if enacted, will allow for patients in the community to be forced to take medication against their will. If Brown (1985) is correct in linking rightist government policies to the fostering of biologism, then we should be able to detect this effect in the balance between biological and psychosocial publications in the psychiatric literature. We can ask whether there is a natural periodicity in the swings between biological and psychosocial research, or whether we can perceive a tendency towards inexorably increasing biologism in recent years that will eventually eclipse psychosocial research. The problem of detecting such a tendency is equivalent to the arguments over climate change, except that the time period available for scrutiny is less than 100 years instead of many millennia. It is worth stating my perception that the pendulum swings in psychiatric fashion in the USA are much more extreme than in the UK. For instance, in the early Woody Allen period a regular visit to a psychoanalyst was a part of everyday life, whereas today psychoanalysis is a beleaguered form of therapy in the USA.

Searching for trends in the psychiatric literature (1) Method

Ideally, it would be desirable to chart the number of research projects in psychiatry funded per year and determine the ratio of psychosocial to biological studies. This is impractical on account of the number of fund-giving organisations that exist around the world. It is necessary to make compromises in order to collect usable data. To identify some of the broad trends in the psychiatric literature I made three decisions. First, I decided to restrict my investigation to two countries only: the USA and the UK. The great bulk of psychiatric research emanates from these two sources. As an indication of their domination, between 1992 and 2001, these two countries contributed more than 50% of mental health publications in the world psychiatric literature (Saxena *et al.*, 2006). Second, I was constrained to limit the data collection to published work, since accessing file-drawer research over the whole field of psychiatry would be an endless task. Third, I decided to scan the publications in just two journals: the *American Journal of Psychiatry* (*AJP*) and the *British Journal of Psychiatry* (*BJP*), since these are comparable general psychiatric journals covering the whole range of psychiatric topics and, hence, are likely to be representative of the research output and current opinion on clinical practice.

There are a number of limitations to this approach, in particular relating to the countries of origin of the authors and the influence of the editor. A proportion of the articles in each of these journals is likely to emanate from countries other than the USA and the UK; there are also likely to be UK papers published in the *AJP* and vice versa. Further, regardless of the quality of the submissions, the editor makes the final decision on acceptance. Given the low acceptance rate for both these journals (in 2007, this was one in five for the *BJP*) it is probable that many high quality papers are being rejected, indicating that the editors are accepting papers they judge to be of most relevance to their readers and to the general scientific community. In a period of intense competition for publication, editors probably mould the character of their journals to a greater extent than in other eras. Therefore, we need to consider whether it is possible for an editor with a strong adherence to a biological approach to shift the balance of a journal significantly. This has to be a possibility, but then it can be argued that candidates for an editorial position on a major journal are bound to be senior colleagues, often with a long track record of their own publications, and their intellectual biases will be well known to the appointments committee. If the committee chooses to appoint a 'biological' editor, this in itself is a reflection of the zeitgeist.

In approaching the task, I had to make decisions about the number of years to sample, the type of article to be included and the criteria for characterising articles as biological or psychosocial. There are precedents for this kind of analysis. Brodie and Sabshin (1973) noted that there had been no surveys of overall psychiatric research trends in the USA for a specific decade, and only a very sparse use of the objective data that was available. They chose to survey all papers published in the *AJP* and *Archives of General Psychiatry* in the decade 1963 to 1972. They selected those they judged to be research articles, and then assigned them to biological, psychological and social categories. The proportion of the 1885 research papers falling into each of the categories was: biological 41%, psychological 35% and social 24%. It is noteworthy that under the psychological rubric they included papers dealing with diagnosis and classification, and screening devices, self-scoring tests and computers. Furthermore they excluded papers on the delivery of mental health services from the research category. As we shall see, I took an opposing position on both these points.

Another group (Pincus *et al.*, 1993) surveyed the same two American journals, but covered a greater time period of three decades, in each of which they selected one year of journal articles: 1969–70, 1979–80 and 1989–90. They detected a significant growth in research in clinical psychobiology during the 1970s, which continued through the 1980s. During this time span there was a reduction in research reports on behavioural and cognitive science, and on health and mental health services. A comparison of the contents of the two journals revealed that the *AJP* had a greater representation of articles on social sciences, diagnosis and nosology and health and mental health services. Pincus and colleagues (1993) noted that the increase in psychobiological articles coincided with the development of neuroimaging techniques and assays for measurement of neuropeptides, receptor physiology and regional glucose metabolism.

Moncrieff and Crawford (2001) confined their study to a single periodical, the *BJP*, and surveyed all issues for the year at the midpoint of each of the ten decades: 1900–2000. They found that the nine descriptive fields to which Pincus *et al.* (1993) assigned articles were insufficiently comprehensive, so expanded them to 15. Moncrieff and Crawford presented a detailed tabulation of the proportion of articles assigned to each of the 15 categories for the period surveyed (1905–1995). They did not apply any statistical tests to their quantitative material, but from inspection of the data concluded that 'biological concerns have been continuously at the heart of the journal' (p. 355). By contrast, 'other systems of understanding and methods of treatment such as psychoanalysis and social psychiatry have generally received little attention' (p. 356).

Since my interest lay in a comparison of the emphasis in American and British psychiatric periodicals, none of the three previous studies was directly informative, but did provide useful guidelines for the classification of articles, which I followed. I decided to cover 55 years, from 1950 to 2005, and to survey a full year of journals for the first and sixth year of each decade. The start date of 1950 was chosen, since in the following decade the first specific psychoactive drugs were introduced to clinical practice.

My survey was more comprehensive than that of previous work, as I included all articles reporting research studies, clinical reports that were not confined to a single case and editorials. My reason for this strategy is that I wished to assess the climate of opinion of the time, which is reflected in more than the published research. I amalgamated the 15 categories of Moncrieff and Crawford (2001) into three major divisions. Basic science, genetics and family studies, psychopharmacology and physical treatments were included under the rubric of 'biological'. Psychology, psychotherapy, psychoanalysis, social psychiatry and epidemiology, social intervention and service provision or organisation constituted the category 'psychosocial'. Instrument development, research methods, statistics, history and philosophy were assigned to a 'neutral' category. Clinical topics were judged by their content to belong to either the biological or psychosocial category. Articles on the psychiatric training of psychiatric professionals, general practitioners and medical students were classified as psychosocial, as were legal aspects of psychiatry, on the basis that these topics reflect social and cultural attitudes and influences. Individual articles that I found difficult to categorise as either biological or psychosocial were classified as neutral.

Searching for trends in the psychiatric literature (2) Findings

The number of articles in the two journals assigned to psychosocial and biological categories and the proportion of psychosocial articles in each year are shown in Table 2.2 for the years from 1951 to 2005. These data are presented graphically in Figure 2.1. In interpreting these graphs, we need to take account of the fact that in 1963 the official publication of the Royal College of Psychiatrists changed its title from the *Journal of Mental Science* to the *British Journal of Psychiatry*. This was more than a cosmetic change, because the content of the periodical had already been changing from brief reports and news items to more detailed accounts of research studies. This is reflected in the increase in the number of articles I could assign to one of the two categories, from 28 during the entire year 1951, to 71 ten years later.

Inspection of the two graphs shows that in 1951 the *AJP* published a small majority of psychosocial articles, whereas the *BJP* published predominantly biological articles. Most of these dealt with aspects of insulin coma therapy,

Table 2.2 Articles assigned to psychosocial (PS) and biological (B) categories in the *British Journal of Psychiatry* and the *American Journal of Psychiatry*

Year	British			American		
	PS	B	%PS	PS	B	%PS
1951	7	21	25.0	52	40	56.5
1956	16	28	36.4	71	68	51.1
1961	24	47	33.8	63	93	40.4
1966	55	40	57.9	109	43	71.7
1971	60	57	51.3	127	52	70.9
1976	61	56	52.1	102	49	67.5
1981	57	66	46.3	69	43	61.6
1986	84	88	48.8	51	53	49.0
1991	97	94	50.8	64	89	41.8
1996	96	71	57.5	95	108	46.8
2001	86	64	57.3	89	167	34.8
2005	95	66	59.0	101	168	37.5

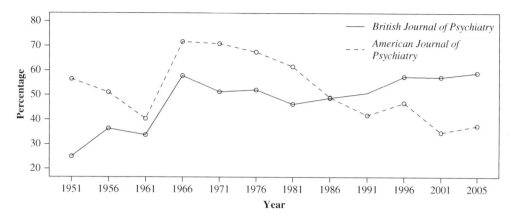

Figure 2.1   Proportion of psychosocial articles in the *British Journal of Psychiatry* and the *American Journal of Psychiatry*

leucotomy, treatment of epilepsy and penicillin for neurosyphilis. During the following decade the proportion of biological articles in the *BJP* gradually fell, with a continuation of the same topics, but also studies on electroconvulsive therapy and the newly introduced psychotropic drugs: chlordiazepoxide, tricyclic antidepressants and antipsychotics. During this decade the proportion of psychosocial articles in the *AJP* declined as controlled and uncontrolled studies of the new psychotropic drugs began to be published.

Then between 1961 and 1966 there was a steep rise in the proportion of psychosocial articles in both journals, the slopes being almost parallel. However, the difference in proportions between these two years' issues was of greater significance for the *AJP* ($\chi^2 = 30.64$, df 1, $p < 0.001$) than for the *BJP* ($\chi^2 = 9.46$, df 1, $p < 0.001$). Both journals maintained the high proportion of psychosocial articles over the next decade, and then there was the beginning of a fall. Brown (1985, p. 149) locates the period of greatest optimism for community psychiatry during the decade and a half from 1960, which exactly coincides with the high plateau for psychosocial articles on the two graphs. Of course, this is also the period during which the Civil Rights Movement in the USA became a prominent political force, the Feminist Movement took off on both sides of the Atlantic, and hippy culture was in the ascendant in the USA and the UK. In 1966, the *AJP* included a special section on Social Psychiatry in one issue, and articles were also published on 'The stresses of the white female worker in the Civil Rights Movement in the South' (Poussaint, 1966) and 'Psychological aspects of the Civil Rights Movement and the Negro professional man' (Beisser and Harris, 1966). These topics constitute further evidence for the influence of the cultural and political environment on the contents of both psychiatric journals, suggested by the timing of the rise revealed by the graphs.

The fall in the proportion of psychosocial articles in the *AJP* continues in an almost linear fashion over the next two decades, reaching its lowest level in the years surveyed (34.8%) in 2001. At this time the *AJP* features almost twice as many articles of a biological nature than psychosocial articles. By contrast, the proportion of psychosocial articles in the *BJP*, after a moderate fall from 57.9% in 1966 to 46.3% in 1981, rises slowly but steadily to 59.0% in 2005, its highest level in the years covered by the survey. By chance the proportions in the two journals are virtually identical in 1986, when the descending graph of the *AJP* crosses the ascending graph of the *BJP*. This occurrence enables us to make a direct comparison of the trends in the two journals between 1986 and 2005, a period of 19 years.

Increasing and decreasing trends for proportions in the data were assessed using the Cochrane–Armitage trend test (Agresti, 1990, pp. 100–2). Analyses were done with STATA 9.1 using the ptrend module (Stata, 2005). In the *BJP*, the trend for psychosocial articles to predominate over biological articles has a slope of 0.027 and a χ^2 of 4.96 (df 1, $p < 0.026$). The slope for the *AJP* is, of course, negative at -0.030, since biological articles predominate, and gives a χ^2 of 6.26 (df 1, $p < 0.012$). It was considered of interest to express the trend for psychosocial articles in the *BJP* as a proportion of the combined number of such articles in both British and American journals. The slope of this trend is -0.038, with a χ^2 of 9.31 (df 1, $p < 0.002$).

We can conclude from this analysis that in terms of the publication of psychosocial articles, the two journals have been moving progressively further apart during the past 19 years. The *BJP* shows a significant increase in the proportion of these articles, while the *AJP* exhibits a significant decrease of approximately the same magnitude. As a result, by 2005 the difference in the composition of the two journals is highly significant.

Conclusions

Before speculating on the factors producing these effects, it is necessary to consider the validity of the approach adopted here. It could be argued that the classification of articles was idiosyncratic, particularly since I did not involve a colleague to assess inter-rater reliability. However, it is possible to cross-check my data from the *AJP* with the data produced by Brodie and Sabshin (1973). They surveyed all the research articles in the *AJP* and *Archives of General Psychiatry* during the decade 1963 to 1972, while I confined my survey to the years 1961, 1966 and 1971 and used a broader remit. Nevertheless, there is a striking similarity between our results. Amalgamating their categories of 'psychological' and 'social' yields a proportion of 59%, compared with 41% for biological articles: my corresponding figures are 61% and 39%. My findings for the *AJP* are also in accord with those of

Pincus *et al.* (1993) for the period 1969 to 1990. Hence it is reasonable to assume that I have not introduced a major source of bias.

We saw that both the *AJP* and *BJP* responded in the same way to the social and political movements of the 1960s. Why should they be showing such divergent trends in the past two decades? There is the possibility of a positive feedback effect amplifying the divergence between the two journals. This means that as a journal becomes more polarised, fewer articles from the minority discipline are even submitted for consideration. However, the trends have to be established in the first place before amplification can occur, and it is here that I invoke the forces of major political movements. The predominant policy in the USA is neoliberalism, which is exerting an increasing influence on this side of the Atlantic (Moncrieff, 2006). However, the UK still has a National Health Service and a Welfare State, even though both have been subject to erosion by privatisation in recent decades. The massive demonstration of public opposition to the Iraq War and the determination of the great majority of the populace to preserve a state health service are indications of a resistance to the tsunami of neoliberalism. The discipline of social psychiatry in the UK has a long history and has maintained a high research output, despite the greater influx of funds into biological psychiatry. In terms of policy and practice, deinstitutionalisation has proceeded as far as in any country in the world, and the development of community psychiatric services, while far from ideal, has not met the kind of setbacks encountered in the USA (Leff *et al.*, 2000). We can conclude that these influences, and others not specifically identified, have maintained the salience of psychosocial psychiatry in the UK, and that the exciting developments in biological research and the power of the pharmaceutical industry are far from eclipsing its light.

Acknowledgement

I am grateful to Dr Alex Leff for his constructive comments on a draft of this chapter.

REFERENCES

Ackner, B., Harris, A. and Oldham, A. J. (1957). Insulin treatment of schizophrenia: a controlled study. *Lancet*, **i**, 607–11.

Agresti, A. (1990). *Categorical Data Analysis*. New York: John Wiley and Sons.

Beisser, A. R. and Harris, H. (1966). Psychological aspects of the Civil Rights Movement and the Negro professional man. *American Journal of Psychiatry*, **123**, 733–8.

Brandon, S., Cowley, P., Mcdonald, C. *et al.* (1984). Electroconvulsive therapy: results in depressive-illness from the Leicestershire trial. *British Medical Journal*, **288** (6410), 22–5.

Brodie, K. H. and Sabshin, M. (1973). An overview of trends in psychiatric research: 1963–1972. *American Journal of Psychiatry*, **130**, 1309–18.

Brown, P. (1985). *The Transfer of Care: Psychiatric Deinstitutionalisation and its Aftermath.* New York: Routledge.

Clare, A. (1980). *Psychiatry in Dissent.* London: Tavistock.

Engel, G. L. (1980). The clinical application of the biopsychosocial model. *American Journal of Psychiatry*, **137**, 535–44.

HMSO (1995). *HC 134–1. House of Commons Health Committee. Priority setting in the NHS purchasing.* First report sessions 1994–5. London: HMSO.

Kandel, E. (2005). *Psychiatry, Psychoanalysis, and the New Biology of the Mind.* Washington, DC: American Psychiatric Publishing.

Kuipers, E., Fowler, D., Garety, P. *et al.* (1998). The London East Anglia randomised controlled trial of cognitive behaviour therapy for psychosis III: follow up and economic evaluation at 18 months. *British Journal of Psychiatry*, **173**, 69–74.

Leff, J. (ed.) (1997). *Care in the Community: Illusion or Reality?* Chichester: Wiley.

Leff, J., Kuipers, L., Berkowitz, R. *et al.* (1985). A controlled trial of social intervention in the families of schizophrenic patients: two year follow-up. *British Journal of Psychiatry*, **146**, 594–600.

Leff, J., Trieman, N., Knapp, M. *et al.* (2000). The TAPS Project: a report on 13 years of research, 1985–1998. *Psychiatric Bulletin*, **24**, 165–8.

Moncrieff, J. (2006). Psychiatric drug promotion and the politics of neoliberalism. *British Journal of Psychiatry*, **188**, 301–2.

Moncrieff, J. and Crawford, M. J. (2001). British psychiatry in the 20th century – observations from a psychiatry journal. *Social Science and Medicine*, **53**, 349–56.

Pincus, H. A., Henderson, B., Blackwood, D. *et al.* (1993). Trends in research in two general psychiatric journals in 1969–1990: research on research. *American Journal of Psychiatry*, **150**, 135–42.

Poussaint, A. V. (1966). The stresses of the white female worker in the Civil Rights Movement in the South. *American Journal of Psychiatry*, **123**, 401–7.

Saxena, S., Paraje, G., Sharan, P. *et al.* (2006). The 10/90 divide in mental health research: trends over a 10-year period. *British Journal of Psychiatry*, **188**, 81–2.

Sedgwick, P. (1982). *Psychopolitics (The Politics of Health).* London: Pluto Press.

Stata (2005) *STATA Statistical Software, Release 9.* College Station, TX: Stata Corporation.

Part I

Theoretical and conceptual foundations

3

Social science, psychiatry and psychosis

Craig Morgan

Introduction

The relationship between psychiatry and the social sciences has frequently been antagonistic. A major assumption underpinning psychiatry is that mental illnesses are at root biological and, as such, are primarily the remit of biomedical science. Within this conceptualisation, social science can at best assume a peripheral role, perhaps in helping to understand environmental influences on the presentation and course of the mental illnesses or in explaining patterns of service use (Kleinman, 1991). As for the key issue of aetiology, the biological sciences provide the framework and method for research; with regard to clinical practice, physical medicine offers the template. This is particularly true for schizophrenia and other psychoses, the disorders assumed to be most determined by biology (e.g., Crow, 2007). During the past two decades, the dominance of biological perspectives within psychiatry has increased, fuelled by rapid advances in genetics and the development of increasingly sophisticated techniques for studying the brain, such as functional magnetic resonance imaging. However, somewhat ironically, these advances are generating evidence that social experiences over the life course can affect gene expression and neurodevelopment (e.g., Meaney, 2001; Teicher et al., 2003), and this is fuelling a renewed interest in the potential role of the social environment in the aetiology of schizophrenia and other psychoses (see Chapters 6–10).

The extent to which psychiatry has stood in direct opposition to the social sciences has fluctuated over time, and at any given point there have been proponents of closer collaboration with sociologists and anthropologists (e.g., Cooper, 1992). There is, moreover, a substantial body of literature from these disciplines addressing key issues relevant to the study of mental illness, including schizophrenia and other psychoses, many of which have had a major influence on our understanding of these complex disorders (e.g., Warner, 2003; Wing and Brown, 1970). It is, then, timely to re-appraise the potential role and contribution of the social sciences. Specifically, what, in the ages of the brain and the genome, is the relevance of the social sciences to the study of schizophrenia and other psychoses? In this chapter, this broad

Society and Psychosis, ed. Craig Morgan, Kwame McKenzie and Paul Fearon. Published by Cambridge University Press. © Cambridge University Press 2008.

question is addressed through a critical review of select examples of social science research and theory concerned with key aspects of mental illness: (1) concepts and social responses; and (2) causes. Before this, it is necessary to begin with some definitions, and to set the question in its historical context.

Social science

The social sciences comprise those disciplines primarily concerned with understanding the social world and our place in it. An over-inclusive list of the disciplines comprising the social sciences might include economics, geography, history, psychology, anthropology and sociology. In this chapter, however, the discussion will be restricted to the latter two of these, anthropology and sociology, primarily because it is the relevance of these two disciplines that has been most intensely disputed. This is not to deny the importance of the other social sciences. The relevance and contribution of psychology is surely indisputable, and history (e.g., Scull, 2005), economics (e.g., Knapp *et al.*, 2006) and geography (e.g., Parr *et al.*, 2004) all continue to generate work of direct relevance to all aspects of mental illness. It is, nonetheless, the claims to relevance and importance of sociological and anthropological approaches to mental illness that have generated the most profound and illuminating debates.

Drawing a clear line of demarcation between sociology and anthropology is far from straightforward. Naturally, they have much in common. The emphasis in each is very much on how social and cultural processes both shape, and are shaped by, individuals in what Skultans and Cox (2000) have referred to as 'an ongoing process of mutual influence' (p. 8). Distinctions between the two reside in the focus and methods of research. A major focus of sociological analyses, for example, is on discrete components of the social world, such as class, sex and ethnicity, in contrast to anthropology, which has more often sought to analyse whole cultures, stressing the interconnectedness of the various aspects of the society under scrutiny. In terms of method, sociology, or at least a significant strand in sociology, has made greater use of quantitative methods to analyse the relationships between the various discrete components of interest, an emphasis no doubt heavily influenced by the positivist beginnings of the discipline (Comte, 1986; Durkheim, 1970). In contrast, the defining method and approach of anthropology is that of participant observation and the interpretative endeavour of the researcher in rendering local cultures accessible and understandable. The emphasis on local meanings and interpretation, which eschews universal laws and objective causal processes, marks a further point of distinction from, at least, quantitative sociology. That said, there has long been an interpretative tradition in sociology, stretching back to Weber (Parkin, 1982) and forward to postmodern sociology, that overlaps considerably with the focus and methods of social anthropology. It is here that the distinctions between the two disciplines blur.

Historical tensions

The relationship between psychiatry and the social sciences has a chequered history, with examples of both fruitful collaboration and periods of extreme animosity, the legacy of which is an ongoing ambivalence of each towards the other (Skultans, 1991). Underpinning this animosity are basic differences in the philosophical assumptions that characterise dominant strands in each discipline concerning the nature of knowledge and scientific enquiry. Psychiatry's position as a sub-specialty of medicine carries with it both an adherence to the methods of the natural sciences – empirical observation, hypothesis testing, objective quantification and classification of phenomena – and a strong tendency to privilege biological explanations of mental phenomena over psychological or social ones. This has created scepticism about the usefulness and relevance of the social sciences to the subject matter of psychiatry, particularly that strand of social science concerned with interpretation and subjective meanings.

More than this, social scientists were at the forefront of the anti-psychiatry movement of the 1960s and 1970s, a movement that attacked the very foundations of psychiatry, questioning the reality of mental illness and branding psychiatry an agent of social control serving the function of silencing difference (Foucault, 1965; Laing, 1960; Szasz, 1960). Psychiatry's response to the charge that it was 'invalidating, medicalising and brutalising the meaning in mental disorder' (Bolton, 1997, p. 255) was both a re-assertion of the legitimacy of its approach to the understanding and treatment of mental illness and a counter-attack accusing its critics of being unscientific and engaging in unfounded theorising (Bolton, 1997; Roth and Kroll, 1986). The acrimonious debate made explicit the underlying philosophical and methodological differences that divide the dominant perspectives in psychiatry and the social sciences. Towards the end of the 1970s, Eisenberg (1977) commented that the gap between psychiatry and the social sciences was almost unbridgeable. The result is a legacy of mistrust that has not been entirely overcome by the many examples of fruitful collaboration between psychiatrists and social scientists, or by the increasing awareness that social and cultural dimensions are crucial to a full understanding of all forms of mental illness (Kleinman, 1987; Leff, 2001). This is the historical subtext to any effort to appraise the contribution of the social sciences to the study of schizophrenia and other psychoses.

The social creation of mental illness

Perhaps the core idea that unified the amorphous perspectives of the 'anti-psychiatry' movement was that mental illness was a myth (Szasz, 1960), a social construction designed to silence difference (Foucault, 1965). The most sociological, and influential, expression of this basic idea came in the work of Thomas Scheff (1966), who applied a labelling theory of deviance to mental illness.

Originally, labelling theory was used to explain why some acts are defined as criminal or deviant and others are not (Becker, 1963). The basic idea is straightforward: deviance is determined not by the nature of the deviant acts, but by societal responses to those acts. Perhaps the most famous statement of this premise is from Howard Becker's seminal book *Outsiders*: 'Social groups create deviance by making rules whose infraction constitutes deviance, and by applying those rules to particular people and labelling them as outsiders' (Becker, 1963, p. 9). Rule breaking is not enough; the rule or norm violation has to be identified and labelled as such, usually by agents of social control (e.g., the police). Scheff (1966) extended this to mental illness, reframing psychiatric symptoms as rule or norm violations. More specifically, he viewed mental illness as a kind of residual rule breaking, i.e., as norm-violating behaviour that cannot be readily ascribed to any other culturally recognised category (Thoits, 1999). Once this 'primary deviance' is labelled, according to the theory, an individual is then treated differentially on the basis of the label and, in the process of being treated differentially, increasingly comes to take on the stereotypical characteristics of, in this case, a mentally ill person, the result being continued and amplified norm violations, i.e., 'secondary deviance'. It is, thus, the application of the label of mental illness that traps an individual into a career as a 'mental patient'.

Some of the classic sociological studies of mental illness present a broadly similar account of how individuals become psychiatric patients. Goffman, in his seminal work *Asylums* (Goffman, 1961), saw the process of becoming a mental patient as a social process, in which a series of actors, including those in positions of authority, e.g., police, and family and friends, convince the patient-to-be that his or her eccentricities and difficulties relating to others are problematic and indicative of mental illness. Gradually, the person comes to accept this self-view as being mentally ill and in need of treatment, and so embarks on what Goffman termed 'the moral career of the mental patient'. A further relevant example is Rosenhan's classic study, 'On being sane in insane places' (Rosenhan, 1973). In the 1970s, Rosenhan, then a professor of psychology at Stanford University, and colleagues gained admission to psychiatric hospitals in the USA by claiming to hear voices saying a single word, such as 'empty', 'hollow' and 'thud'. After admission, all 'pseudo-patients' then behaved normally. All but one was given a diagnosis of schizophrenia; most were treated with powerful medication and kept in hospital for a number of weeks. What is interesting from a labelling point of view is that, once applied, aspects of the 'pseudo-patients'' behaviour and past were viewed through the prism of the label, for example, note taking was seen as pathological 'writing behaviour'.

So, it is society, through its labelling of certain behaviours as mental illness, that creates mental illness; the chronic course of a mental illness career is the product of secondary deviance, of those labelled fulfilling the stereotypical expectations of the labellers. This is not a benign view of mental illness as just one among many historical constructions of unusual behaviour. At its heart is a critique of the perceived damaging consequences of the application of such labels. Psychiatry is not a profession engaged in identifying and treating distressing mental disorders; it is an agency of social control, policing forms of undesirable behaviour. Mental illness is not 'in' the person, it is created by society (Thoits, 1999, p. 136).

The reality of mental illness

There are many well documented problems with this theory as applied to mental illness, and labelling theory is much less influential now than it was. To begin with, labelling theory (and indeed many sociological critiques of psychiatry) tends to aggregate all forms of mental disorder into a single category, and then apply arguments uniformly. This, at the very least, and being charitable, obscures the fact that the theory fits more with some and less with other forms of mental disorder. Eisenberg (1977) is less charitable: 'The aggregation into the single category, 'mental illness', of psychiatric disorders that differ in manifestations, course and pathogenesis is reminiscent of medieval treatises on 'fevers' and 'pestilences'.' (p. 903.) Furthermore, the implication that deviant behaviours will stop if they are not labelled is simply not true of serious mental illness; most clinicians will know of patients who have experienced psychotic symptoms for many years before finally coming into contact with professional services (Morgan et al., 2006). Recent studies of the social construction of certain non-psychotic mental illnesses, including multiple-personality disorder (Hacking, 1998), PTSD and ADHD (Horwitz, 2001), explicitly exclude the psychoses (Hacking, 2002).

The key problem here is the denial of the reality of mental illness. In the context of her recent study of American psychiatry, anthropologist Tanya Luhrman (2000) addresses this head on: 'Madness is real, and it is an act of moral cowardice to treat it as a romantic freedom. Most people who end up in a psychiatric hospital are deeply unhappy and seriously disturbed, and many of them lead lives of humiliation and deep pain.' (p. 12.) This is not now seriously disputed. It is, moreover, possible to reject the idea of mental illness as a socially created myth without rejecting the weaker argument that the specific diagnostic concepts used to make sense of the phenomena of mental illness are social constructs. In a straightforward sense, all scientific concepts are social constructs (or 'constrained fictions' (Eisenberg, 1988)) developed to make sense of the world, and their value can be judged purely in terms of their utility. Current challenges to the diagnostic category of schizophrenia (Bentall, 2003), for example, do not discount the reality of abnormal and deeply distressing experiences, but rather question whether conceptualising these as a distinct disease entity is of heuristic value.

Being mentally ill

However, and the above notwithstanding, the focus of labelling theory (and other sociological and anthropological approaches) on the consequences of social responses to primary deviance (mental illness) has contributed much to our understanding of how social forces shape the manifestation, course and outcome of mental illness, including schizophrenia. At the very least, it has helped to focus attention on how social responses to mental illness and the mentally ill shape the course of specific disorders, such that what seem like intrinsic features of the illness are actually socially driven. It is now clear, for example, that some of the chronic negative behaviours that were deemed intrinsic to schizophrenia were products of the impoverished institutional environments in which patients were treated (Wing and Brown, 1970). It is notable that Kraepelin formulated the concept of dementia praecox, a core feature of which is expectation of gradual mental and functional decline or degeneration, on the basis of observations of large numbers of patients housed in long-stay asylums. Barrett (1998a,b) has argued that an expectation of degeneration and chronicity remains at the core of the concept of schizophrenia. Does this contribute to therapeutic pessimism and, for many, become a kind of self-fulfilling prophecy?

One of the surprising findings from the WHO Ten Country Study was that outcomes were better in developing countries than in developed countries, despite the greater access to more effective treatments in developed countries (Jablensky et al., 1992). The explanation most commonly proposed for this (an explanation supported by work carried out by Nancy Waxler in Sri Lanka (Waxler, 1977)) is that severe mental illness in developing countries is less stigmatised and traditional remedies focus on reintegration of the affected individual into the social group. The expectation is of recovery, and so this promotes recovery. In developed countries, in contrast, the expectation of chronicity (as evident in the very concept of schizophrenia) promotes chronicity. As ever, there is a need for caution, and recent commentators have questioned the validity of the WHO findings in light of more recent outcome studies in developing countries (Patel et al., 2006).

The impact of labelling on social outcomes has been the focus of the most recent research within this area (reflecting also an acceptance that labelling theory has little to say about the initial onset of mental illness) (Link and Phelan, 1999; Phelan and Link, 1999). This suggests that the difficulties that sufferers experience in terms of finding work, accessing decent accommodation and sustaining supportive social networks are not simply a result of the direct effects of the illness, but also result from the reactions of others, particularly stigma and discrimination (Thornicroft, 2006). Furthermore, there is increasing interest in the concepts of social inclusion (Morgan et al., in press) and social reintegration (Ware et al., in press) in formulating interventions to promote more positive social, and clinical, outcomes for those with severe and long standing mental health problems. It is not just conceptual and theoretical social science work that is relevant here. There has been an increasing recognition of the value of qualitative research methods in understanding the lived experiences of those with a mental illness, their interactions with mental health services and the social processes that exclude them from mainstream society (e.g., Morgan *et al.*, 2004). There is not room here to go into detail, but there is a vast body of research in sociology and anthropology documenting how social and cultural contexts impact on the expression and management of mental illness, a body of work that is of clear relevance here (for example, see Horwitz and Schied, 1999; Kleinman, 1991). Research in the social sciences, thus, has an important contribution to make to our understanding of how social contexts shape the course and outcome of schizophrenia and other psychoses, and how we can intervene to moderate these contexts and improve long-term outcomes. What about aetiology?

Social causation

From the inception of the discipline, sociologists have been interested in the social patterning and determinants of health and illness. This body of work, following Thoits (1999), can be considered under two headings: (1) structural strain theory and (2) social stress theory. A key feature of both these strands of research, in contrast to that already described, is that they leave uncontested the categories of mental illness and work with them, attempting to explain their distribution and causes. In this, they overlap with social epidemiology (Berkman and Kawachi, 2000).

Structural strain theory

Put simply, structural strain theory locates the origins of illness in the organisation of society (Thoits, 1999). One of the earliest and most influential studies within this tradition is Durkheim's study on suicide (Durkheim, 1970). Durkheim observed that suicide was unequally distributed across societies, with rates being higher, for example, in Protestants compared with Catholics and Jews and in unmarried people compared with married people. Further, he observed that suicide rates were particularly elevated during periods of marked economic upheaval. It is not necessary to dwell on the many methodological problems with this study. For our purposes, the explanations he proposed to account for these patterns provide a useful illustration of sociological explanations of behaviour that operate at the level of social structure.

To take one example, Durkheim argued that groups and societies differ in their degree of social integration (i.e., the degree to which people are attached and bound together in social groups), and that it was the degree and nature of integration that explained variations in suicide rates. For instance, according to

Durkheim, sudden changes in individuals' social positions, at times of economic flux, could provoke confusion and what he termed 'normlessness', leading to despair and suicide (anomic suicide). In short, the causes of suicide, a deeply personal act, reside not in individuals but in wider social forces.

Since Durkheim there has been a strong tradition within medical sociology that seeks to explain the social patterning of disease in terms of social structure and an individual's place within it. A classic example is the study by Faris and Dunham (1939). In this, the authors plotted the addresses of all patients admitted with mental disorders to four state and eight private hospitals in Chicago over a 12-year period on a census map of the city. They found considerable variance in the rates of mental illness according to place of residence, with the highest rates being in those districts characterised by social disorganisation, squalid housing, poverty and excess crime rates. This finding was particularly marked for schizophrenia, where the range was from 700 per 100 000 in city centre districts to 100 per 100 000 in the peripheral residential districts. The areas with the highest rates were those with: a high level of social mobility, a high proportion of foreign-born residents, a large proportion of the population living in single rooms or hostels, a high proportion who were unmarried, and a high proportion of people living below the official poverty line. Twenty years later, Hollingshead and Redlich (1958) published details of research considering the relationship between social class and mental illness. They found that patients with schizophrenia were over-represented in the lower socioeconomic classes. The association reported in these two classic studies has been replicated fairly consistently since, such that a class gradient for schizophrenia is evident. What has not been so clear, however, is why this gradient exists.

For some time, research along these lines was very much marginal, partly because the true nature of the association was unclear – the debate centring on the direction of causation. Recently, however, there has been a resurgence of interest in the study of macroscopic-level social variables and their relationship with forms of mental illness. For example, there has been a renewed interest in the association between urban living and schizophrenia. Recent research has added weight to the suggestion that living in urban settings substantially increases the risk of schizophrenia. Perhaps the most intriguing recent study is that of Pedersen and Mortensen (2001), which utilised data from large population registers in Denmark covering a total of 1.9 million people. Investigating the relationship between place of residence and schizophrenia, they found a dose–response relationship between length of residence in an urban setting and risk of later schizophrenia: in short, the longer a person lived in increasingly urbanised areas, the greater the risk for developing schizophrenia (Pedersen and Mortensen, 2001).

However, what it is about living in cities that increases risk is far from clear. It has been argued that this is one area where the data are stronger than the explanatory hypotheses (McGrath and Scott, 2006; see also Chapter 6). Nevertheless, one candidate is social fragmentation, which returns us full circle to the work of Durkheim (1970) and Faris and Dunham (1939). Of particular relevance here is the more recently developed concept of social capital, a concept drawn directly from the social sciences (Putnam, 2000). In so far as researchers have attempted to apply this to the study of mental illness, most have drawn specifically on Putnam's formulation of social capital as a collective resource that inheres in the social ties and connections of local communities (McKenzie and Harpham, 2006; Putnam, 2000). As yet, this research is very much in its infancy, and findings are currently thin. There are, however, some indications that eco-logical-level measures of social capital (e.g., voter turnout), and, indeed, other measures of social integration (e.g., ethnic density), are associated with popula-tion-level variations in the incidence of psychosis (Boydell *et al.*, 2001). This is clearly a potentially fruitful area for further research, one that will benefit from close collaboration with social scientists.

The key problem with structural strain theory, as hinted at above, is one of mechanism. In other words, 'Structural theorists generally do not elaborate the ways in which broad social structures . . . become actualised in the lives of specific individuals, and thus they do not clarify how or why macro-social trends can produce psychological distress or disorder.' (Thoits, 1999, p. 133.) Implicitly, the mechanism is stress, that is, the social structure causes stress for certain groups. Indeed, for structural strain theory to make sense, there has to be a linking mechanism that connects social structure and individual pathology. This links and overlaps with social stress theory.

Social stress theory

The concept of stress was first introduced into the medical sciences in the 1930s by the psychologist, Hans Selye (Pearlin, 1999; Selye, 1978). (It originated in engineer-ing and metallurgy as a means of quantifying the effects of external forces on metals (Wheaton, 1999).) Selye saw stress as the body's physiological response to stressors, by which he meant anything that represented an insult or threat to the body, such as extreme heat or cold (i.e., anything provoking a stress response) (Thoits, 1999). His model of stress was developed on the basis of experiments with laboratory animals and comprises four components: (1) stressors; (2) factors that mediate the impact of stressors on the body (e.g., personality, social support networks); (3) the general adaptation syndrome (see below); and (4) responses, positive or negative (Wheaton, 1999, p. 178). Selye conceptualised the three stages of physical response to stressors that animals pass through as the general adaptation syndrome. Briefly, the three stages are: (1) alarm reaction, (2) resistance and (3) exhaustion – they constitute a process during which the body is physiologically aroused and prepared to resist the threat (i.e., fight or flight), and which, if continued for a sufficient period, leads to exhaustion and illness. Indeed, Selye's research suggested that prolonged exposure to stressors would almost certainly lead to illness in laboratory animals. Conceptually, if not in detail, this is the basic framework for current views about how social stressors impact on individuals to increase risk of mental illness.

The social sciences have made considerable use of the concept of stress in attempting to understand the relationship between social and environmental factors and illness in human beings. Studies of stress have proliferated and there are now an astonishing number of papers considering the effects of stress (Helman, 2000). The concept of stress has seeped into the wider culture and is now almost ubiquitous, and provides a near universal lay explanation for a variety of illnesses (Helman, 2000).

Forms of social adversity are, then, reconceptualised as stressors. The primary means by which social scientists have operationalised social stress at an individual level, and studied its effect on physical and mental illness, is through the study of life events and chronic ongoing difficulties. Life events, as a marker for social stress, have been found to correlate with the onset and course of a range of illnesses – asthma, breast cancer, lupus, myocardial infarction, headaches, irritable bowel syndrome, dementia, gastrointestinal disorders, diabetes, Crohn's disease and, of course, the full range of mental health problems, from insomnia to chronic schizophrenia (see Thoits, 1999). What is relevant here is the different ways in which life events have been studied. The methodological literature on this is well known but is worth revisiting, as the issues remain relevant to current attempts to investigate the effect of social factors on the risk of psychosis.

One of the earliest attempts to study stress and its impact on human health using major life events was by Holmes and Rahe (1967). They sought to investigate the relationship between major life events (i.e., major changes in people's lives that require extensive behavioural readjustments) and illness, injury and death, hypothesising that events could impair a person's capacity to cope or adapt, leaving them vulnerable (Thoits, 1999). To investigate this, they developed the Social Readjustment Scale (Holmes and Rahe, 1967), which contained a list of 43 major events, ordered in importance to create an index of life change units (determined by asking respondents to judge how much readjustment each event required) (Thoits, 1999). While Holmes and Rahe (1967) found strong associations between life change unit scores and risk of illness, the Social Readjustment Scale, as a measure of adverse social experiences, is problematic for a number of reasons, not least because the potential range of events is predetermined. Further, studies simply correlating the number of life events, measured in this way, and morbidity or mortality fail to take account of the type and meaning of events and of individuals' coping resources and strategies. That is, they do not take into consideration the range of potential conditioning factors (as Selye called them) that mediate the effects of stress on the organism. This applies to subsequent instruments that have adopted more of a checklist approach to the study of life events (e.g., the List of Threatening Experiences Scale, Brugha *et al.*, 1985).

Many of these limitations were addressed and overcome by the seminal work of George Brown (a social anthropologist) and Tirril Harris (a psychologist and psychoanalyst). The approach of Brown and Harris (1978), though well known, is worth considering in detail, as it provides a template for social science research that can inform our understanding of the impact of complex social processes on the aetiology of schizophrenia and other psychoses. Of central importance is the emphasis on meaning.

Brown and Harris, in their initial study of depression among working class women in London, conducted detailed in-depth interviews focusing not only on life events, but also chronic ongoing difficulties, such as marital and financial problems (Brown and Harris, 1978). Their approach has been developed and refined over the years and, arguably, represents the gold standard of social research in psychiatry. The most significant advance was that they developed a method to take account of the meaning of events. To get around the potential problems of relying solely on subjective interpretations of the impact and meaning of life events, Brown and Harris rated the contextual meaning of events, essentially the level of threat that most others in a similar situation would experience. The importance of this in achieving a more accurate assessment of the significance of life events (or any adverse experience) cannot be underestimated. The impact of the death of a relative, for example, is evidently dependent on the closeness of the relationship.

The approach developed by Brown and Harris has provided some detailed insights into the relationship between social stressors (as defined by life events and ongoing difficulties) and depression. While confirming the basic relationship between life events and ongoing difficulties and depression, they further demonstrated that: (1) the relationship is strongest for negative events, particularly those involving loss, entrapment and humiliation; (2) the association remains when only events pre-onset are considered; (3) the six-month period pre-onset is important; (4) social circumstances and supportive resources mediate the risk, the risk being highest among those women with three children aged under 11 and who lack supportive networks and relationships; and (5) positive, fresh-start events can promote recovery (Harris, 2001).

Social experience and psychosis

The conceptual and methodological lessons from the study of life events and depression are clearly relevant to ongoing efforts to understand how social experiences over the life course affect risk for schizophrenia and other psychoses. As noted, consistent correlations have been documented between psychosis and social class, urban living and migration (Cantor-Graae and Selten, 2005; Fearon and Morgan, 2006; van Os, 2004). However, all that these findings do is hint at a potential role for social experience, and Suchman's (1967) comment, if perhaps overstating the case, remains relevant:

> Nothing is as sterile as demographic group comparisons. Results analysed in relation to such categories as sex, age, race, marital status, occupation and geographical region are an essential part of the book keeping of modern society. In and of themselves, however, these rates offer little by way of explanation ... These may be convenient, easily studied labels for sub-dividing populations, but they are not dynamic social ideas and cannot, except in a very limited way, represent the kind of social phenomenon that may cause disease or anything else. (Quoted in Cooper, 1992, p. 595)

There is a clear need for research to move from analyses of demographics to detailed consideration of the social phenomena that may underlie these broad associations.

These issues are further illustrated with the example of trauma. A number of recent reports from large population surveys suggest that those who experience psychotic symptoms are more likely to have experienced traumatic life events, particularly during childhood (e.g., Bebbington *et al.*, 2004; Janssen *et al.*, 2004; Spauwen *et al.*, 2006). However, despite grand claims made by some (Read *et al.*, 2005), the data are inconsistent with regard to the impact of trauma, which traumas are relevant, and during which time period. This is not surprising, given the widely different ways in which trauma has been assessed. Many have relied simply on yes or no responses to single questions concerning specific traumas, such as sexual abuse (e.g., Bebbington *et al.*, 2004). These studies are important in pointing to the potential relevance of early adversity and trauma; the findings equally point to the need for detailed studies that take account of the age, severity, meaning and duration of abuse or trauma. Detailed assessments, similar to that devised by Brown and Harris for adult life events, have been developed by social scientists for the study of early life experiences and, indeed, have been used in the study of other disorders, including depression (e.g., Bifulco *et al.*, 1991). Further, it appears that more detailed interviews in this area generate more valid data, an issue of crucial importance given concerns about recall bias in retrospective studies of psychosis and childhood trauma (Morgan and Fisher, 2007; see Chapter 7). When more detailed social science methodologies are employed, as in the use of the Experience Sampling Method to assess the impact of daily hassles on psychotic symptoms, valuable insights are provided (see Chapter 9). Moreover, such experiences need to be contextualised; that is, we need to investigate how such individual-level processes interact with features of the wider social environment in which the individual lives (see Chapter 4).

Conclusion

Kleinman (1991) has commented that a substantial amount of social science has been absorbed into medical research where it is often the unrecognised base of epidemiology, health services research and social medicine. There remains, however, scepticism about the potential value of the social sciences, particularly those concerned with interpretations and meaning and that predominantly utilise qualitative methods. Lingering suspicions, in part created by a denial of the reality of mental illness by many social scientists in the 1960s and 1970s, unfortunately obscure the potential value of social science perspectives and methods. This is unfortunate because our understanding of the aetiology of psychosis, of how social and cultural contexts shape the course and outcome of psychosis, and interactions with mental health services, will be greatly enhanced by closer engagement with the social sciences.

REFERENCES

Barrett, R. J. (1998a). Conceptual foundations of schizophrenia: I. Degeneration. *Australian and New Zealand Journal of Psychiatry*, **32** (5), 617–26.

Barrett, R. J. (1998b). Conceptual foundations of schizophrenia: II. Disintegration and division. *Australian and New Zealand Journal of Psychiatry*, **32** (5), 627–34.

Bebbington, P. E., Bhugra, D., Brugha, T. *et al.* (2004). Psychosis, victimisation and childhood disadvantage. *British Journal of Psychiatry*, **185**, 220–6.

Becker, H. (1963). *Outsiders: Studies in the Sociology of Deviance*. New York: Free Press.

Bentall, R. (2003). *Madness Explained: Psychosis and Human Nature*. London: Allen Lane.

Berkman, L. F. and Kawachi, I. (eds) (2000). *Social Epidemiology*. Oxford: Oxford University Press.

Bifulco, A., Brown, G. W. and Adler, Z. (1991). Early sexual abuse and clinical depression in adult life. *British Journal of Psychiatry*, **159**, 115–22.

Bolton, D. (1997). Encoding of meaning: deconstructing the meaning/causality distinction. *Philosophy, Psychiatry and Psychology*, **4**, 255–67.

Boydell, J., van Os, J., McKenzie, K. *et al.* (2001). Incidence of schizophrenia in ethnic minorities in London: ecological study into interactions with environment. *British Medical Journal*, **323** (7325), 1336–8.

Brown, G. and Harris, T. (1978). *The Social Origins of Depression*. London: Tavistock.

Brugha, T., Bebington, P., Tennant, C. *et al.* (1985). The list of threatening experiences: a subset of 12 life event categories with considerable long-term contextual threat. *Psychological Medicine*, **15**, 189–94.

Cantor-Graae, E. and Selten, J. P. (2005). Schizophrenia and migration: a meta-analysis and review. *American Journal of Psychiatry*, **162** (1), 12–24.

Comte, A. (1986). *The Positive Philosophy*. London: Bell and Sons.

Cooper, B. (1992). Sociology in the context of social psychiatry. *British Journal of Psychiatry*, **161**, 594–8.

Crow, T. (2007). How and why genetic linkage has not solved the problem of psychosis: review and hypothesis. *American Journal of Psychiatry*, **164**, 13–21.

Durkheim, E. (1970). *Suicide: A Study in Sociology*. London: Routledge and Kegan Paul.

Eisenberg, L. (1977). Psychiatry and society: a sociobiologic synthesis. *New England Journal of Medicine*, **296**, 903–10.

Eisenberg, L. (1988). The social construction of mental illness. *Psychological Medicine*, **18**, 1–9.

Faris, R. and Dunham, H. (1939). *Mental Disorders in Urban Areas*. Chicago: University of Chicago Press.

Fearon, P. and Morgan, C. (2006). Environmental factors in schizophrenia: the role of migrant studies. *Schizophrenia Bulletin*, **32**, 405–8.

Foucault, M. (1965). *Madness and Civilisation: A History of Insanity in the Age of Reason*. New York: Random House.

Goffman, E. (1961). *Asylums*. New York: Anchor.

Hacking, I. (1998). *Rewriting the Soul: Multiple Personality and the Sciences of Memory*. New Jersey: Princeton University Press.

Hacking, I. (2002). *Mad Travellers: Reflections on the Reality of Transient Mental Illnesses*. Boston: Harvard University Press.

Harris, T. (2001). Recent developments in understanding the psychosocial aspects of depression. *British Medical Bulletin*, **57**, 17–32.

Helman, C. G. (2000). *Culture, Health and Illness*, 4th edn. Oxford: Butterworth Heinemann.

Hollingshead, A. and Redlich, R. C. (1958). *Social Class and Mental Illness*. London: Wiley.

Holmes, T. H. and Rahe, R. H. (1967). The social readjustment rating scale. *Journal of Psychosomatic Research*, **11**, 213–18.

Horwitz, A. V. (2001). *Creating Mental Illness*. Chicago: Chicago University Press.

Horwitz, A. V. and Schied, T. L. (eds) (1999). *A Handbook for the Study of Mental Health: Social Contexts, Theories and Systems*. Cambridge: Cambridge University Press.

Jablensky, A., Sartorius, N., Ernberg, G. *et al.* (1992). Schizophrenia: manifestations, incidence and course in different cultures. A World Health Organization ten-country study. *Psychological Medicine. Monograph Supplement*, **20**, 1–97.

Janssen, I., Krabbendam, L., Bak, M. *et al.* (2004). Childhood abuse as a risk factor for psychosis. *Acta Psychiatrica Scandinavica*, **109**, 38–45.

Kleinman, A. (1987). Anthropology and psychiatry: the role of culture in cross-cultural research on illness. *British Journal of Psychiatry*, **151**, 447–54.

Kleinman, A. (1991). *Rethinking Psychiatry: From Cultural Category to Personal Experience*. New York: The Free Press.

Knapp, M., Thorgrimsen, L., Patel, A. *et al.* (2006). Cognitive stimulation therapy for people with dementia: cost-effectiveness analysis. *British Journal of Psychiatry*, **188**, 574–80.

Laing, R. D. (1960). *The Divided Self*. Harmondsworth: Penguin.

Leff, J. (2001). *The Unbalanced Mind*. London: Weidenfeld and Nicolson.

Link, G. A. and Phelan, J. C. (1999). The labelling theory of mental disorder (II): the consequences of labelling. In *A Handbook for the Study of Mental Health: Social Contexts, Theories and Systems*, ed. A. V. Horwitz and T. L. Schied. Cambridge: Cambridge University Press, pp. 361–76.

Luhrman, T. H. (2000) *Of Two Minds: An Anthropologist Looks at American Psychiatry*. New York: Vintage.

McGrath, J. and Scott, J. (2006). Urban birth and risk of schizophrenia: a worrying example of epidemiology where the data are stronger than the hypotheses. *Epidemiologia e Psichiatria Sociale*, **15**, 243–6.

McKenzie, K. and Harpham, T. (eds) (2006). *Social Capital and Mental Health*. London: Jessica Kingsley.

Meaney, M. J. (2001). Maternal care, gene expression, and the transmission of individual differences in stress reactivity across generations. *Annual Review of Neuroscience*, **24**, 1161–92.

Morgan, C. and Fisher, H. (2007). Environmental factors in schizophrenia: childhood trauma: a critical review. *Schizophrenia Bulletin*, **33** (1), 3–10.

Morgan, C., Mallett, R., Hutchinson, G. *et al.* (2004). Negative pathways to psychiatric care and ethnicity: the bridge between social science and psychiatry. *Social Science and Medicine*, **58**, 739–52.

Morgan, C., Abdul-Al, R., Lappin, J. *et al.* (2006). Clinical and social determinants of duration of untreated psychosis in the ÆSOP first-episode psychosis study. *British Journal of Psychiatry*, **189** (5), 446–52.

Morgan, C., Burns, T., Fitzpatrick, R. *et al.* (in press). Social exclusion and mental health: conceptual and methodological review. *British Journal of Psychiatry*.

Parkin, F. (1982). *Max Weber*. London: Routledge.

Parr, H., Philo, C. and Burns, N. (2004). Social geographies of rural mental health: experiencing inclusions and exclusions. *Transactions of the Institute of British Geographers*, **29**, 401–19.

Patel, V., Cohen, A., Thara, R. *et al.* (2006). Is the outcome of schizophrenia really better in developing countries? *Revista Brasileira Psiquiatria*, **28** (2), 129–52.

Pearlin, L. J. (1999). Stress and mental health: a conceptual overview. In *A Handbook for the Study of Mental Health: Social Contexts, Theories and Systems*, ed. A. V. Horwitz and T. L. Schied. Cambridge: Cambridge University Press, pp. 161–75.

Pedersen, C. and Mortensen, P. (2001). Evidence of a dose–response relationship between urbanicity during upbringing and schizophrenia risk. *Archives of General Psychiatry*, **58**, 1039–46.

Phelan, J. C. and Link, G. A. (1999). The labelling theory of mental disorder (I): the role of social contingencies in the application of psychiatric labels. In *A Handbook for the Study of Mental Health: Social Contexts, Theories and Systems*, ed. A. V. Horwitz and T. L. Schied. Cambridge: Cambridge University Press, pp. 139–50.

Putnam, R. (2000). *Bowling Alone*. New York: Simon and Schuster.

Read, J., van Os, J., Morrison, A. P. *et al.* (2005). Childhood trauma, psychosis and schizophrenia: a literature review with theoretical and clinical implications. *Acta Psychiatrica Scandinavica*, **112**, 330–50.

Rosenhan, D. L. (1973). On being sane in insane places. *Science*, **179**, 250–8.

Roth, M. and Kroll, P. (1986). *The Reality of Mental Illness*. Cambridge: Cambridge University Press.

Scheff, T. J. (1966). *Being Mentally Ill: A Sociological Theory*. Chicago: Aldine Publishing Company.

Scull, A. (2005). *Madhouse: A Tragic Tale of Megalomania and Modern Medicine*. New Haven: Yale University Press.

Selye, H. (1978). *Stresses of Life*. Maidenhead: McGraw-Hill.

Skultans, V. (1991). Anthropology and psychiatry: the uneasy alliance. *Transcultural Psychiatry*, **28**, 5–24.

Skultans, V. and Cox, J. (2000). Introduction. In *Anthropological Approaches to Psychological Medicine: Crossing Bridges*, ed. V. Skultans and J. Cox. London: Jessica Kingsley, pp. 7–40.

Spauwen, J., Krabbendam, L., Lieb, R. *et al.* (2006). Impact of psychological trauma on the development of psychotic symptoms: relationship with psychosis proneness. *British Journal of Psychiatry*, **188**, 527–33.

Suchman, E. A. (1967). Social stress and cardiovascular disease: appraisal and implications for theoretical development. *Millbank Memorial Fund Quarterly*, **45**, 109–13.

Szasz, T. (1960). The myth of mental illness. *American Psychologist*, (15 Feb.), 113–18.

Teicher, M. H., Andersen, S. L., Polcari, A. *et al.* (2003). The neurobiological consequences of early stress and childhood maltreatment. *Neuroscience and Behavioral Reviews*, **27**, 33–44.

Thoits, P. A. (1999). Sociological approaches to mental illness. In *A Handbook for the Study of Mental Health: Social Contexts, Theories and Systems*, ed. A. V. Horwitz and T. L. Schied. Cambridge: Cambridge University Press, pp. 121–38.

Thornicroft, G. (2006). *Shunned*. Oxford: Oxford University Press.

van Os, J. (2004). Does the urban environment cause psychosis? *British Journal of Psychiatry*, **184**, 287–8.

Ware, N., Hopper, K., Tugenberg, T. *et al.* (2007). Connectedness and citizenship: redefining social integration. *Psychiatric Services*, **58**, 469–74.

Warner, R. (2003). *Recovery from Schizophrenia: Psychiatry and the Political Economy*, 3rd edn. London: Routledge.

Waxler, N. (1977). Is mental illness cured in traditional societies? A theoretical analysis. *Culture, Medicine and Psychiatry*, **1**, 233–53.

Wheaton, B. (1999). The nature of stressors. In *A Handbook for the Study of Mental Health: Social Contexts, Theories and Systems*, ed. A. V. Horwitz and T. L. Schied. Cambridge: Cambridge University Press, pp. 176–97.

Wing, J. and Brown, G. (1970). *Institutionalism and Schizophrenia*. London: Cambridge University Press.

4

Conceptualising the social world

Dana March, Craig Morgan, Michaeline Bresnahan and Ezra Susser

Introduction

The social world has long been of interest to those concerned with the aetiology, course and outcome of psychosis. In the middle decades of the twentieth century, the relationship between aspects of the social world and the causes of psychosis was the subject of a number of influential studies (e.g., Faris and Dunham, 1939; Hare, 1956; Hollingshead and Redlich, 1958). It provided a rich subject for sociologists and others, as well as an important theme for psychiatric epidemiology. While the findings consistently indicated higher rates of serious mental illness in the most socially disadvantaged and marginalised groups, unresolved disputes about the causal direction of these associations contributed to a declining interest in the role of social factors in the aetiology of schizophrenia and other psychoses. Eclipsed for a period of time by other types of investigation – largely individually oriented and biological – the social world has appeared once again in our causal field. In recent years, a growing body of research has revived the notion that social factors play some role in the full sequence of causes of psychosis.

Conceptualising the social world, the subject of this chapter, is a critical first step in attempting to understand the aetiological role of social factors. The formulation of our research questions, interpretation of data and refinement of our hypotheses rely on our conception of the social world. This chapter draws on ideas developed in a previous era to suggest a theoretically informed rubric for conceptualising components of the social world to make them amenable to investigation, the focus being specifically on aetiology. We address the necessity of considering distinctions between processes and conditions, levels of organisation and place and time.

History and currency

The importance and prominence attached to social factors as potential contributing causes of psychotic disorders has fluctuated over the past century. For example, during

Society and Psychosis, ed. Craig Morgan, Kwame McKenzie and Paul Fearon. Published by Cambridge University Press. © Cambridge University Press 2008.

the latter half of the nineteenth and the first half of the twentieth centuries, the causes of mental disorders were thought by some to be largely sociocultural in nature, a perspective that perhaps reflected a wider concern with the socially corrosive effects of large-scale processes – primarily industrialisation, urbanisation and migration. A number of studies from this era found striking differences between social groups and across social contexts in the prevalence of schizophrenia and other psychoses (for a review of select domains, see Murphy, 1961). To test theories that social arrangements might be of aetiological significance, sociologists and social psychiatrists attempted to capture and study markers of these dynamic social processes. Various constructs, such as social disorganisation and social isolation, crystallised from sociological theories and informed the construction of social variables that were examined quantitatively.

Perhaps the best known of these early studies is Faris and Dunham's *Mental Disorders in Urban Areas* (1939), a pioneering investigation carried out in Chicago in the 1930s. The study examined the relationship between the functional psychoses and social organisation, a construct that emerged from theories put forward to under-stand the relationship between urban environs and social problems. Congruent with the Chicago school of sociology, a dominant force in shaping the zeitgeist of socio-logical research at the time, Faris and Dunham theorised social isolation and compro-mised communication as sociological explanations of mental disorders. Application of the concentric zone model of urban organisation – developed a decade earlier by their mentor, sociologist Ernest Burgess, in a study of Chicago (Park *et al.*, 1925) – allowed Faris and Dunham to test their theories empirically. In this model, inner urban zones consisted of the most disorganised communities, characterised by isolation and poor communication among their residents. Social organisation increased as the circles radiated from the epicentre (see Figure 4.1). Faris and Dunham hypothesised an inverse relationship between social organisation and rates of mental disorder, i.e., that inner urban zones would have higher rates of mental disorder.

Mining available data to test this hypothesis empirically, Faris and Dunham conceived of social organisation as a function of social interaction within a given context, and examined variables that characterised communities in such terms. Context was captured by characteristics of a community's built environment as measured by residence type (e.g., rooming-house, rental, etc.). Social interaction was approximated by variables comprising population characteristics, both fixed (e.g., country of birth) and dynamic (e.g., mobility and government assistance status), framed in terms of the community (e.g., percent minority). Consistent with their hypothesis, a distinct social patterning of schizophrenia – though not manic-depression – emerged; the highest rates of schizophrenia were found in the most socially disorganised areas.

As many commentators have subsequently pointed out, these findings do not necessarily implicate social disorganisation in the aetiology of schizophrenia. They

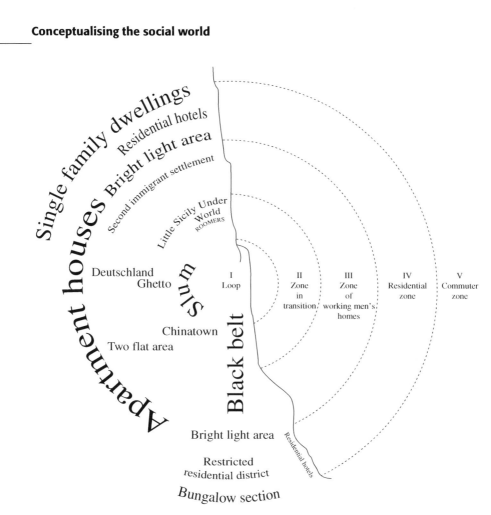

Figure 4.1   The concentric zone model devised by Ernest Burgess in a 1920s study of Chicago (adapted from Faris and Dunham, 1939)

may also reflect a downward drift of those with schizophrenia into areas characterised by disorganisation and instability. Faris and Dunham considered downward drift as one of a number of potential explanations of their findings, but concluded that drift could not fully account for their results. In fact, their analysis encompassed a whole range of social phenomena – including the notion of ethnic density, explored in greater detail below. For our purposes, one of the most salient aspects of the work of Faris and Dunham, which helped lay the foundation for psychiatric epidemiology and shape quantitative sociological investigations with the refinement of the ecological study design, is their sophisticated attempt to conceptualise and measure aspects of the social environment.

In terms of conceptualising the social world, the work of Faris and Dunham highlights two critical points still relevant to the study of social factors. First, theory should inform constructs, which in turn, bear on our definition and measurement of variables. Second, to achieve an understanding of the full range and sequence of causes of illness, social factors should be considered in concert with other variables. When Faris and Dunham carried out their work in Chicago, causal factors were viewed as being located in three primary domains: constitutional, psychological and sociological.

The ecological notion of aetiology held by Faris and Dunham and their contemporaries eventually gave way to a focus on what they termed constitutional factors. In the past 25 years, the primary focus in mainstream epidemiology and medicine has been on biological and genetic determinants of health. Social factors have often been relegated to the realm of the invariant and potentially confounding; downstream causes, more proximal to the individual, have been prioritised.

In the current era, in which interest in social factors has been revived, we are charged with understanding what and how social conditions and experiences over the life course may contribute to the aetiology of psychosis (see Part II). In this, there is much that can be learned from the early literature. The concepts put forward by researchers in that era, like Faris and Dunham, inform a key guiding principle: conceptualising the social world should be infused with theory and attentive to history. Beyond the theory, we are also challenged to define and measure constructs of interest. Below, we outline a logic and strategy – informed by an ecological perspective – that can be used to build an understanding, and capture the complexities, of the social world.

Processes and conditions

Organisation of the social world calls for consideration of the relationship between processes and conditions. Processes refer to phenomena marked by changes that lead to a particular result. Conditions are characteristics that evidence changes in our world; they are indices of processes. At any given moment, they capture a state resulting from processes. Conditions can be caused by one or more processes. Any condition resulting from processes can be defined operationally and measured, at least in theory. While this chapter focuses on social processes resulting in conditions that may be considered aetiologically important exposures, it is important to bear in mind that social processes are embodied and give rise to changes in states of health. It is through the process of embodiment that social processes and conditions play a causative role.

A number of steps are required. First, we need to form theories about the aetiological role of processes and conditions and how they are embodied. We then need to capture conditions quantitatively by forming constructs and variables intended to measure these relevant operationally defined constructs. These steps are dependent and inter-related. Formulating our hypotheses and empirically testing our theories relies on our constructs and variables, and forming our constructs and variables depends on our theories and hypotheses.

Consider, for example, socioeconomic status (SES), a common exposure and confounder in psychiatric epidemiology. Socioeconomic status is a complex condition that results from many dynamic processes. However, most studies treat SES crudely as a unidimensional and static condition. The conception of SES varies by location; in Europe, occupation forms the basis for SES, while income or education is used in the USA (Braveman *et al.*, 2005). Moreover, the point at which SES is measured is a crucial consideration; changes in SES over the life course affect risk of various outcomes – a finding well documented for physical health outcomes (e.g., Davey Smith *et al.*, 1997). Various indicators of SES capture different aspects of the construct, and thus have limitations in terms of measuring SES as a social cause of illness (Galobardes *et al.*, 2006). Many measures of SES lack the proper grounding in social theory, which, in effect, divorces SES as a condition from the processes that gave rise to it.

We can take this further. Wittingly or not, the choice of occupation or education as a marker for SES will reflect past theoretical formulations. Concern with social status and position within the overall social structure has been a focus of sociological interest for the past century. Many of the most influential thinkers produced detailed theories relevant to understanding social structure and its influence on action. For instance, Marx's formulation of social class as a function of an individual's relationship to the means of production underpins the use of occupation (i.e., economic position) as the basis for determining SES – even if current systems of classification include more social classes than a Marxist theoretical orientation permits. In contrast, the use of education, income and wealth as markers of SES reflects Weberian notions that social position is influenced partly by 'social honour' and 'styles of living' in specific communities. Understanding *that* social factors, like those captured by SES, affect health is well established (e.g., Marmot and Wilkinson, 1999). Understanding *how*, which requires theory, is our current challenge (Lynch and Kaplan, 2000). Ultimately, our choice of theory, which shapes our constructs and our variables, must be guided by a broad conception of aetiology, encouraging us to consider the mechanistic role of social factors.

Indeed, the role of social factors was examined rigorously within the context of the selection–causation debate (e.g., Dohrenwend *et al.*, 1992). A clear social class gradient exists for schizophrenia; those with the disorder are much more likely to be of low SES. Preoccupation with whether SES is a cause or consequence of the disorder has ultimately led to a focus on parental – primarily paternal – social class at birth. With parental social class, however, the evidence for a gradient is inconsistent; it appears that SES affects the risk of schizophrenia in children only from the lowest social classes or with other indicators of adversity (Byrne *et al.*, 2004;

Wicks *et al.*, 2005). The point is that an emphasis on the role of SES diverted attention from conceptualising and investigating other aspects of the social world. Creative efforts to translate concepts of social stratification into environmental exposures have not been taken up in larger contexts (Link *et al.*, 1986). Overall, theoretical considerations have been generally absent from debates in the recent literature about the relationship between SES and psychosis.

Recognition of these and other problems has led to recent calls for a refined approach to SES that is both outcome and social group specific. Braveman and colleagues (2005) recommend granting consideration to: plausible pathways and mechanisms, gathering all potentially relevant socioeconomic information, specifying the measured components of SES and systematically considering the potential effects of unmeasured socioeconomic factors. An important step forward is the recognition that most of our current measures capture a condition at a given moment. As the product of complex processes, a condition is subject to change over time. The challenge is to develop concepts and methodological tools that are better equipped to approximate social processes and their dynamics over time.

Levels of organisation

There are myriad ways in which the social world and related processes have been understood and studied in relation to health and illness by researchers working from within a range of academic disciplines. The scope of this chapter limits consideration of that work. Our focus is instead on the provision of a framework, with illustrative examples, built on the idea that the social world can be conceptualised and studied at different levels of organisation, from the microscopic to the macroscopic.

In our world, phenomena take on different properties as they become increasingly complex. There are different levels at which certain properties of phenomena emerge; they constitute the units of analysis in our research studies. While the concept of levels of organisation is not new – it was formally introduced into epidemiology by Mervyn Susser in the 1970s (Susser, 1973) – it was taken up in the mainstream only in the last decade (Diez-Roux, 1998). It forms a useful organising framework for this discussion.

Central to this framework is the notion that phenomena can be arranged in a hierarchy of increasing complexity. Each level of organisation is a more complex whole consisting of less complex parts. Each whole is one level of organisation higher than its component parts, and creates the context in which its component parts exist. A part on one level of organisation is a whole on a lower level of organisation, and a whole on one level of organisation is a part on a higher level of organisation (March and Susser, in press; Susser *et al.*, 2006, pp. 441–60). For

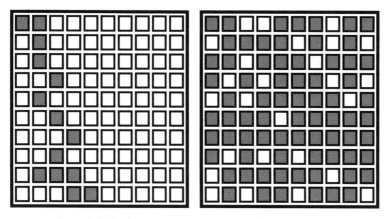

Low ethnic density   High ethnic density

Figure 4.2 Ethnic density. The black squares represent a given minority group; the white squares represent the majority group. Low ethnic density, depicted by the left square, is the situation in which the minority group constitutes a small proportion of the total number in a given area. High ethnic density, depicted by the right square, is the situation in which the minority group constitutes a high proportion of the total number in a given area.

instance, individuals are the constituent parts of the wholes of neighbourhoods, and neighbourhoods are the constituent parts of the wholes of towns.

Each whole has characteristics or properties that are distinct from those of its constituent parts. The characteristics of neighbourhoods differ from the characteristics of their constituent individuals. For instance, ethnicity is a characteristic of an individual, while ethnic density (e.g., the proportion of a given ethnicity in a given area; see Figure 4.2) is a characteristic of a neighbourhood. While individual ethnicity contributes to the ethnic density of the neighbourhood in which an individual resides, ethnic density is a property that emerges at a group level – in this instance, the neighbourhood. Characteristics at each of these levels are interdependent and can have both independent and interlinked effects.

Individual ethnicity may have effects on health that are independent of the ethnic density of a neighbourhood. Perhaps more important, however, are the combined effects of individual ethnicity and ethnic density. Though the nature of the combined effects is unknown, we can consider two possibilities and their implications. A finding that the effects conferred by individual ethnicity and ethnic density are additive, such that being a minority and living in a minority neighbourhood both confer increased risk, is consistent with an aetiological role of the social *or* physical environments. A finding that the combined effects of individual ethnicity and ethnic density are interactive, such that being a minority and living in a neighbourhood of the majority ethnicity confers increased risk, is more consistent with an aetiological role primarily for the social environment. In keeping with studies conducted by

Faris and Dunham (1939) and others (e.g., Rabkin, 1979), a recent study conducted in south London by Boydell and colleagues (2001) supports the latter. The risk of schizophrenia increased for African-Caribbean and black African groups as they formed a decreasing proportion of the local population. This suggests an interaction between ethnic density and individual ethnicity (Boydell *et al.*, 2001). Moreover, it underscores the importance of conceptualising the social world and experience at different levels of organisation and investigating interactions between them.

Further, variation in factors at a given level of organisation might not explain variation in factors at another level of organisation. Indeed, the factors that cause variation in the rates of disorder across populations may be different from the factors that cause variation in disease risk among individuals within a population (Schwartz and Diez-Roux, 2001; Susser *et al.*, 2006). Alternatively phrased, the causes of incidence rates are not necessarily the causes of cases in a given population. For example, a factor such as municipal services may vary across cities. Indeed, it may partially explain the variation of incidence rates of a given illness across cities. However, municipal services may not vary within a city, and would not explain variation in illness among individuals within a city. Restricting our studies to the detection of factors that cause inter-individual variation precludes detecting the impact of factors at other levels; explaining variation in rates of disorder at other levels of social organisation is essential to uncovering the full range and sequence of causes of psychosis.

The number of levels of social organisation is, in theory, considerable, beginning with the global population, and descending through levels such as societies, regions, towns, neighbourhoods, families and, ultimately, individuals. It is impossible to encompass all levels in one study. An essential step in any particular investigation of social factors, therefore, is to select the levels of organisation considered most important to the aetiological question at hand. For Faris and Dunham, the community level constituted the most important level of organisation. Since they were interested in testing a social disorganisation theory, their work examined community characteristics and rates of serious mental illness, as opposed to individual characteristics and cases of psychosis.

These points, and the utility of this organising framework, can be illustrated with specific examples. Here we consider two levels: the societal and the individual. These examples further allow for discussion of the importance of theory in driving the ways in which we seek to make sense of the social world and consider its impact on the risk of psychosis.

Urbanicity and schizophrenia

One of the most consistent findings in the epidemiology of schizophrenia is that those who live in cities are at greater risk (see Chapter 6). Given that social drift is less likely in view of recent evidence (Krabbendam and van Os, 2005), how do we explain this finding? Are people who live in cities more likely to be exposed to known risk factors? Or is the reservoir of risk found in some characteristic of cities, such as the physical and human geography or social structure? Most recent research has operationalised urbanicity using population density (e.g., Pedersen and Mortensen, 2001). However, there have been very few attempts to move beyond this broad and relatively crude measure to examine specific hypotheses about either the structure of cities or experiences of living in cities. There have been few studies of the physical environments of cities, including levels of pollution and other potentially toxic exposures, though it appears that the risks conferred by urban areas persist even when there is movement to a rural area (Pedersen and Mortensen, 2006), indicating the family as a potentially important reservoir of risk (March and Susser, 2006).

The relatively small amount of extant research that transcends the crude urban–rural distinction emphasises the need for more theoretically informed studies (e.g., van Os *et al.*, 2000). In one example, Kirkbride and colleagues have shown that risk of schizophrenia varies both within and between urban centres (Kirkbride *et al.*, 2007). This is illustrated in Figure 4.3, which provides the relative risks by neighbourhood for a large inner-city area in south-east London. The darker shades represent higher relative risks for schizophrenia. It is not necessary to understand the statistical models generating these data to see the clear variation even within a densely populated urban centre – a finding that clearly mirrors the work of Faris and Dunham (1939).

Two important conclusions follow. The first is that social factors must be considered across different levels of organisation. The second is that future research needs to be more theoretically and conceptually informed if meaningful hypotheses are to be generated and tested.

Migration and psychosis

As robust and consistent as the association between urbanicity and schizophrenia is the association between migrant or ethnic minority status and psychosis in Western Europe (Cantor-Graae and Selten, 2005; Fearon and Morgan, 2006; see Chapter 10). As with the association between urbanicity and schizophrenia, we are faced with the task of attempting to explain this association. Most commentators point to the social environment, broadly construed. A number of candidate explanatory factors have been proposed, including socioeconomic disadvantage, social isolation, social defeat and discrimination (Cantor-Graae and Selten, 2005; Fearon and Morgan, 2006). The findings from the study by Boydell and colleagues (2001), for example, hint at a protective role for social cohesion in areas with high ethnic density. However, once again, the question remains unanswered: is migrant

a) Area of study: south-east London, UK   b) Posterior probability of relative risk greater than 1.0

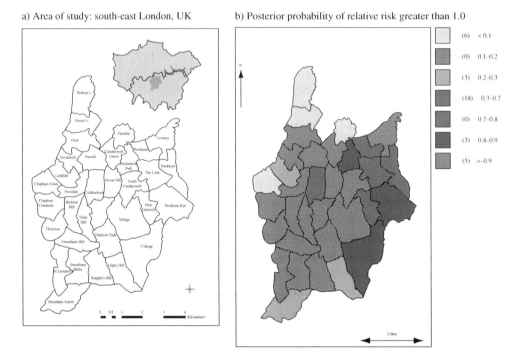

Figure 4.3   Variation in incidence of schizophrenia by neighbourhood in south-east London, UK (modified from Kirkbride *et al.*, 2007). Explanatory note: Figure 4.3 shows the Bayesian posterior probabilities of a rate ratio exceeding 1.0 in any given ward, having been adjusted for individual-level sex, age and ethnicity (where 1.0 represents the mean incidence rate of the study area). Bayesian posterior probabilities of greater than 0.8 indicate good evidence of areas with raised incidence rates, not explained by individual characteristics. Conversely, Bayesian posterior probabilities of less than 0.2 indicate good evidence of wards with rate ratios of less than 1.0 (i.e., where the incidence rate is significantly lower than the study area rate). Taken as a whole, the map indicates that the incidence of schizophrenia is not homogenous by neighbourhood, even after adjustment for the aforementioned individual-level risk factors. (We are very grateful to James Kirkbride for providing this explanatory note.)

status or ethnicity, in this context, a proxy marker for exposure to known or hypothesised social factors, or are more specific factors operating, relating perhaps to processes of acculturation or discrimination in areas of low ethnic density?

There is a need to move beyond simply employing demographic labels, such as SES, to investigate the impact of lived experiences. For this, concepts capable of capturing or at least approximating the relevant social processes need to be developed and employed. Discrimination, for example, is a multifaceted concept that assumes varied forms (e.g., economic, institutional, interpersonal, legal, direct or indirect), is expressed in different ways (e.g., non-verbal, verbal, violent) and occurs in a range of domains (e.g., in the family, at school, at work, in interactions with public servants) and at different levels (e.g., individual, neighbourhood, region). There have been some attempts to investigate aspects of discrimination and risk of psychosis in migrant and ethnic minority groups (Karlsen et al., 2005). Studies employing clear conceptual frameworks, and, where possible, taking account of the impact of duration, timing and severity of discrimination, are necessary to move from broad associations to meaningful understanding. In addition, as noted above, there is a need to distinguish the effects that operate at the level of the individual (e.g., interpersonal discrimination) from those that operate at the level of the group (e.g., ethnic density) (for a relevant analysis see Kirkbride et al., in press).

The ecological and atomistic fallacies

Care must be taken to guard against two common inferential mistakes involving multiple levels of organisation. The ecological fallacy is familiar to most investigators. It results from making comparisons across populations and inferring causation at the individual level (Susser, 1973; Susser et al., 2006). For example, Faris and Dunham (1939) found that populations living in more socially organised areas had lower rates of schizophrenia. Social organisation may have caused rates in populations to vary, but could not account for inter-individual variation within a given population, since everyone within that population has the same exposure.

The equally important converse fallacy, sometimes referred to as the atomistic fallacy, is less familiar (Susser, 1973). It results from comparing individuals and inferring causation at the group level. Suppose we find that cannabis use is associated with the development of schizophrenia in individuals. While cannabis use might contribute to variation among individuals in risk of schizophrenia, differences in community prevalence of cannabis use may not explain variation in rates of schizophrenia across populations. From determinants of variation among individuals, we cannot reliably infer a corresponding ecological determinant of variation across populations.

Measurement and analysis

Companion considerations to inference are those of measurement and analysis. The most rigorous studies of the social world measure it directly at the relevant levels of organisation and compare rates of disorder across varying contexts. However, these studies are exceptional. It is much more common to add measures thought to reflect social context indirectly to studies of individuals. We may, for example, ask individuals about the characteristics of their neighbourhood, rather than actually measuring the characteristics of the neighbourhood itself. Moreover, studies are rarely designed with sufficient variation at higher levels of organisation, such as the city (March and Susser, in press).

With the advent of multilevel modelling, analytic approaches do not compel researchers to assign greater importance to individual-level factors than to societal-level factors (Diez-Roux, 1998). Given the requisite data, it is possible to analyse group-level as well as individual-level variation within the same study. There are emerging examples of this in relation to psychosis (e.g., Kirkbride *et al.*, in press). Still, it must be acknowledged that study designs and statistical methods are better developed for studying variation across individuals than across contexts.

Place and time

A further consideration in conceptualising the social world is the place in, and time over, which processes occur. Social processes occur in a given place and over a given period of time. In what place and over what time is important in understanding aetiology. It structures the dimensions of our causal field.

Understanding the place in which social factors exist is part and parcel of determining their relevance to aetiology. Place structures social factors; space constitutes one important aspect of place. For example, in neighbourhoods with few physical spaces conducive to social interaction – whether they do not exist in the built environment, or they exist and are either in disrepair or are unsafe – there may be more social isolation. The significance of place as it bears on social factors was illustrated clearly in the work of Faris and Dunham, and has certainly been the subject of a large and growing body of scientific literature.

As emphasised earlier, it is necessary to measure characteristics of place so that our understanding of social factors can be enhanced. Aspects of place can assume the form of conditions that one could measure at a given level of organisation across contexts. Like SES, however, measurement of place to enhance our understanding of social factors can be, in part, context specific. Some characteristics of place that might bear on social factors as causes of illness in New York City may well differ from those in, for example, Nottingham. Drawing on theory and empirical work, researchers interested in social factors should take care to consider properly the characteristics of the areas under investigation and how they shape the social processes that occur in that particular space.

Social processes also occur over time. At a given moment, we are interested in a particular social condition or a particular set of social conditions consequent to social processes that occur over time. Because social conditions that exist at one time may affect states of health later on (i.e., latent effects), we must consider the passage of time and its relationship to social conditions of aetiological interest. Even when we focus on social conditions at a particular moment, we should always be mindful of dynamic interplay, and the resulting possibilities of both time-sensitive and cumulative effects. The deeper meanings of social processes (e.g., segregation, assimilation) that are currently being investigated cross-sectionally (e.g., ethnic density) may emerge when considered longitudinally.

In attempting to understand aetiological processes in psychosis and other disease outcomes, time also has several levels. On one level, time means at what point or across what period in history. On another level, time means at what point or across what period in an individual life course. It is likely that age, period and cohort effects all exist for psychosis, indicating the importance of considering historical time and its effects on aetiological processes, including the distribution of risk factors. Consider one of a number of examples from the schizophrenia literature. Takei and colleagues (1996) examined data on a Scottish national sample of patients (6301 males and 5047 females) diagnosed with schizophrenia, first admitted between 1966 and 1990. Adjustment for age and period effects indicated a 55% and 39% respective reduction in the incidence of schizophrenia in males and females born between 1923 and 1973. The authors posit a diminishing intensity of environmental factors as one possible explanation of their findings (Takei *et al.*, 1996), a suggestion that has been the source of some debate. Nonetheless, findings like these highlight the importance of the social world and the need to consider historical time in aetiological studies. Consideration of historical time is critical to contextualising data, particularly data that have been collected in the past, perhaps even generations ago. Understanding history helps us to understand the types and magnitude of social processes that might be causally significant.

We also know that the individual life course must be considered when determining the effect of exposures on outcomes. It may be, for example, that susceptibility to adult life stresses is influenced by early childhood adversity (see Chapter 7). Alternatively phrased, time, over both the life course and history, affects our conception of potentially important social factors as causes of changes in states of health. Time, both life-course and historical, can shape the meaning of social processes and hence their relevance to aetiology. For instance, at one moment during the life course, social isolation may be more important than at other times. During the process of transition from childhood to adulthood, one potentially critical period of psychosis risk, social isolation may exert particularly negative effects. Likewise, there may be periods in history in a given place that social isolation is greater and thus more aetiologically operative than others.

New directions

One of the most pressing problems in conceptualising the social world is bringing together all elements of the rubric set forth in the previous sections of this chapter. Uniting these would require consideration of the relevant processes and conditions, levels of organisation and place and time, in order to generate a greater understanding of aetiology.

One relevant process is segregation. Movement in and out of cities and ethnic density are related to the process of segregation. Both theory and technology are currently being developed to enrich our understanding of segregation and, thereby, related processes and conditions. Sociologists Sean Reardon and David O'Sullivan have put forward a line of thinking and companion analytic tools that foster an understanding of the conception and measurement of segregation, both as a process and as a condition – a pattern of spatially uneven distribution of groups in a region (Reardon and O'Sullivan, 2004). Their thinking reaches beyond the concept of ethnic density to account for the spatial patterning of population distributions. Reardon and O'Sullivan have developed an index of the proportion of a group in a particular space that accounts for the distribution of the proportion therein (Reardon and O'Sullivan, 2004). Their work provides more resolution by granting both specificity and a dynamic dimension to our understanding of one of the processes that evinces the condition we know as 'ethnic density'.

In one recent analysis, Reardon and colleagues applied this approach to the 100 largest metropolitan areas in the USA between 1990 and 2000. They considered the scale on which, as well as the time over which, racial residential segregation occurred. By considering the spatial distribution of the percentage composition of minority groups (i.e., ethnic density), they found that racial residential segregation occurred on different scales. Over the decade examined, black–white segregation on a macroscopic scale remained virtually unchanged, while it declined on a microscopic scale (Reardon et al., 2007). Examining segregation on different scales, akin to examining segregation at different levels of organisation, provides a more nuanced understanding of the spatial distribution of population groups and the social processes exerting effects thereon.

Reardon and colleagues examined the process of segregation without relating it to any outcome. Their work, however, helps us to understand the possibilities for rendering the social world amenable to aetiological investigation. In demonstrating a means of determining where, when and on what scale the process of segregation operates, they show how other processes, such as immigration, affect ethnic density, thereby extending our understanding of how immigration might be related to both urbanicity and ethnic density. Understanding ethnic density as a function of segregation may prove useful in terms of determining whether the ethnic density effect, which has spawned a line of research addressing its relation to psychosis, varies across contexts. For instance, does ethnic density as a neighbourhood or community characteristic mean something different for migrants in ethnic enclaves than for native ethnic minorities who are segregated by law or by an extreme structuring of their opportunities to live in more integrated areas? Indeed, understanding the processes that give rise to the conditions that we might find aetiologically relevant presents an immediate challenge if we are to pursue social factors in a meaningful fashion, fully considering processes and conditions, levels of organisation and place and time.

Conclusion

Much recent research investigating the relationship between social conditions and experiences and risk of psychosis has focused on individual-level factors, often measured fairly crudely. The very nature of the studies from which the data are culled is partly responsible. Many have utilised large population-based register data or already existing cohorts, where the available variables are not within the control of the investigators. However, such studies have been of crucial importance in re-establishing social contexts as relevant to the aetiology of psychosis. These should be supplemented with more detailed investigations.

The social sciences can inform a more complete conceptualisation and measurement of individual-level risk factors. However, individual-level factors occur in a social context, which needs to be conceptualised, measured and modelled with respect to a given outcome or set of outcomes. Carefully conceptualising and measuring the social world, while time consuming and difficult, is essential if we are to understand the aetiology of psychosis. For psychosis, as with a host of other illnesses, the social world must be considered fully and integrated with other evidence to achieve a broader, ecological understanding of aetiology.

REFERENCES

Boydell, J., van Os, J., McKenzie, K. *et al.* (2001). Incidence of schizophrenia in ethnic minorities in London: ecological study into interactions with environment. *British Medical Journal*, **323** (7325), 1336–8.

Braveman, P., Cubbin, C., Egerter, S. *et al.* (2005). Socioeconomic status in health research: one size does not fit all. *Journal of the American Medical Association*, **294** (22), 2879–88.

Byrne, M., Agerbo, E., Eaton, W. *et al.* (2004). Parental socio-economic status and risk of first admission with schizophrenia – a Danish national register based study. *Social Psychiatry and Psychiatric Epidemiology*, **39** (2), 87–96.

Cantor-Graae, E. and Selten, J. (2005). Schizophrenia and migration: meta-analysis and review. *American Journal of Psychiatry*, **162** (1), 12–24.

Davey Smith, G., Hart, C., Blane, D. *et al.* (1997). Lifetime socioeconomic position and mortality: prospective observational study. *British Medical Journal*, **314** (7080), 547.

Diez-Roux, A. (1998). Bringing context back into epidemiology: variables and fallacies in multilevel analyses. *American Journal of Public Health*, **88**, 216–22.

Dohrenwend, B., Levav, I., Shrout, P. *et al.* (1992). Socioeconomic status and psychiatric disorders: the causation-selection issue. *Science*, **255** (5047), 946–52.

Faris, R. and Dunham, H. (1939). *Mental Disorders in Urban Areas*. Chicago: The University of Chicago Press.

Fearon, P. and Morgan, C. (2006). Environmental factors in schizophrenia: the role of migrant studies. *Schizophrenia Bulletin*, **32** (3), 405–8.

Galobardes, B., Shaw, M., Lawlor, D. *et al.* (2006). Indicators of socioeconomic position (part 1). *Journal of Epidemiology and Community Health*, **60** (1), 7–12.

Hare, E. (1956). Mental illness and social conditions in Bristol. *Journal of Medical Science*, **102**, 349–57.

Hollingshead, A. and Redlich, F. (1958). *Social Class and Mental Illness*. New York: John Wiley and Sons.

Karlsen, S., Nazroo, J., McKenzie, K. *et al.* (2005). Racism, psychosis and common mental disorder among ethnic minority groups in England. *Psychological Medicine*, **35** (12), 1795–803.

Kirkbride, J. B., Fearon, P., Morgan, C. *et al.* (2007). Neighbourhood variation in the incidence of psychotic mental disorders in Southeast London. *Social Psychiatry and Psychiatric Epidemiology*, **42** (6), 438–45.

Kirkbride, J., Morgan, C., Fearon, P. *et al.* (in press). Neighbourhood-level effects on psychoses: towards a new psychiatric paradigm. *Psychological Medicine*.

Krabbendam, L. and van Os, J. (2005). Schizophrenia and urbanicity: a major environmental influence – conditional on genetic risk. *Schizophrenia Bulletin*, **31** (4), 795–9.

Link, B., Dohrenwend, B. and Skodol, A. (1986). Socio-economic status and schizophrenia: noisome occupational characteristics as a risk factor. *American Sociological Review*, **51** (2), 242–58.

Lynch, J. and Kaplan, G. (2000). Socioeconomic position. In *Social Epidemiology*, ed. L. Berkman and I. Kawachi. New York: Oxford University Press, pp. 13–35.

March, D. and Susser, E. (2006). Invited commentary: taking the search for causes of schizophrenia to a different level. *American Journal of Epidemiology*, **163** (11), 979–81.

March, D. and Susser, E. (in press). Developing perspective: social context and developmental psychopathology. In *Genetic and Environmental Influences on Developmental Psychopathology*, ed. J. Hudziak. Arlington, VA: APPI Press.

Marmot, M. and Wilkinson, R. (eds) (1999). *Social Determinants of Health*. Oxford: Oxford University Press.

Murphy, H. (1961). Social change and mental health. *The Milbank Memorial Fund Quarterly*, **39** (3), 385–445.

Park, R., Burgess, E. and McKenzie, R. (1925). *The City*. Chicago: The University of Chicago Press.

Pedersen, C. and Mortensen, P. (2001). Evidence of a dose–response relationship between urbanicity during upbringing and schizophrenia risk. *Archives of General Psychiatry*, **58** (11), 1039–46.

Pedersen, C. and Mortensen, P. (2006). Are the cause(s) responsible for urban–rural differences in schizophrenia risk rooted in families or individuals? *American Journal of Epidemiology*, **163** (11), 971–8.

Rabkin, J. (1979). Ethnic density and psychiatric hospitalization: hazards of minority status. *American Journal of Psychiatry*, **136** (12), 1562–6.

Reardon, S. and O'Sullivan, D. (2004). Measures of spatial segregation. *Sociological Methods*, **34**, 1221–62.

Reardon, S. F., Farrell, C. R., Matthews, S. *et al.* (2007). *Race and Space in the 1990s: Changes in the Spatial Scale of Racial Residential Segregation, 1990–2000*. Paper presented at the annual meeting of the Population Association of America, New York, NY, USA, March, 2007. Available at: www.pop.psu.edu/mss/pubs.htm.

Schwartz, S. and Diez-Roux, A. (2001). Commentary: causes of incidence and causes of cases – a Durkheimian perspective on Rose. *International Journal of Epidemiology*, **30** (3), 435–9.

Susser, E., Schwartz, S., Morabia, A. *et al.* (2006). *Psychiatric Epidemiology: Searching for the Causes of Mental Disorders*. New York: Oxford University Press.

Susser, M. (1973). *Causal Thinking in the Health Sciences*. New York: Oxford University Press.

Takei, N., Lewis, G., Sham, P. *et al.* (1996). Age-period-cohort analysis of the incidence of schizophrenia in Scotland. *Psychological Medicine*, **26** (5), 963–73.

van Os, J., Driessen, G., Gunther, N. *et al.* (2000). Neighbourhood variation in incidence of schizophrenia. Evidence for person–environment interaction. *British Journal of Psychiatry*, **176**, 243–8.

Wicks, S., Hjern, A., Gunnell, D. *et al.* (2005). Social adversity in childhood and the risk of developing psychosis: a national cohort study. *American Journal of Psychiatry*, **162**, 1652–7.

5

Genes and the social environment

Jennifer H. Barnett and Peter B. Jones

Introduction

Understanding the contributions of both genes and environments is essential to unravelling the aetiology of psychosis. In this chapter, we consider how genes might interact with aspects of the social environment in the genesis of psychiatric disorders. We describe evidence for such interactions from early adoption studies to recent investigations using modern molecular genetic techniques. We discuss the principal methodological issues of such research, and the need for clarification of the mechanisms of gene–environment interaction. Finally we consider the challenges that increasing knowledge of epigenetics will bring to the field.

History and overview of the field

Schizophrenia and other psychotic illnesses are undoubtedly highly heritable. For schizophrenia, the risk of the disorder in first-degree relatives is perhaps 5%, compared with 0.5% for the relatives of controls (Kendler and Diehl, 1993). Concordance rates for schizophrenia are 42–50% in monozygotic (identical) twins and 0–14% in dizygotic (fraternal) twins (Cardno and Murray, 2003); heritability estimates for most psychotic disorders hover around 80–85% (Cardno et al., 1999). Since concordance in monozygotic twins is not 100%, genes cannot be 'sufficient' causes for psychosis, though they may be 'necessary', and unaffected relatives may pass on an increased risk for disorder (Gottesman and Bertelsen, 1989). This high heritability does not rule out the importance of environments in the aetiology of psychosis, nor of gene–environment interactions; in fact, gene–environment interactions contribute to the heritability estimates produced by quantitative genetic studies (Moffitt et al., 2005).

The importance of gene–environment interactions in schizophrenia has been clear from the very earliest quantitative genetic studies, especially those using adoption designs (e.g., Heston, 1966; Kety et al., 1971). Adoption studies allow

Society and Psychosis, ed. Craig Morgan, Kwame McKenzie and Paul Fearon. Published by Cambridge University Press. © Cambridge University Press 2008.

the unique separation of genetic and environmental influences, by comparing adoptive siblings who have genetic risk (inferred from psychiatric disorder in the biological parents) with those who do not, or by studying the effects of genetically high-risk children raised in environmentally high-risk or low-risk adoptive families. There are several limitations to adoption designs, including the tendency for adoptive families to preclude high levels of exposure to risk factors such as deprivation and poverty (Rutter and Silberg, 2002). Nonetheless, adoption studies have produced important illustrations of gene–environment interaction. Heston's classic studies demonstrated that children with biological parents with schizophrenia who were adopted away were at approximately the same risk for schizophrenia as those brought up by parents with schizophrenia (Heston, 1966). More recent studies from Finland have confirmed that the environmental sources of risk for schizophrenia have little effect in the absence of genetic risk. Tienari *et al.* (2004) found that in the adopted-away children of parents with schizophrenia, adoptive-family rearing behaviour is predictive of later schizophrenia, but has no effect on risk for children with no familial liability. This is also the case for individual symptoms. Wahlberg *et al.* (1997) showed that thought disorder was more likely in the offspring of parents with schizophrenia adopted into families where the mother showed communication difficulties. In contrast, there was no increased risk for thought disorder in children with genetic risk raised in families where the mother showed low levels of communication disturbance or in children with no genetic risk raised in families with high communication difficulties.

A classic example of gene–environment interaction is phenylketonuria (Plomin *et al.*, 1997). Phenylketonuria is a single-gene recessive disorder present in about 1 in 10 000 live births, which, if untreated, leads to mental retardation. The mutation is in the gene that produces the enzyme phenylalanine hydroxylase; individuals who are homozygous for the mutation cannot effectively break down phenylalanine in their food. If children with the disorder are not prevented from eating foods that contain phenylalanine, its metabolic products build up and damage the developing brain. Because retardation can be prevented by a relatively simple environmental intervention (a diet low in phenylalanine), newborn babies are routinely screened for the mutation. Phenylketonuria is, therefore, a model gene–environment interaction, where the phenotype of mental retardation results directly from the combination of a genetic mutation and exposure to phenylalanine in the diet.

Recently, psychiatric research has been revolutionised by molecular genetics, such as the hunt for candidate genes for schizophrenia (Owen *et al.*, 2004). Although this has been slow to start, the falling cost and increasing technological and statistical sophistication of molecular genetics makes the search for gene–environment interactions that can be assessed at the molecular level both inevitable and irresistible. Perhaps because of the difficulties of determining the specific brain effects of a myriad of environmental effects (Petronis, 2004), molecular genetic research has somewhat dominated this field. However, the search for gene–environment interactions depends crucially on the development of similarly sophisticated means of measuring environmental risk.

Definitions of relevant terms and concepts

Molecular genetic studies group individuals according to *genotype* (their genetic constitution) or *phenotype* (their displayed characteristics, such as the presence or absence of a psychotic disorder). Individuals differ in genotype owing to variation at a particular point on a gene. Such variation could include a *single nucleotide polymorphism* (SNP) (a one-letter change in the coding sequence), or a *variable number tandem repeat* (VNTR) sequence, where a short segment of DNA is repeated any number of times. If the form of the gene (or *allele*) on both chromosomes is identical, the individual is said to be *homozygous* for that allele. If the two copies differ, the individual is *heterozygous*.

Gene–environment correlation occurs where a gene influences the likelihood of exposure to an environment. This is plausible for many putative environmental risk factors in schizophrenia. There is evidence that genetic factors influence exposure to obstetric complications (Marcelis *et al.*, 1998) and to life events (Kendler *et al.*, 1993). Genetics also influence the likelihood of abusing alcohol, cannabis and other illicit substances (Tsuang *et al.*, 1996). Gene–environment correlation can also occur where environment factors cause genetic variation. A well known example of this is the high prevalence of sickle-cell carriers in countries where malaria is endemic. Individuals who are heterozygous for the sickle-cell mutation have a slight survival advantage in such countries because they are somewhat protected against the malaria parasite (Carlson, 1999). Since homozygous sickle-cell carriers have a shortened lifespan, in countries where malaria is not an issue, the sickle-cell trait will tend to be bred out of the population.

Gene–environment correlation is likely in schizophrenia because the children of parents with schizophrenia are the potential recipients of two correlated risks: they may inherit genes that increase risk for schizophrenia, and they will also be brought up in a family environment that may be affected by schizophrenia. This process is known as *passive correlation* of gene and environment, where children (passively) inherit environments that are correlated with their genetic make-up. In contrast, *evocative correlations* occur where the environment is itself affected by the child's genotype, for example where genetic factors influence a child's personality in a way that elicits poor parenting behaviours. It has been suggested that the evidence linking parenting with an increased risk for schizophrenia in the offspring may be interpreted in this way (Jones *et al.*, 1994). A third type, *active correlation*, occurs when individuals seek out or create environments that correlate with their genetic propensities, for example, by choosing friends with similar talents or interests as their own.

Gene–environment correlations are described where genetics influence exposure to environments. In contrast, *gene–environment interactions* occur where there is genetic control of sensitivity to the environment (Kendler and Eaves, 1986), for example where the effects of an environmental risk factor are moderated by genetic predisposition. Conversely, they might also include situations where the expression of a person's genetic constitution is affected by the environment. Genes and environment might operate in a number of ways to cause schizophrenia: they might be *additive*, where the risks for schizophrenia genes and environments simply add to one another's effects in determining risk for schizophrenia, or *multiplicative*, such that genetic risks are multiplied by environmental exposures, or vice versa. An alternative is a model of *gene–environment synergism*, where exposure to both genetic and environmental factors would be required, to produce the disorder.

These are models of interaction at a biological, or causal, level. Statistically speaking, however, an interaction occurs when the effect of genotype on disease risk depends on the level of exposure to an environmental factor or vice versa. Unfortunately, this definition depends on how risks are measured, for example, as an odds ratio or a rate difference: the practical implication of this is that psychiatric researchers may fall foul of claiming (statistical) interactions that would simply not exist if their data were scaled in a different way (Clayton and McKeigue, 2001). Unawareness of these statistical hazards might be a serious impediment to the field. Nonetheless, it need not affect the validity of discussing the principles of gene–environment interactions.

Recent studies of gene–environment interaction

Classical and molecular forms of genetic epidemiology have complemented one another in contributing to the current surge in interest in gene–environment interactions. In recent years, a number of studies have demonstrated the likelihood of gene–environment interactions for many long-established environmental risk factors, by studying their effects in genetically sensitive designs.

Malaspina *et al.* (2001) investigated rates of traumatic brain injury and mental illness in families with at least two first-degree relatives diagnosed with schizophrenia, schizoaffective disorder or bipolar disorder. They found that head injury was associated with mental illness in families with a history of schizophrenia, but not in those with a history of bipolar disorder. Interestingly, head injury was more common even among the healthy relatives of patients with schizophrenia, suggesting some synergism between genetic liability for schizophrenia and for head injury.

Gene–environment synergism was also the subject of a recent study (van Os et al., 2003), which investigated whether familial liability and urbanicity, an established environmental risk factor in schizophrenia (Krabbendam and van Os, 2005), coparticipate to cause psychosis. In this large general population study from the Netherlands, subjects were screened for DSM-III-R psychotic disorders and were also asked about psychotic symptoms and psychiatric treatment in all first-degree relatives. Each place of residence was classified into a five-level urbanicity rating, depending on the number of addresses within the geographical area surrounding the residence.

As expected, both urbanicity and familial liability significantly increased the risk for psychotic disorder. However, the effect of urbanicity was much larger in those with familial liability. The authors estimated that 60–70% of the cases of psychosis could be explained by the synergism between urbanicity and familial liability in this sample. This study demonstrates the continuing utility of quantitative genetic epidemiology in establishing possible modes of gene–environment interaction, which may subsequently become the subject of molecular genetic studies.

Yet another putative environmental risk factor for schizophrenia, foetal hypoxia (Clarke et al., 2006), was the subject of an interesting neuroimaging study by Cannon et al. (2002). They examined the brain structure of subjects with schizophrenia or schizoaffective disorder, their unaffected siblings and a group of healthy unrelated controls. They also studied the hospital birth records of all the subjects and compared the brain structures of those who had experienced obstetric complications that led to foetal hypoxia. In this sample, foetal hypoxia was not more common in patients or siblings than in controls. Foetal hypoxia was associated with reduced grey matter and increased cerebral spinal fluid throughout the cortex among patients and their siblings, but no such relationship existed in controls. The existence of the relationship in the healthy siblings suggests that the effect of foetal hypoxia on brain structure may be greater in those with a genetic liability for schizophrenia, suggesting a classical gene–environment interaction.

In the brave new world of molecular genetic studies, one has proven particularly fruitful in demonstrating statistical interactions between specific genes and environments. The Dunedin birth cohort consists of around a thousand individuals followed from birth through to adult life. The sample is relatively small but remains almost intact, with 96% of the original participants taking part at the age 26 follow-up. The study has provided evidence for gene–environment interactions linking genes involved in neurotransmission, environmental exposures during the course of development and psychiatric phenotypes. Although only one of these relates to psychosis per se, all three shed interesting light on the advantages and difficulties of gene–environment interactions in psychiatric outcomes.

In the first study, the authors questioned why some children who are maltreated grow up to develop antisocial behaviour while others do not. Abnormalities in the gene encoding monoamine oxidase A (MAOA), an enzyme that breaks down neurotransmitters, including dopamine, noradrenalin and serotonin, have been linked with antisocial behaviour in human beings (Brunner *et al.*, 1993) and aggressive behaviour in mice (Cases *et al.*, 1995). Caspi and colleagues (2002) hypothesised that variation in the MAOA gene might underlie the apparent differences in antisocial behaviour seen in maltreated children. Since the MAOA gene is located on the X chromosome it may be especially important in the development of boys, who have only one copy.

In the Dunedin study, boys who had the high-activity form of the MAOA gene did not show increased antisocial outcomes when exposed to childhood maltreatment. However, boys with the low-activity MAOA form who were exposed to childhood maltreatment showed increased risk for a number of antisocial outcomes, including conduct disorder in adolescence, convictions for violence and antisocial personality in adult life. There was a dose–response relationship such that greater levels of maltreatment were associated with greater increases in risk for violent outcomes.

A subsequent study has replicated this result in 514 white male twins in the USA (Foley *et al.*, 2004), where childhood adversity was measured in terms of interparental violence, parental neglect and inconsistent discipline, and the main outcome was conduct disorder. This study went further in attempting to determine the nature of causality of the relationship, by examining whether it might be due to a gene–environment correlation, rather than a true interaction. Two possible models of correlation were suggested: an evocative one, where the child's genotype would affect the likelihood of experiencing adversity. This model was tested by studying the association between the child's exposure to adversity and maternal antisocial personality symptoms (indicative of genetic antisocial liability). A passive model, where an indirect influence of child's genotype on experienced adversity operates via correlated parental characteristics was also tested, by assessing whether MAOA genotype predicted exposure to childhood adversity. In fact, neither type of correlation could explain their findings, leading the authors to conclude that the most likely model was a true interaction, whereby the risk associated with MAOA genotype was qualitatively different in different environments.

The second gene–environment interaction reported in the Dunedin sample concerns an interaction between stressful life events, the serotonin transporter gene and risk for depression (Caspi *et al.*, 2003). Individuals who had experienced more stressful life events (such as work, health or relationship stressors) in the past five years were more likely to be depressed at age 26 and more likely to have suicidal thoughts or to have attempted suicide. There was an interaction between life events and genotype: individuals with one or two copies of the short form of the serotonin transporter gene were much more likely to show depression symptoms in response to life events than individuals who were homozygous for the long form of the gene.

There have been several attempts to replicate the interaction of life events and the serotonin transporter gene in predicting depression. Replications or partial replications have been reported among children (Kaufman *et al.*, 2004), adolescents (Sjoberg *et al.*, 2006) and adults (Wilhelm *et al.*, 2006; Zalsman *et al.*, 2006). The two largest and most statistically powerful studies, however, failed to replicate the effect among Australian twins aged 19–78 years (Gillespie *et al.*, 2005) and a British cohort of adults aged 41–80 (Surtees *et al.*, 2006).

One reason for the mixed results may be that serotonin transporter polymorphism is actually triallelic in function (Hu *et al.*, 2006). There is a functional SNP present on the long allele, making one version of the long allele functionally equivalent to the short allele. This may have confounded earlier reports, and a recent study that took into account this triallelic nature did find the proposed interaction between genotype and life events in causing depression (Zalsman *et al.*, 2006).

An alternative explanation is that publication bias is present (Zammit and Owen, 2006), since several small positive studies have been published but the only large studies have had negative results, making interpretation of the weight of evidence problematic. Moreover, since no genetic or environmental risk factors operate in a vacuum, it is inevitable that other gene–gene or gene–environment interactions will be reported that will themselves interact with effects already described. A recent follow-up of Kaufman's study (Kaufman *et al.*, 2004) reported a significant three-way interaction between the serotonin transporter gene, a second gene that may be associated with depression and life events (Kaufman *et al.*, 2006). Such three-way or four-way interactions are biologically plausible but bring further complexities in terms of sample size, replicability and interpretation.

An environmental exposure that may be of particular importance in the triggering or emergence of psychiatric disorders is illicit drug use. While drug use may itself be under genetic influence (Kendler and Prescott, 1998; Tsuang *et al.*, 1996), exposure to alcohol, cannabis and other drugs is extremely common, if not almost universal, among patients with psychotic disorders (McCreadie, 2002; Regier *et al.*, 1990). Most research in this field has examined the possible effects of cannabis (Arseneault *et al.*, 2004) but other drugs are also of considerable interest in the aetiology of psychiatric disorders. Roiser *et al.* (2005) assessed whether the effects of habitual 3,4-methylene-dioxymethamphetamine (Ecstasy) use on depression and emotional processing varied according to the serotonin transporter gene polymorphism. They found that individuals with the short allele who had used Ecstasy showed abnormal emotional processing, and showed a trend towards higher depression scores, when compared with other genotypes and individuals who had not used Ecstasy.

Returning to psychosis, a third report from Dunedin (Caspi *et al.*, 2005) suggested an interaction between genetic and environmental risk factors in causing schizophreniform disorders. The gene in question, catechol-O-methyltransferase (COMT), is potentially important in psychiatric research because, like MAOA, it is involved in the metabolism of dopamine and other neurotransmitters in the brain. In fact, COMT is relatively restricted in its effects to the prefrontal cortex (Gogos *et al.*, 1998), making it especially relevant to schizophrenia. Several studies have reported an association between the Val (high activity) allele and schizophrenia (Egan *et al.*, 2001), but recent meta-analyses have questioned the association (e.g., Fan *et al.*, 2005).

The environmental factor, early cannabis use, has been reliably associated with increase risk for schizophrenia (Andreasson *et al.*, 1987), although it is not yet known whether cannabis itself causes schizophrenia, or whether some other causal pathway is acting (Arseneault *et al.*, 2004). In the Dunedin study, individuals were assessed at age 26 on three outcomes: meeting criteria for DSM-IV schizophreniform disorder within the past year; having experienced minor psychotic-like symptoms, such as hallucinations or delusions; and informant reports on hallucinatory and paranoid behaviour. Study participants had previously (at ages 13, 15 and 18) been asked whether they used cannabis: a quarter of the sample were classed as adolescent-onset cannabis users because they had used cannabis before the age of 15 or were using it at least monthly by the age of 18.

These adolescent-onset cannabis users had an overall increased risk of adult psychosis, while individuals who began using cannabis in adulthood did not. There was an interaction between cannabis use and COMT genotype, such that the increased risk for psychosis was greatest in those adolescent-onset users who had the Val/Val genotype. The effect could not be explained by the adolescent use of other drugs such as amphetamines and hallucinogens or by psychotic symptoms predating the onset of cannabis use. It appeared specific to COMT (no such effects were found with MAOA or serotonin transporter genes) and to adolescent-onset cannabis use (no such interaction was found with other environmental risk factors, such as life events or maltreatment).

However, the effect may not have been specific to psychotic symptoms: COMT genotype and cannabis use also interacted in predicting later depression in the sample. This may reflect the large overlap of psychotic and depressed symptoms in clinical populations (Hafner *et al.*, 2005) or may reflect common neurobiological pathways underpinning psychotic and affective disorders.

A recent experimental study has partially replicated this result. Henquet *et al.* (2006) gave patients with psychotic disorders, their unaffected relatives and healthy controls a single dose of Δ^9-tetrahydrocannabinol (the principal component of cannabis) and assessed the effect of COMT genotype on the cognitive and psychotic effects of the drug. They found that Val allele carriers who had high trait liability to psychosis were most sensitive to the effects of the drug, in terms of both psychotic-like experiences and cognitive impairments.

As described above, the COMT gene is of special interest to schizophrenia because it appears to have relatively circumscribed effects in the brain: COMT knockout mice show a threefold increase in frontal dopamine levels but little change in other regions (Gogos *et al.*, 1998). This specificity suggests that functions that rely on prefrontal cortical activity may be particularly affected by COMT genotype. Egan *et al.* (2001) reported that carriers of the Met allele perform better on tasks requiring prefrontally-mediated executive functions than Val carriers, and use their prefrontal cortex more efficiently, showing less prefrontal cortical activation at the same level of task performance.

The cognitive effects of COMT are interesting because subtle cognitive impairments are present in schizophrenia many years before psychosis develops (Jones *et al.*, 1994) and appear to worsen in the period leading up to the onset of psychosis (Kurtz, 2005). Executive functions mediated by the prefrontal cortex continue to develop throughout adolescence and into early adulthood (De Luca *et al.*, 2003), probably reflecting the continuing grey and white matter changes that occur in the prefrontal cortex during puberty as the frontal lobes become optimally functional (Giedd, 2004; Sowell *et al.*, 1999). In a recent study (Barnett *et al.*, 2007) we hypothesised that since COMT is especially important in the prefrontal cortex, and since the prefrontal cortex is developing during puberty, the effects of COMT genotype on cognitive functions might be greater in children who were undergoing puberty than those of the same age who not yet entered puberty.

We tested this hypothesis in a large sample of children born in 1991 and 1992 in the south west of England, members of the Avon Longitudinal Study of Parents and Children (ALSPAC) cohort (Golding *et al.*, 2001). The COMT genotype was obtained for over 8000 children and the effect of genotype was assessed on 14 measures of cognitive function, including working memory, verbal and motor inhibition, attentional control, and IQ, assessed at ages 8 and 10 years. Pubertal development was reported by the parents at age 9 years 8 months; around 18% of children were reported to show some signs of entering puberty at this time.

In girls, there was no effect of COMT genotype on cognitive function. However, in boys, there was an association between genotype and several measures of cognitive function. The predicted interaction with puberty was also present, such that in boys who had already entered puberty those with the Met/Met genotype had an average IQ ten points higher than those of the Val/Val genotype. This large effect is interesting both in terms of normal brain development and in its relevance for psychosis, supporting a neurodevelopmental model of schizophrenia where genetic and environmental liabilities interact with normal brain development to catalyse the symptoms of psychosis (Weinberger, 1987).

Methodological issues in gene–environment interactions

Thus far, relatively few interactions between specific genes and specific environmental risk factors have been reported in the field of psychiatry. Of those that have been reported, none have yet been replicated enough for the interaction to be established beyond reasonable doubt. A number of methodological reasons underlie this, not least the relative youth of the field. Only in the last couple of years has the hunt for candidate genes for schizophrenia shown plausible contenders (Owen *et al.*, 2005). We may expect that the next few years will produce an explosion in reports of gene–gene and gene–environment interactions in schizophrenia and other disorders.

One serious issue in these studies will be the specificity of the genetic and environmental risks. The search for candidate genes for schizophrenia has demonstrated that even after multiple replications of association between a disorder and a gene or region on the chromosome, the precise location of the causal variant or variants can remain elusive (Harrison and Weinberger, 2005).

In measuring environment risk, reported replications often reflect similar, but not identical, assessment procedures. These may include minor differences, for example in the rating scale used, or major ones, such as differences in phenotype, age at assessment of phenotype or timing of risk exposure. Attempted replications of the serotonin transporter gene, life events and depression described above include a variety of environmental risk factors including childhood maltreatment, unemployment and chronic disease, measured at a variety of ages, and with phenotypes ranging from diagnoses of major depression and suicidality, to scores on a number of depression scales.

Differences in environmental and phenotypic measures are understandable given that many gene–environment studies will necessarily be opportunistic, taking advantage of large datasets such as birth cohorts where much of the phenotypic and environmental exposure data will already have been collected. This reflects the very large sample sizes that will be needed to detect gene–environment interactions in psychiatric disorders. Since psychosis is itself relatively rare, and since the genetic complexity of the disorder is such that the risk for psychosis remains low even in individuals with a known familial risk, the magnitude of the undertaking in searching for gene–environment interactions is clear.

How close the genetic and environmental exposures must be to the original report to be considered a replication is a question of biological plausibility. To be statistically plausible, such studies must be valid with respect to the issues of multiple testing and publication bias. Multiple testing becomes a problem as soon as more than one genetic locus, environmental risk or phenotype is investigated. Realistically, it is likely that many studies will now investigate a large number of candidate genes and environmental exposures, and perhaps also several phenotypes within the same study. Gene–environment interactions that produce statistically significant results are presumably more likely to be submitted and accepted for publication than studies with only negative results. This massive publication bias is well documented in the literature surrounding gene–disease associations (Ioannidis *et al.*, 2001) and can seriously undermine attempts to evaluate data agnostically using systematic reviews and meta-analysis.

Future challenges

An important challenge will be the elucidation of specific models by which gene and social environment may interact in causing a disease. Shanahan and Hofer (2005) suggest four possible models for this interaction. In the first, an environmental factor acts as a trigger for disease in moderating the expression of a genotype. This is a diathesis–stress model of disorder and fits with much of the evidence described above, including the examples from the Dunedin study. In a related but reverse model, an environmental factor instead acts as compensation for a genetic risk. An example of this is the possibility of staving off dementia through increased physical or mental activity (Lautenschlager and Almeida, 2006). The third model is similar but emphasises the role of social control as the environmental factor protecting against genetic risk. This may apply to the interaction between COMT genotype and adolescent cannabis use: in societies or eras where cannabis is not readily available to adolescents, cases of psychosis might be prevented. Finally, social context may interact with genotype to produce positive, rather than negative, mental health outcomes. Almost all of the research described in this chapter is based firmly upon the first model. It is likely that consideration of other models would significantly help our understanding of how the social environment interacts with genetic liability for psychosis.

A further conceptual challenge will be to study the role of epigenetic factors in psychiatric disorders. Epigenetic mechanisms are stable and potentially heritable effects that do not involve a change in DNA sequence. They include processes such as DNA methylation, imprinting and parent-of-origin effects.

An example of a parent-of-origin effect is Prader–Willi syndrome, a genetic condition for which the symptoms include overeating, hypogonadism, short stature and mild learning disabilities, as well as an increased risk of psychosis (Boer et al., 2002). Prader–Willi syndrome is caused by a partial deletion on the paternal copy of chromosome 15q (Robinson et al., 1991). If the deletion is on the maternal copy, the child instead develops Angelman syndrome (Smith et al., 1992), where the phenotype is quite different and includes ataxia, severe learning disabilities, epilepsy, microencephaly and a characteristic facial appearance.

A second epigenetic mechanism, DNA methylation, is a concrete example of how the environment can affect gene expression. In an elegant series of studies, Meaney and colleagues have demonstrated in rats that early life events, such as maternal care, have long-standing effects on stress responsivity. For example, the offspring of high-care mothers are less fearful and show more modest endocrine responses to stress (Caldji et al., 1998; Liu et al., 1997). These behavioural differences persist into adulthood and result from increased glucocorticoid receptor expression in the hippocampus and enhanced glucocorticoid feedback sensitivity (Meaney, 2001). The mechanism of these individual differences in offspring involves differences in DNA methylation. Cross-fostering of offspring into litters with low or high maternal care reverses the differences in DNA methylation, such that the offspring's phenotype depends entirely on the environment in which it was raised (Weaver et al., 2004). Moreover, the changes can be transmitted to subsequent generations (Francis et al., 1999). The studies, therefore, provide an explanation at the molecular level of how early environment affects adult temperament.

Modification of gene expression by epigenetic mechanisms plays a crucial role in human brain development and is, therefore, likely to be important in the development of schizophrenia (Keverne et al., 1996). One putative risk factor for schizophrenia that may have an epigenetic origin is paternal age. Cases of schizophrenia are more common in the offspring of older men, even when other possible explanations such as maternal age, socioeconomic status, family history, ethnicity and marital status are controlled for (e.g., El-Saadi et al., 2004; Zammit et al., 2003). It may be that new mutations are inherited by the offspring of older fathers. However, epigenetic mechanisms, including errors in the imprinting patterns of paternally inherited alleles, or reduced DNA methylation activity in the production of sperm, might also explain the association (Malaspina, 2001).

A better understanding of the role of epigenetics may cause us to reconsider our knowledge of the importance of both genetic and environmental risk factors in schizophrenia. For example, epigenetic factors, rather than environmental risks, may account for part of the discordance for schizophrenia in monozygotic twins. Indeed, it has been suggested that the current consensus that schizophrenia results from genetic vulnerability plus adverse environment is mistaken, and should be replaced with a model where epigenetic factors are of paramount importance (Petronis, 2004).

The increasing power of genetic approaches means that it will now become possible to measure commensurately complex interactions between genes and the social environment. Understanding their implications and the new biology they describe are key goals for the behavioural sciences and for psychiatry. Devising testable hypotheses in this new landscape, and interrogating them with statistical precision, are, perhaps, our biggest challenges.

REFERENCES

Andreasson, S., Allebeck, P., Engstrom, A. *et al.* (1987). Cannabis and schizophrenia. A longitudinal study of Swedish conscripts. *Lancet*, **2**, 1483–6.

Arseneault, L., Cannon, M., Witton, J. *et al.* (2004). Causal association between cannabis and psychosis: examination of the evidence. *British Journal of Psychiatry*, **184**, 110–17.

Barnett, J. H., Heron, J., Ring, S. M. *et al.* (2007). Gender-specific effects of the catechol-O-methyltransferase Val108/158Met polymorphism on cognitive function in children. *American Journal of Psychiatry*, **164**, 142–9.

Boer, H., Holland, A., Whittington, J. *et al.* (2002). Psychotic illness in people with Prader–Willi syndrome due to chromosome 15 maternal uniparental disomy. *Lancet*, **359**, 135–6.

Brunner, H. G., Nelen, M., Breakefield, X. O. *et al.* (1993). Abnormal behavior associated with a point mutation in the structural gene for monoamine oxidase A. *Science*, **262**, 578–80.

Caldji, C., Tannenbaum, B., Sharma, S. *et al.* (1998). Maternal care during infancy regulates the development of neural systems mediating the expression of fearfulness in the rat. *Proceedings of the National Academy of Sciences of the USA*, **95**, 5335–40.

Cannon, T. D., van Erp, T. G., Rosso, I. M. *et al.* (2002). Fetal hypoxia and structural brain abnormalities in schizophrenic patients, their siblings, and controls. *Archives of General Psychiatry*, **59**, 35–41.

Cardno, A. and Murray, R. M. (2003). The 'classical' genetic epidemiology of schizophrenia. In *The Epidemiology of Schizophrenia*, ed. R. M. Murray, P. B. Jones, E. Susser, J. van Os and M. Cannon. Cambridge: Cambridge University Press, pp. 194–219.

Cardno, A. G., Marshall, E. J., Coid, B. *et al.* (1999). Heritability estimates for psychotic disorders: the Maudsley twin psychosis series. *Archives of General Psychiatry*, **56**, 162–8.

Carlson, J. (1999). Inborn resistance to malaria. In *Malaria: Molecular and Clinical Aspects*, ed. M. Wahlgren and P. Perlmann. Amsterdam: Harwood Academic Publishers, pp. 363–78.

Cases, O., Seif, I., Grimsby, J. *et al.* (1995). Aggressive behavior and altered amounts of brain serotonin and norepinephrine in mice lacking MAOA. *Science*, **268**, 1763–6.

Caspi, A., McClay, J., Moffitt, T. E. *et al.* (2002). Role of genotype in the cycle of violence in maltreated children. *Science*, **297**, 851–4.

Caspi, A., Sugden, K., Moffitt, T. E. *et al.* (2003). Influence of life stress on depression: moderation by a polymorphism in the 5-HTT gene. *Science*, **301**, 386–9.

Caspi, A., Moffitt, T. E., Cannon, M. *et al.* (2005). Moderation of the effect of adolescent-onset cannabis use on adult psychosis by a functional polymorphism in the

catechol-O-methyltransferase gene: longitudinal evidence of a gene X environment interaction. *Biological Psychiatry*, **57**, 1117–27.

Clarke, M. C., Harley, M. and Cannon, M. (2006). The role of obstetric events in schizophrenia.
Schizophrenia Bulletin, **32**, 3–8.

Clayton, D. and McKeigue, P. M. (2001). Epidemiological methods for studying genes and
environmental factors in complex diseases. *Lancet*, **358**, 1356–60.

De Luca, C. R., Wood, S. J., Anderson, V. *et al.* (2003). Normative data from the CANTAB. I:
development of executive function over the lifespan. *Journal of Clinical and Experimental
Neuropsychology*, **25**, 242–54.

Egan, M. F., Goldberg, T. E., Kolachana, B. S. *et al.* (2001). Effect of COMT Val108/158Met
genotype on frontal lobe function and risk for schizophrenia. *Proceedings of the National
Academy of Sciences of the USA*, **98**, 6917–22.

El-Saadi, O., Pedersen, C. B., McNeil, T. F. *et al.* (2004). Paternal and maternal age as risk factors
for psychosis: findings from Denmark, Sweden and Australia. *Schizophrenia Research*,
67, 227–36.

Fan, J. B., Zhang, C. S., Gu, N. F. *et al.* (2005). Catechol-O-methyltransferase gene Val/Met
functional polymorphism and risk of schizophrenia: a large-scale association study plus meta-
analysis. *Biological Psychiatry*, **57**, 139–44.

Foley, D. L., Eaves, L. J., Wormley, B. *et al.* (2004). Childhood adversity, monoamine oxidase a
genotype, and risk for conduct disorder. *Archives of General Psychiatry*, **61**, 738–44.

Francis, D., Diorio, J., Liu, D. *et al.* (1999). Nongenomic transmission across generations of
maternal behavior and stress responses in the rat. *Science*, **286**, 1155–8.

Giedd, J. N. (2004). Structural magnetic resonance imaging of the adolescent brain. *Annals of the
New York Academy of Sciences*, **1021**, 77–85.

Gillespie, N. A., Whitfield, J. B., Williams, B. *et al.* (2005). The relationship between stressful life
events, the serotonin transporter (5-HTTLPR) genotype and major depression. *Psychological
Medicine*, **35**, 101–11.

Gogos, J. A., Morgan, M., Luine, V. *et al.* (1998). Catechol-O-methyltransferase deficient mice
exhibit sexually dimorphic changes in catecholamine levels and behavior. *Proceedings of the
National Academy of Sciences of the USA*, **95**, 9991–6.

Golding, J., Pembrey, M. and Jones, R. (2001). ALSPAC – the Avon Longitudinal Study of Parents
and Children. I. Study methodology. *Paediatric and Perinatal Epidemiology*, **15**, 74–87.

Gottesman, I. I. and Bertelsen, A. (1989). Confirming unexpressed genotypes for schizophrenia.
Risks in the offspring of Fischer's Danish identical and fraternal discordant twins. *Archives of
General Psychiatry*, **46**, 867–72.

Hafner, H., Maurer, K., Trendler, G. *et al.* (2005). Schizophrenia and depression: challenging the
paradigm of two separate diseases – a controlled study of schizophrenia, depression and
healthy controls. *Schizophrenia Research*, **77**, 11–24.

Harrison, P. J. and Weinberger, D. R. (2005). Schizophrenia genes, gene expression, and neuro-
pathology: on the matter of their convergence. *Molecular Psychiatry*, **10**, 804.

Henquet, C., Rosa, A., Krabbendam, L. *et al.* (2006). An experimental study of catechol-O-
methyltransferase Val[158]Met moderation of Δ-9-tetrahydrocannabinol-induced effects on
psychosis and cognition. *Neuropsychopharmacology*, **31**, 2748–57.

Heston, L. L. (1966). Psychiatric disorders in foster home reared children of schizophrenic mothers. *British Journal of Psychiatry*, **112**, 819–25.

Hu, X. Z., Lipsky, R. H., Zhu, G. *et al.* (2006). Serotonin transporter promoter gain-of-function genotypes are linked to obsessive-compulsive disorder. *American Journal of Human Genetics*, **78**, 815–26.

Ioannidis, J. P., Ntzani, E. E., Trikalinos, T. A. *et al.* (2001). Replication validity of genetic association studies. *Nature Genetics*, **29**, 306–9.

Jones, P., Rodgers, B., Murray, R. *et al.* (1994). Child development risk factors for adult schizophrenia in the British 1946 birth cohort. *Lancet*, **344**, 1398–402.

Kaufman, J., Yang, B. Z., Douglas-Palumberi, H. *et al.* (2004). Social supports and serotonin transporter gene moderate depression in maltreated children. *Proceedings of the National Academy of Sciences of the USA*, **101**, 17316–21.

Kaufman, J., Yang, B. Z., Douglas-Palumberi, H. *et al.* (2006). Brain-derived neurotrophic factor–5-HTTLPR gene interactions and environmental modifiers of depression in children. *Biological Psychiatry*, **59**, 673–80.

Kendler, K. S. and Diehl, S. R. (1993). The genetics of schizophrenia: a current, genetic-epidemiologic perspective. *Schizophrenia Bulletin*, **19**, 261–85.

Kendler, K. S. and Eaves, L. J. (1986). Models for the joint effect of genotype and environment on liability to psychiatric illness. *American Journal of Psychiatry*, **143**, 279–89.

Kendler, K. S. and Prescott, C. A. (1998). Cannabis use, abuse, and dependence in a population-based sample of female twins. *American Journal of Psychiatry*, **155**, 1016–22.

Kendler, K. S., Neale, M., Kessler, R. *et al.* (1993). A twin study of recent life events and difficulties. *Archives of General Psychiatry*, **50**, 789–96.

Kety, S. S., Rosenthal, D., Wender, P. H. *et al.* (1971). Mental illness in the biological and adoptive families of adopted schizophrenics. *American Journal of Psychiatry*, **128**, 302–6.

Keverne, E. B., Fundele, R., Narasimha, M. *et al.* (1996). Genomic imprinting and the differential roles of parental genomes in brain development. *Developmental Brain Research*, **92**, 91–100.

Krabbendam, L. and van Os, J. (2005). Schizophrenia and urbanicity: a major environmental influence – conditional on genetic risk. *Schizophrenia Bulletin*, **31**, 795–9.

Kurtz, M. M. (2005). Neurocognitive impairment across the lifespan in schizophrenia: an update. *Schizophrenia Research*, **74**, 15–26.

Lautenschlager, N. T. and Almeida, O. P. (2006). Physical activity and cognition in old age. *Current Opinion in Psychiatry*, **19**, 190–3.

Liu, D., Diorio, J., Tannenbaum, B. *et al.* (1997). Maternal care, hippocampal glucocorticoid receptors, and hypothalamic-pituitary-adrenal responses to stress. *Science*, **277**, 1659–62.

Malaspina, D. (2001). Paternal factors and schizophrenia risk: de novo mutations and imprinting. *Schizophrenia Bulletin*, **27**, 379–93.

Malaspina, D., Goetz, R. R., Friedman, J. H. *et al.* (2001). Traumatic brain injury and schizophrenia in members of schizophrenia and bipolar disorder pedigrees. *American Journal of Psychiatry*, **158**, 440–6.

Marcelis, M., van Os, J., Sham, P. *et al.* (1998). Obstetric complications and familial morbid risk of psychiatric disorders. *American Journal of Medical Genetics*, **81**, 29–36.

McCreadie, R. G. (2002). Use of drugs, alcohol and tobacco by people with schizophrenia: case-control study. *British Journal of Psychiatry*, **181**, 321–5.

Meaney, M. J. (2001). Maternal care, gene expression, and the transmission of individual differences in stress reactivity across generations. *Annual Review of Neuroscience*, **24**, 1161–92.

Moffitt, T. E., Caspi, A. and Rutter, M. (2005). Strategy for investigating interactions between measured genes and measured environments. *Archives of General Psychiatry*, **62** (5), 473–81.

Owen, M. J., Williams, N. M. and O'Donovan, M. C. (2004). The molecular genetics of schizophrenia: new findings promise new insights. *Molecular Psychiatry*, **9**, 14–27.

Owen, M. J., Craddock, N. and O'Donovan, M. C. (2005). Schizophrenia: genes at last? *Trends in Genetics*, **21**, 518–25.

Petronis, A. (2004). The origin of schizophrenia: genetic thesis, epigenetic antithesis, and resolving synthesis. *Biological Psychiatry*, **55**, 965–70.

Plomin, R., DeFries, J. C., McClearn, G. E. *et al.* (1997). *Behavioral Genetics*, 3rd edn. New York: Freeman.

Regier, D. A., Farmer, M. E., Rae, D. S. *et al.* (1990). Comorbidity of mental disorders with alcohol and other drug abuse. Results from the Epidemiologic Catchment Area (ECA) Study. *Journal of the American Medical Association*, **264**, 2511–18.

Robinson, W. P., Bottani, A., Xie, Y. G. *et al.* (1991). Molecular, cytogenetic, and clinical investigations of Prader–Willi syndrome patients. *American Journal of Human Genetics*, **49**, 1219–34.

Roiser, J. P., Cook, L. J., Cooper, J. D. *et al.* (2005). Association of a functional polymorphism in the serotonin transporter gene with abnormal emotional processing in Ecstasy users. *American Journal of Psychiatry*, **162**, 609–12.

Rutter, M. and Silberg, J. (2002). Gene–environment interplay in relation to emotional and behavioral disturbance. *Annual Review of Psychology*, **53**, 463–90.

Shanahan, M. J. and Hofer, S. M. (2005). Social context in gene–environment interactions: retrospect and prospect. *Journal of Gerontology Series B – Psychological Sciences and Social Sciences*, **60**, 65–76.

Sjoberg, R. L., Nilsson, K. W., Nordquist, N. *et al.* (2006). Development of depression: sex and the interaction between environment and a promoter polymorphism of the serotonin transporter gene. *International Journal of Neuropsychopharmacology*, **9**, 443–9.

Smith, J. C., Webb, T., Pembrey, M. E. *et al.* (1992). Maternal origin of deletion 15q11–13 in 25/25 cases of Angelman syndrome. *Human Genetics*, **88**, 376–8.

Sowell, E. R., Thompson, P. M., Holmes, C. J. *et al.* (1999). In vivo evidence for post-adolescent brain maturation in frontal and striatal regions. *Nature Neuroscience*, **2**, 859–61.

Surtees, P. G., Wainwright, N. W., Willis-Owen, S. A. *et al.* (2006). Social adversity, the serotonin transporter (5-HTTLPR) polymorphism and major depressive disorder. *Biological Psychiatry*, **59**, 2241–9.

Tienari, P., Wynne, L. C., Sorri, A. *et al.* (2004). Genotype–environment interaction in schizophrenia-spectrum disorder. *British Journal of Psychiatry*, **184**, 216–22.

Tsuang, M. T., Lyons, M. J., Eisen, S. A. *et al.* (1996). Genetic influences on DSM-III-R drug abuse and dependence: a study of 3,372 twin pairs. *American Journal of Medical Genetics*, **67**, 473–7.

van Os, J., Hanssen, M., Bak, M. *et al.* (2003). Do urbanicity and familial liability coparticipate in causing psychosis? *American Journal of Psychiatry*, **160**, 477–82.

Wahlberg, K-E., Wynne, L. C., Oja, H. *et al.* (1997). Gene–environment interaction in vulnerability to schizophrenia: findings from the Finnish Adoptive Family Study of Schizophrenia. *American Journal of Psychiatry*, **154**, 355–62.

Weaver, I. C., Cervoni, N., Champagne, F. A. *et al.* (2004). Epigenetic programming by maternal behavior. *Nature Neuroscience*, **7**, 847–54.

Weinberger, D. R. (1987). Implications of normal brain development for the pathogenesis of schizophrenia. *Archives of General Psychiatry*, **44**, 660–9.

Wilhelm, K., Mitchell, P. B., Niven, H. *et al.* (2006). Life events, first depression onset and the serotonin transporter gene. *British Journal of Psychiatry*, **188**, 210–15.

Zalsman, G., Huang, Y. Y., Oquendo, M. A. *et al.* (2006). Association of a triallelic serotonin transporter gene promoter region (5-HTTLPR) polymorphism with stressful life events and severity of depression. *American Journal of Psychiatry*, **163**, 1588–93.

Zammit, S. and Owen, M. J. (2006). Stressful life events, 5-HTT genotype and risk of depression. *British Journal of Psychiatry*, **188**, 199–201.

Zammit, S., Allebeck, P., Dalman, C. *et al.* (2003). Paternal age and risk for schizophrenia. *British Journal of Psychiatry*, **183**, 405–8.

Part II

Social factors and the onset of psychosis

6

Society, place and space

Jane Boydell and Kwame McKenzie

Introduction

This chapter will discuss the impact of society, place and space on the incidence of psychosis. It will briefly introduce the history of social causation theory before using the well established effect of urban residence on the incidence of psychosis in general, and schizophrenia in particular, as a lens through which to consider the possibilities for, and problems with, this research field. The reasons why the socioenvironmental context seems likely to be important will be described. Recent attention has focused on the idea that neighbourhood factors might exert an effect beyond their individual equivalents. For example, the social cohesion of a neighbourhood might have an effect on rates of psychosis above and beyond that of individual social networks. These possibilities, and the challenges associated with them, will be discussed.

History

Prior to the rise of modern medicine, the cause of disease was attributed to a variety of spiritual or mechanical factors, such as the elements, humours or miasma – bad air arising out of dirt and decaying organic matter. Early public health research, built on these theories, took the environment, in particular poor areas, to be aetiologically relevant. Risk was related to place; populations, rather than individuals, were considered more vulnerable because of where they lived rather than because of their own behaviour. Pioneers of public health in the mid-nineteenth century targeted sanitation of the slums, not education on personal hygiene, considering this to be the most important way of improving health (Porter, 1997, p. 411).

This ecological approach to health, however, was soon undermined by the development of new concepts; of particular importance was the discovery of disease-causing micro-organisms, and the rise of germ theory (Porter, 1997, p. 415). The importance of these developments was twofold: first, they changed

Society and Psychosis, ed. Craig Morgan, Kwame McKenzie and Paul Fearon. Published by Cambridge University Press. © Cambridge University Press 2008.

the target of investigation from the community as a whole to pathological agents in the community; and second, they moved the place for investigation of aetiology away from the community and into the laboratory (and the individual).

Germ theory was useful, but had its problems. For instance, not everybody exposed to infection contracts a disease. Exposure, though necessary, is not always sufficient to produce illness. Because of this and other deficiencies, the so-called 'epidemiological triangle' approach was developed. This renewed interest in the environment but still did not bring it back centrally into the causal pathway. It posited that disease is the product of an interaction between an agent, the host and the environment. The host and environment determine exposure and susceptibility. An example would be methicillin-resistant *Staphylococcus aureas* (MRSA) infection, which is a current scourge of UK hospitals. The environment has a part to play, in that poor hospital hygiene increases the chance of infection being spread. However, the weakest people in a hospital, whose immune systems are not functioning fully (e.g., post-operative patients, the old and infirm), are most likely to develop an infection. The risk of MRSA infection, therefore, depends on the presence of the bug in the hospital, the hospital environment and individual vulnerability.

Although the epidemiological triangle works well for infectious disease, it is more difficult to apply to chronic illnesses, such as psychotic disorders. The problem is that there is often no specific agent or exposure. There is a web of causation. Disorders develop through the complex interactions of many factors over time, which form interlocking chains of events (Krieger, 1994). Here, the environment is important, but only as a site for risk factors or behaviours that increase risk. The general move has been towards the individualisation of risk and away from the ecological basis of risk that was the genesis of public health.

However, some theories have continued to emphasise the importance of society and community. They have thrived because there are significant differences in rates of illness between groups, which are not explained by known risk factors (e.g., residents in urban and rural areas), and because some social groups seem to be at increased risk for a number of disparate disorders (e.g., migrants). There are some general theories of susceptibility that do not identify single or even multiple risk factors associated with specific disorders, but seek to understand why some social groups are generally more at risk than others for a range of illnesses. One incarnation is the fundamental social cause hypothesis (Link and Phelan, 1996). This attempts to explain why disparities in illness remain between socioeconomic groups despite adequate public health interventions. In the words of Link and Phelan (1995, p. 80), '... social factors such as socioeconomic status and social support are likely 'fundamental causes' of disease . . . because they embody access to important resources, affect multiple disease outcomes through multiple mechanisms, and consequently maintain an association with disease even when intervening mechanisms change.'

In the nineteenth century, the higher mortality and morbidity rates in the lower social classes were primarily due to infectious disease. Public health interventions, such as sanitation and vaccination, had a significant impact on disparities resulting from infections, but the differences in life expectancy between the social classes remained. Over time, the reasons for these disparities were no longer infectious disease, but became chronic diseases, such as cardiac problems (Link and Phelan, 1996). The theory of fundamental social causes aims to identify factors, such as education, access to prevention messages and access to healthcare, that work together to produce health disparities. Such fundamental causes are lodged in the fabric of society rather than in the individual. This theory has heralded a recent return to ecological considerations of aetiology (Diez-Roux, 1998).

A further move in this direction has been the social capital literature (McKenzie and Harpham, 2006). Social capital is a way of understanding communities and how their structure and function affect rates of mental illness. It is a group of concepts that includes individual and ecological factors. These may prove to be powerful predictors of rates of mental illness and outcome, but the concepts and methodologies are still under revision and there is significant work needed before any conclusions can be drawn (McKenzie and Harpham, 2006, pp. 151–7). What is exciting is that the use of multilevel modelling techniques has allowed social capital to be measured at ecological and individual levels in the same data sets. This has made it possible to disentangle the impact of the social environment on the individual from the impact on the group (McKenzie and Harpham, 2006, pp. 86–109).

Conceptualising society, place and space

Over time, society, place and space have been conceptualised in a number of different ways (see Chapter 4). The environment has been considered as a cause of illness at a population level and at an individual level, and as a vector of risk factors at an individual level.

Psychiatrists and social scientists have a long history of interest in the impact of society, place and space on the aetiology of mental illness. For instance, Durkheim (1951) developed theories that linked social structure and suicide (see Chapter 3); Faris and Dunham (1939) investigated the social organisation of cities and mental health (see Chapter 4); and Leighton (1982), Freeman (1994) and others (e.g., McKenzie et al., 2002) have been interested in the impact of societal and socio-cultural change on mental health.

There have been a number of attempts to describe society and social structure. Economic variables have been considered significant. They have included concepts of wealth, income inequality and poverty; both absolute poverty (money needed to sustain life) and relative poverty (the money needed to be able to have a normal life within a society). Many types of inequality cluster together – the financially poor are often disadvantaged in accessing high quality education, decent housing, and so on. These socially structured inequalities have been studied through concepts such as social class, poverty and social exclusion. Socioenvironmental stressors, such as crowding, crime and fear, have been less well conceptualised and studied, at least in relation to mental illness.

Social context is considered so important in the understanding of symptoms and illness that it has been written into psychopathological definitions and diagnoses. But it is often unclear what that context is; whether it should be considered as acting on individuals or whether it should be considered to be truly ecological (i.e., acting at a group level). Because of this, it is difficult to know how far this understanding helps us in developing healthy communities. A classic example of this is urbanisation. On a population level, the most important risk factor for psychosis is being born and brought up in a city. We will use this as a model for the investigation of how society, place and space may affect aetiology.

Methodological issues

To understand theories of how urbanisation may cause mental illness, one has to accept some simple premises. The first is that psychosis often develops over a life course, with a balance of propsychotic (i.e., risk-increasing) and antipsychotic (i.e., risk-reducing) factors moving individuals up or down a scale of risk (Figure 6.1).

Propsychotic and antipsychotic risk factors are complex and exist at a number of discrete levels. For instance, a non-exhaustive list of levels would be molecular, genetic, individual, interpersonal and environmental (Figure 6.2). Investigation of the cause of psychosis is complicated by the fact that each of these levels is

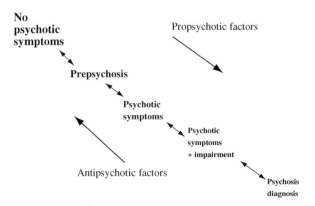

Figure 6.1   Life course journey to a diagnosis of psychosis

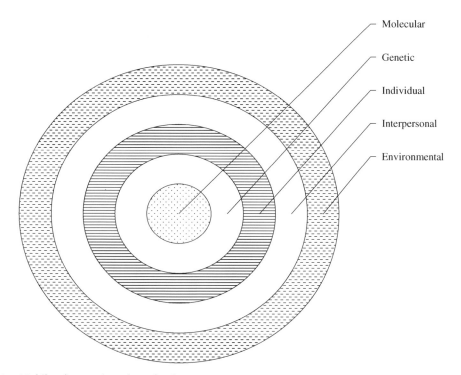

Molecular

Genetic

Individual

Interpersonal

Environmental

Figure 6.2   Multilevel causation of psychosis

governed by different scientific rules and so different tools are needed for assessment (Susser and Susser, 1996).

It is perhaps easier to understand this by considering the case of smoking and
premature death. Those who smoke have an increased risk of developing a variety
of cancers and cardiovascular disease. The rates of illness in groups who smoke are
increased. To build an evidence-based strategy to decrease the impacts of smoking
on health, we may want initially to investigate the mechanisms through which
smoking has its effects. The mechanisms can be interrogated in a number of ways
and at a number of levels, as follows:

- *Molecular level*   How do nicotine and tar affect the contents of a cell?
- *Metabolic level*   How do cell death and disruption affect other bodily systems?
- *Individual level*   Why does the individual smoke, why can't the individual stop
  and what can the individual do to decrease the risk that
  smoking causes?
- *Group level*   Why do certain social groups smoke more than others?
- *Societal level*   Why do some societies have higher rates of smoking than
  others and what can be done legislatively to decrease the rate
  of harm from smoking?

Investigations at each of these levels have the same aim – to examine the mechanisms linking smoking to illness. However, the analytical tools needed, and the relevant theory and scientific rules at each level, are different, as are the inferences that can be made from the research. Using the tools and methodology of molecular biology to investigate societal-level factors is unlikely to work very well. Similarly, we are unlikely to understand an individual's metabolic pathophysiology by using a systems theory of group dynamics. Investigating smoking legislation and tariffs may give an indication of why the rate of smoking is higher in one country than another, it may give information on why there are consequent increases in, for instance, cardiovascular illness in one area or another, but it does not give information on an individual's risk of harm if he or she is a smoker or why one person smokes and another does not.

The possible impact of a factor at any level is constrained by the higher level. To understand causation, we need not only to measure the impact of a factor at a given level, but also to understand the interaction with other levels.

There are particular difficulties in studying geographical variations in mental health. In such ecological studies, the exposure (risk factor) is measured at the group level (population or subpopulation) and the outcome is usually the proportion of the group who develop the disease. These aggregated data have some advantages in that there is less random error, more power and less selection bias, but also the disadvantage that one can never be certain that those who developed the disease were those who were exposed. Grouped results tell us about the group but not necessarily about the individuals within the group. For instance, if there was an association between the incidence of schizophrenia and the rate of crime in an area, it could not be assumed that being a victim of crime would increase an individual's risk of developing the disorder. Making such individual-level inferences from ecological-level data is termed the 'ecological fallacy'. Further, any systematic differences between areas or groups in the recording or classification of exposure or disease will bias the results in ecological studies. It is also sometimes difficult to identify ecological confounders and effect modifiers, as populations might differ in many ways, such as diet, alcohol consumption and attitudes that may affect the outcome (disease) being measured. Nevertheless, ecological studies are of great value in generating hypotheses and investigating phenomena that only exist at a group level. We now turn to the specific example of urbanicity and psychosis.

Urbanisation literature review

Incidence rates in rural and urban areas

Faris and Dunham (1939) reported that first-admission rates of schizophrenia were particularly high in certain areas of inner-city Chicago, and decreased towards the periphery (see Chapter 4 for a detailed summary). Furthermore, there were considerable differences within the inner city itself, with rates being higher in the more disorganised areas, irrespective of deprivation and ethnicity. Faris and Dunham suggested that the nature of living conditions in certain neighbourhoods, particularly extended isolation, produced abnormalities of behaviour and mentality, which subsequently led to increased rates of schizophrenia. A number of other early studies (reviewed by Freeman (1994)) also demonstrated clearly that the rates of schizophrenia increase towards city centres in Western societies.

The generally accepted view for most of the twentieth century was that the high rates of schizophrenia in the inner city could be accounted for by the drift of people with, or beginning to develop, schizophrenia into the more urbanised and anonymous areas (the 'social drift' hypothesis). A variant on this theme suggested non-balanced migration, i.e., that as a city develops, the more able move out to better areas, leaving a residual population in the centre with a high risk of psychiatric disorders (previously called the 'social residue' theory). The idea that causal agents are associated with urbanisation (the 'breeder' hypothesis) was largely dismissed. It has only been relatively recently that these ideas have been revisited.

In a study looking back at the nineteenth century, Fuller Torrey et al. (1997) used the comprehensive 1880 census of the 'insane' in the USA to examine the association between urbanicity and severe mental illness. They calculated prevalence rates for different degrees of urbanicity, characterised as follows:

- *Urban*   30 largest cities;
- *Semi-urban*   50% or more people living in towns of greater than 4000 people;
- *Semi-rural*   25–50% living in towns of 4000 or more people;
- *Rural*   1–25% living in towns of greater than 4000 people;
- *Completely rural* no-one living in a town of greater than 4000 people.

Fuller Torrey et al. (1997) found a strong linear trend, with the prevalence in urban areas being 66% higher than in completely rural areas. This study is fascinating, despite its limitations, because a gradient was found between areas that would all be considered rural today.

Most recent research has come from Northern Europe where good quality national records have made large-scale epidemiological studies possible. In the first of these, Lewis et al. (1992) investigated the association between place of upbringing and incidence of schizophrenia using data from a cohort of over 49 000 male Swedish conscripts, linking it to the Swedish national psychiatric register. They found a strong significant linear trend. The highest rate of clinically diagnosed schizophrenia was in those who had mostly lived in cities (Stockholm, Göteborg, Malmö) while they were growing up (odds ratio (OR) 1.65). There were intermediate rates in towns with populations greater than 50 000 (OR 1.39), and towns with populations less than 50 000 (OR 1.28), compared with baseline country areas. A similar though weaker trend was found for other psychoses. Adjusting for family finances, parental divorce and family psychiatric history (whether a relative is 'on medication for nervous trouble') had little effect on these findings. Adjusting for cannabis use and any psychiatric disorder at conscription reduced but did not eliminate the associations. The authors concluded that causal environmental factors are implicated, as the association remained after adjusting for family history, a proxy measure of genetic risk. However, this study could not distinguish between place of birth, place of upbringing and place of residence at onset.

Mortensen *et al.* (1999) investigated the effect of place of birth on risk of admission with schizophrenia in a large Danish population-based cohort of 1.75 million people. The relative risk of schizophrenia for those born in Copenhagen, compared with those born in rural areas, was 2.40 (95% confidence interval (CI) 2.13–2.7). There was also a clear dose–response relationship for urbanicity: the larger the town of birth, the greater the risk, a finding not explained by a family history of schizophrenia. Mortensen and colleagues further calculated the population-attributable risk (the proportion of the risk of schizophrenia in the whole population that can be accounted for by a particular factor, assuming causality) for urban birth. This was 34.6%, a much larger figure than the 9% and 7% respectively for having a mother or father who suffered from schizophrenia. Like the original study of Faris and Dunham (1939), Mortensen and colleagues found the incidence of manic-depression to be fairly evenly distributed across rural and urban areas.

Peen and Decker (1997) also reported a significant positive correlation between admission rates for clinically diagnosed schizophrenia and degree of urbanisation. They also investigated whether differences in the availability of psychiatric services were to blame but concluded that they were not, as the average length of hospital admission and average number of readmissions did not differ between urban and rural areas.

There are, of course, problems with using admission data to measure incidence and in relying on national case registers of clinical diagnoses. These strategies enable wide coverage but gloss over the possibility that bias due to different routes to care and diagnostic practices may have affected the results. Such bias can be decreased by studying all incident cases, whether admitted or not, in specified populations. Allardyce *et al.* (2001) compared all incident cases of psychosis from two areas in the UK, a largely rural part of south-west Scotland and urban south London. The incidence of schizophrenia was 61% higher in the urban area compared with the rural area. Intriguingly, the urban excess was more marked in males than females.

The studies of the last decades move us on from considering the urban effect as possibly due to social drift. Dauncey and colleagues (1993), who examined where patients had lived five years before their first admission in Nottingham, were unable to find evidence for systematic geographic drift. Though it could be argued that the drift had occurred in previous generations, the magnitude of this movement would need to have been extremely high to explain the findings. For example, in the Danish study, Mortensen and colleagues (1999) calculated that nearly 50 000 children born in the capital city and its suburbs needed to have a parent who transmitted a genetic risk equal to that transmitted by a parent with diagnosed schizophrenia, to account for the urban excess. Social drift in the current or previous generation could also not explain the cumulative effect of urban exposure throughout childhood. This is also relevant for the social residue theory (that those at greater risk are left behind in an area as it becomes less desirable).

Krabbendam and van Os (2005) reviewed more recent studies. They report an effect of urbanicity on rates of schizophrenia (i.e., an overall pooled effect size) of 1.72 (95% CI 1.53–1.92), with many showing a dose–response relationship. The effect seems to be greater in younger people and more recent birth cohorts (Haukka et al., 2001; Marcelis et al., 1998) and for schizophrenia. On the basis of their review, Krabbendam and van Os (2005) estimated that urbanicity accounts for around 30% of schizophrenia, assuming causality, in Western countries.

Urban birth, upbringing or residence

Urbanisation, then, is strongly associated with the incidence of schizophrenia. However, it is unclear whether its effects operate at the time of gestation and birth, throughout the pre-morbid lifespan of the individual, or around the time of onset of the illness.

For many years the only published study that had separated place of birth and place of upbringing was that carried out by Astrup and Ödegard (1961), which found a stronger effect of city upbringing on the incidence of schizophrenia in those who had moved. More recently, a re-analysis of the Danish population cohort study (Pedersen and Mortensen, 2001) addressed this issue. This study found that schizophrenia risk increased both with the number of years (between 0 and 20 years) that an individual lived in an urbanised area and with increasing degree of urbanisation. Compared with those who had always lived in the most rural areas, the relative risk for those who had spent their entire childhood in the capital was 2.75 (95% CI 2.31–3.28).

In contrast, Marcelis et al. (1999) investigated the risk of early onset psychosis in a cohort of all people born between 1972 and 1978. They found no additional risk for urban residence at the time of onset of psychosis above that of urban birth and upbringing. The evidence for an early effect, therefore, is strong, but an effect of urbanisation around the time of onset cannot be completely ruled out.

It is now recognised that psychotic symptoms are relatively common in 'healthy' people and that there is possibly a continuum between no symptoms and a psychotic illness. Van Os *et al.* (2001) examined psychiatric symptoms in a large Dutch study of the general population. Psychotic-like symptoms (isolated delusions or hallucinations) were found in 17.5% of the community sample, largely in people who had never presented to psychiatric services. Furthermore, such symptoms increased with increasing urbanisation, but to a lesser extent than for schizophrenia (10–20% higher in urban areas).

Possible explanations for the risk-increasing effect of cities

Classical causation theory states that we need to demonstrate a correlation, a correct temporal sequence and that no third explanatory variable exists that effects the urban environment and schizophrenia, before concluding that there is a causal link. Most explanations identify the urban environment as either a vector of risk, for instance, by increasing rates of infection, or as a potentiator of known risk factors. But critical analysis demonstrates that the association between urbanicity and schizophrenia is not explained by known risk factors. One problem is that most risk factors have been investigated at the individual level. How plausible, then, are the various proposed explanations?

Individual level (1) Biological explanations

Genetic risk

Although genetic risk itself does not explain the urban–rural difference, as explained above, there is new evidence of gene–environment synergism. Van Os *et al.* (2004) found that people with a family history of schizophrenia, or any severe mental illness, were more likely to develop schizophrenia if they lived in cities.

Obstetric complications

Eaton *et al.* (2000) tested the hypothesis that the urban–rural difference is mediated by obstetric complications in a Danish case-control study. They again found that birth in Copenhagen was a strong risk factor for schizophrenia. Obstetric complications that were prospectively measured had a moderate sized relationship to early onset schizophrenia, but the relationship of urbanicity to schizophrenia was unaffected by adjusting for obstetric complications. Similarly, Harrison *et al.* (2003) found that adjusting for obstetric complications did not significantly reduce the excess incidence of schizophrenia associated with urban birth or upbringing in Sweden.

Data from Holland suggest that malnutrition during pregnancy (Hoek *et al.*, 1998) increases the risk of schizophrenia, though this finding has yet to be replicated. Again, it is conceivable that mothers in poor inner-city areas have poorer nutrition, but there is no empirical evidence that this explains the urban effect.

Infectious disease and season of birth

More people with schizophrenia are born in late winter and early spring than at other times of the year. Some believe that this reflects exposure to infectious disease at the time of foetal brain development. Since many infections are passed on more readily in crowded areas, researchers have questioned whether the season of birth effect is greater in urban than rural settings, with several early studies reporting positive results (e.g., O'Callaghan *et al.*, 1995).

Takei *et al.* (1995) tested the hypothesis that winter birth and urban birth potentiate each other in a sample of first-admission patients with schizophrenia who were born between 1936 and 1963 in England and Wales. They calculated that city birth was only associated with an increased risk of schizophrenia in those born in autumn (OR 1.19, 95% CI 1.06–1.35) and winter (OR 1.21, 95% CI 1.08–1.36) but not summer or spring. Verdoux *et al.* (1997) found a greater season of birth effect in densely populated areas in France (20% excess for >136 inhabitants per km^2). However, a Danish study did not find any interaction between urbanicity and season of birth (Mortensen *et al.*, 1999) or urbanicity and exposure to influenza (Westergaard *et al.*, 1999). Similarly, large population-based studies in Finland (Suvisaari *et al.*, 2000) and the Netherlands (Marcelis *et al.*, 1998) did not find a significant interaction between season and place of birth.

Overall, it seems that the urban effect operates independently of season of birth. The season of birth effect is not only seen in highly populated areas, but there is some evidence, mainly from the UK, Ireland and France, that the two might interact.

Drug use

There is increasing evidence that drug use, particularly cannabis use, can increase the incidence of schizophrenia, which raises the question of whether this could confound the association between urbanisation and schizophrenia. Boydell *et al.* (2006) found that the incidence of schizophrenia rose dramatically in south-east London in the 1980s and 1990s at a time of greatly increased cannabis use. Furthermore, the proportion of people presenting with first-onset schizophrenia who used cannabis had increased disproportionately compared with people presenting with other psychiatric disorders. However, it is unlikely that drug abuse can account for the entire urban effect as the early studies were carried out before recreational drug use was so prevalent. Furthermore, this issue was also addressed in the Swedish conscript study by Lewis *et al.* (1992), and the effect of urban upbringing remained after adjusting for cannabis use. Nevertheless, a high prevalence of drug use in urban centres may contribute, especially to the observed increasing effect in younger birth cohorts.

Individual level (2) Socioenvironmental explanations

Social class

It has been suggested that social class at birth or during childhood might confound the urban–rural difference. Thus, Ohta *et al.* (1992) did not find a significant urban–rural difference in Nagasaki and attributed this to there being few social class differences between areas. Castle *et al.* (1993) carried out a case-control study in south London and found that people with schizophrenia were more likely to have been born in socially deprived areas and to have fathers with manual occupations. Byrne *et al.* (2004), in a population-based case-control study of 7700 people with schizophrenia, found evidence of lower social class at onset but limited evidence of lower social class at birth. In Dublin, Mulvany *et al.* (2001) found no evidence of an effect of social class at birth. Harrison *et al.* (2001) found evidence that birth into a deprived area was associated with an increased risk of schizophrenia; particularly so if the child was of lower social class. The evidence, therefore, is mixed, and it is unlikely that the entire urban effect can be attributed to social class. Indeed, some of the positive findings have come from countries where there is a higher standard of living in cities than in the rural areas; furthermore, in the Swedish conscript study of Lewis *et al.* (1992), the urban effect remained after adjusting for 'family finances'.

Psychosocial stress

Three prospective studies have found an association between life events and onset of psychosis (Bebbington *et al.*, 1993; Malla *et al.*, 1990; Neuchterlein *et al.*, 1989). It is possible that adverse life events may be more common in the inner city, but again there is no direct evidence that this explains the increased urban risk of schizophrenia. Indeed, given that the effect for life events is greater in affective psychosis than schizophrenia, this hypothesis would have predicted an increased urban incidence of manic-depression, which, as we noted earlier, has not generally been found.

Social isolation

Hare (1956) found that social isolation was associated with an increased risk of schizophrenia in his early studies in Bristol. There has been a recent resurgence of interest in this theory. Thornicroft *et al.* (1993) noted that clustering of individuals with schizophrenia in deprived areas occurs only in urban areas and suggested that social isolation is an important mediator of this. However, it is difficult to distinguish between cause and effect in this context. Related to these ideas is the theory that disruption of social networks decreases an individual's capacity to cope with psychosocial stress and increases the risk of schizophrenia.

Van Os *et al.* (2000) found evidence for person–environment interaction in Holland. People who were single had a slightly higher risk of developing psychosis if they lived in a neighbourhood with fewer single people, compared with a neighbourhood with many other single people. The authors suggested that single status might give rise to perceived (or actual) social isolation if most other people were living with a partner. The question of whether social isolation might increase the risk of schizophrenia (or whether a close relationship might be protective) is also raised by Jablensky (1997), who showed that marriage had a protective effect, and that this was not simply a consequence of better adjusted males being more able to marry.

Ecological explanations

Non-random differences in rates of psychosis have been demonstrated between neighbourhoods. These are not accounted for by differences in the structure of these communities in terms of age, sex and ethnicity (Kirkbride *et al.*, 2006). This suggests that characteristics of the communities might be important.

Silver *et al.* (2002) used the Epidemiological Catchment Area survey to investigate the effect of neighbourhood-level social factors after adjusting for individual-level equivalents. They found that individual socioeconomic status did predict risk of schizophrenia but that neighbourhood deprivation did not confer an additional risk. Another community-level factor, the proportion of people moving in and out of an area, was associated with the rate of schizophrenia even after controlling for confounders, such as ethnicity, living alone, income and education.

Allardyce *et al.* (2005) investigated the effects of social fragmentation, deprivation and urbanicity in a study of 5800 first-admission cases covering the whole of Scotland. Social fragmentation (defined as a composite measure of mobility in the previous year, single-person households, unmarried persons and privately rented households) had the strongest association with psychosis (OR 12.84, 95% CI 5.71–28.88); deprivation also exerted a strong effect (OR 5.29, 95% CI 1.49–18.75). However, after adjusting for fragmentation and deprivation, there was only a non-significant trend towards an association between urbanicity and schizophrenia. This study, however, could not control for individual-level factors. Boydell *et al.* (2004) found an effect of neighbourhood inequality on the incidence of schizophrenia. After controlling for individual deprivation there was an increased rate of schizophrenia with increasing neighbourhood inequality, but only in more deprived areas.

The findings of increased incidence of schizophrenia in deprived, unequal areas with a high proportion of single-person households and high levels of population mobility, leads to hypotheses about social cohesion and social capital (as outlined above).

Mechanisms

The investigation of social aetiology has been in abeyance for some time. There are few theories on how individual or neighbourhood-level factors operate. The urban environment may simply increase the possibility of individuals encountering known risk factors. It may increase the impact of known risk factors or it may produce new risk factors for an individual. These effects may act singly or in concert.

At an ecological level, the urban environment may increase the likelihood of schizophrenia developing. For instance, the lower levels of social cohesion and higher levels of fear and vigilance that characterise city life may increase the proportion of people who proceed along a life course towards the development of psychosis. Alternatively the structure and functioning of the urban environment may decrease investment in education and the social safety net, thus potentially contributing to a greater vulnerability to mental distress in a population. Recently, it has been suggested that social cohesion in the area in which a person develops might be relevant, as this might induce a cognitive bias, for example, towards paranoid ideation in low cohesion areas (Krabbendam and van Os, 2005).

Summary and challenges for future research

Recent research has confirmed the area-level findings from the 1930s and 1950s. Urbanicity is a clear risk factor for schizophrenia, to a lesser extent for other psychotic disorders, and to a lesser extent again for psychotic symptoms in the healthy population. The best estimate is that 30% of the population risk for schizophrenia is attributable to urban residence.

After urbanicity, the strongest evidence is that high levels of residential mobility in a neighbourhood are associated with higher rates of psychosis, but further research is needed to determine the direction of causation. This will be a common theme for all future area-based research, if arguments over reverse causality are to be overcome. The difficulty is that, as psychosis is relatively rare, large areas and numbers of areas are needed to gather sufficient cases, and that, together with the intensive interviewing of the cases needed to determine the presence of individual-level risk factors, makes a definitive study extremely expensive. However, the main difficulty with the research is that there has been surprisingly little work on the concept of a city. Studies have generally aimed to try to quantify, rather than understand, the association between the urban environment and schizophrenia.

Perhaps we have now reached the point where we have to consider what urbanisation is rather than trying to interrogate it through the current risk factors. Further studies of simple proxy measures, like population density, are unlikely to yield much more useful information. There also needs to be some clarity as to whether studies are investigating individual-level effects, ecological-level effects or interactions at different levels. The history of ideas of causation should help us understand the importance of a conceptual framework in understanding not only what our findings could mean but also how they can inform intervention.

Conclusion

Investigation of the urban effect demonstrates how difficult it is to understand the impact of society, place and space on the rates of psychosis. Even when we try to be more specific and focus on urbanisation, there is a clear need for further solid conceptual work to be undertaken before we are able to move forward. The renewed interest in societal factors is important, but there will need to be considerably more research if we are to make progress on ideas that have been around for at least 70 years. It may seem as though we have come full circle with causal theories targeting society, place and space, rather than individuals, but this is not the case. There are better analytical tools available, and methodologies that allow us to look across several levels of causation. The use of such methods, combined with more sophisticated conceptualisations of urban living, promises to yield important insights into the aetiology of psychosis.

REFERENCES

Allardyce, J., Kelly, J., van Os, J. et al. (2001). A comparison of the incidence of schizophrenia in rural Dumfries and Galloway and urban Camberwell. *British Journal of Psychiatry*, **179**, 335–9.

Allardyce, J., Gilmour, H., Atkinson, J. et al. (2005). Social fragmentation, deprivation and urbanicity. *British Journal of Psychiatry*, **187**, 401–6.

Astrup, C. and Ödegard, O. (1960). Internal migration and mental illness in Norway. *Psychiatric Quarterly Supplement*, **34** (suppl.), 116–30.

Bebbington, P., Wilkins, S., Jones, P. et al. (1993). Life events and psychosis. Initial results from the Camberwell Collaborative Psychosis Study. *British Journal of Psychiatry*, **162**, 72–9.

Boydell, J., van Os, J., McKenzie, K. *et al.* (2004). The association of inequality with the incidence of schizophrenia – an ecological study. *Social Psychiatry and Psychiatric Epidemiology*, **39** (8), 597–9.

Boydell, J., van Os, J., Caspi, A. *et al.* (2006). Trends in cannabis use prior to first presentation with schizophrenia, in south-east London between 1965 and 1999. *Psychological Medicine*, **36** (10), 1441–6.

Byrne, M., Agerbo, E., Eaton, W. *et al.* (2004). Parental socio-economic status and risk of first admission with schizophrenia: a Danish national register based study. *Social Psychiatry and Psychiatric Epidemiology*, **39** (2), 87–96.

Castle, D., Scott, K., Wessely, S. *et al.* (1993). Does social deprivation during gestation and early life predispose to later schizophrenia? *Social Psychiatry and Psychiatric Epidemiology*, **28**, 1–4.

Dauncey, K., Giggs, J., Baker, K. *et al.* (1993). Schizophrenia in Nottingham: lifelong residential mobility of a cohort. *British Journal of Psychiatry*, **163**, 613–19.

Diez-Roux, A. V. (1998). Bringing context back into epidemiology: variables and fallacies in multilevel analysis. *American Journal of Public Health*, **88** (2), 216–22.

Durkheim, E. (1951). *Suicide*. New York: Free Press.

Eaton, W., Mortensen, P. and Frydenberg, M. (2000). Obstetric factors, urbanization and psychosis. *Schizophrenia Research*, **43**, 117–23.

Faris, R. and Dunham, H. (1939). *Mental Disorders in Urban Areas*. Chicago: University of Chicago Press.

Freeman, H. (1994). Schizophrenia and city residence. *British Journal of Psychiatry*, **164** (suppl. 23), 39–50.

Fuller Torrey, E., Bowler, A. and Clark, K. (1997). Urban birth and residence as risk factors for psychoses: an analysis of 1880 data. *Schizophrenia Research*, **25**, 169–76.

Hare, E. (1956). Mental illness and social conditions in Bristol. *Journal of Mental Science*, **102**, 349–57.

Harrison, G., Gunnell, D., Glazebrook, C. *et al.* (2001). Association between schizophrenia and social inequality at birth: case-control study. *British Journal of Psychiatry*, **179**, 346–50.

Harrison, G., Fouskakis, D., Rasmussen, F. *et al.* (2003). Association between psychotic disorder and urban place of birth is not mediated by obstetric complications or childhood socio-economic position: a cohort study. *Psychological Medicine*, **33** (4), 723–31.

Haukka, J., Suvisaari, J., Varilo, T. *et al.* (2001). Regional variation in the incidence of schizophrenia in Finland: a study of birth cohorts born from 1950 to 1969. *Psychological Medicine*, **31** (6), 1045–53.

Hoek, H. W., Brown, A. S. and Susser, E. (1998). The Dutch famine and schizophrenia spectrum disorders. *Social Psychiatry and Psychiatric Epidemiology*, **33** (8), 373–9.

Jablensky, A. (1997). The 100-year epidemiology of schizophrenia. *Schizophrenia Research*, **28**, 111–25.

Kirkbride, J., Fearon, P., Morgan, C. *et al.* (2006). Heterogeneity in incidence rates of ÆSOP study. *Archives of General Psychiatry*, **63**, 250–8.

Krabbendam, L. and van Os, J. (2005). Schizophrenia and urbanicity: a major environmental influence – conditional on genetic risk. *Schizophrenia Bulletin*, **31** (4), 795–9.

Krieger, N. (1994). Epidemiology and the web of causation: has anyone seen the spider? *Social Science and Medicine*, **39** (7), 887–903.

Leighton, A. H. (1982). *Caring for Mentally Ill People: Psychological and Social Barriers in Historical Context*. New York: Cambridge University Press.

Lewis, G., David, A., Andreasson, S. *et al.* (1992). Schizophrenia and city life. *Lancet*, **340**, 137–40.

Link, B. G. and Phelan, J. C. (1995). Social conditions as fundamental causes of disease. *Journal of Health and Social Behavior*, **Extra Issue**, 80–94.

Link, B. G. and Phelan, J. C. (1996). Understanding sociodemographic differences in health – the role of fundamental social causes. *American Journal of Public Health*, **86** (4), 471–3.

Malla, A., Cortese, L., Shaw, T. S. *et al.* (1990). Life events and relapse in schizophrenia: a one year prospective study. *Social Psychiatry and Psychiatric Epidemiology*, **25**, 221–4.

Marcelis, M., Navarro-Mateu, F., Murray, R. *et al.* (1998). Urbanization and psychosis: a study of 1942–1978 birth cohorts in the Netherlands. *Psychological Medicine*, **28** (4), 871–9.

Marcelis, M., Takei, N. and van Os, J. (1999). Urbanization and risk for schizophrenia: does the effect operate before or around the time of illness onset? *Psychological Medicine*, **29**, 1197–203.

McKenzie, K. and Harpham, T. (2006). *Social Capital and Mental Health*. London: Jessica Kingsley Publishers.

McKenzie, K., Whitley, R. and Weich, S. (2002). Social capital and mental illness. *The British Journal of Psychiatry*, **181**, 280–3.

Mortensen, P., Pedersen, C., Westergaard, T. *et al.* (1999). Effects of family history and place and season of birth on the risk of schizophrenia. *New England Journal of Medicine*, **340** (8), 603–8.

Mulvany, F., O'Callaghan, E., Takei, N. *et al.* (2001). Effect of social class at birth on risk and presentation of schizophrenia: a case-control study. *British Medical Journal*, 323, 1398–401.

Nuechterlein, K. H., Goldstein, M. J., Ventura. J. *et al.* (1989). Patient-environment relationships in schizophrenia – information-processing, communication deviance, autonomic arousal, and stressful life events. *British Journal of Psychiatry Supplement*, **155** (suppl.), 84–9.

O'Callaghan, E., Cotter, D., Colgan, K. *et al.* (1995). Confinement of winter birth excess in schizophrenia to the urban born and its gender specificity. *British Journal of Psychiatry*, **166**, 51–4.

Ohta, Y., Nakane, Y., Nishihara, J. *et al.* (1992). Ecological structure and incidence rates of schizophrenia in Nagasaki City. *Acta Psychiatrica Scandinavica*, **86** (2), 113–20.

Pedersen, C. B. and Mortensen, P. B. (2001). Urbanization and schizophrenia: evidence of a cumulative negative effect of urban residence during upbringing. *Archives of General Psychiatry*, **58** (11), 1039–46.

Peen, J. and Dekker, J. (1997). Admission rates for schizophrenia in the Netherlands: an urban/ rural comparison. *Acta Psychiatrica Scandinavica*, **96** (4), 301–5.

Porter, R. (1997). *The Greatest Benefit to Mankind*. London: HarperCollins.

Silver, E., Mulvey, E. and Swanson, J. (2002). Neighbourhood structural characteristics and mental disorder: Faris and Dunham revisited. *Social Science and Medicine*, **55** (8), 1457–70.

Susser, M. and Susser, E. (1996). Choosing a future for epidemiology II: from black boxes to Chinese boxes and eco-epidemiology. *American Journal of Public Health*, **86**, 674–7.

Suvisaari, J. M., Haukka, J. K., Tanskanen, A. J. *et al.* (2000). Decreasing seasonal variation of births in schizophrenia. *Psychological Medicine*, **30**, 315–24.

Takei, N., Sham, P., O'Callaghan, E. *et al.* (1995). Schizophrenia increased risk associated with winter and city birth. *Journal of Epidemiology and Community Health*, **49**, 106–7.

Thornicroft, G., Bisoffi, G., De Salva, D. *et al.* (1993). Urban–rural differences in the associations between social deprivation and psychiatric service utilization in schizophrenia and all diagnoses: a case-register study in Northern Italy. *Psychological Medicine*, **23**, 487–96.

van Os, J., Driessen, G., Gunther, N. *et al.* (2000). Neighbourhood variation in incidence of schizophrenia. Evidence for person–environment interaction. *British Journal of Psychiatry*, **176**, 243–8.

van Os, J., Hanssen, M., Bijl, R. V. *et al.* (2001). Prevalence of psychotic disorder and community level of psychotic symptoms: an urban–rural comparison. *Archives of General Psychiatry*, **58** (7), 663–8.

van Os, J., Pedersen, C. and Mortensen, P. (2004). Confirmation of synergy between urbanicity and familial liability in the causation of psychosis. *American Journal of Psychiatry*, **161** (12), 2312–14.

Verdoux. H., Takei, N., de Saint Mathurin, R. C. *et al.* (1997). Seasonality of birth in schizophrenia: the effect of regional population density. *Schizophrenia Research*, **23** (2), 175–80.

Westergaard, T., Mortensen, P., Pedersen, C. *et al.* (1999). Exposure to prenatal and childhood infections and the risk of schizophrenia. *Archives of General Psychiatry*, **56**, 993–8.

7

Childhood adversity and psychosis

Helen Fisher and Tom Craig

Introduction

Back in the 1950s and 1960s, it was popular to insinuate that the development of mental health problems, particularly schizophrenia, was a result of being brought up in a disturbed family (see Chapter 8). Unfortunately, this led to a family-blaming culture based on little evidence, which, not surprisingly, was met with anger from relatives' support groups. Subsequently, few psychosis researchers have explored potential risk factors relating to the family. However, in the past few years there has been a resurgence of research into how the family environment and adverse childhood experiences may be linked to later development of psychosis (see also Chapter 8). This area of research appears to have come almost full circle and careful consideration of recent research is essential if simplistic and potentially harmful conclusions are to be avoided. In this chapter, we focus on childhood adversity, and begin with a review of the most commonly researched aspects of early adversity and trauma.

Summary of existing literature

Separation from parents or loss of at least one parent

Recent investigations employing reasonably robust methodologies have found a twofold to threefold increased risk of adult psychosis in those who experienced long-term separation from, or death of, at least one parent during childhood, independent of a variety of confounders, including a parental history of mental illness (e.g., Morgan et al., 2007). Moreover, an increased risk of psychosis has been found in those who lived in a single-parent household during childhood (Wicks et al., 2005) and in those who spent time in institutional care (Bebbington et al., 2004). It remains unclear, however, whether these associations reflect a direct effect of parental separation and loss on risk of psychosis, or whether such events are proxy indicators for associated adversity, such as family conflict and socioeconomic disadvantage.

Society and Psychosis, ed. Craig Morgan, Kwame McKenzie and Paul Fearon. Published by Cambridge University Press. © Cambridge University Press 2008.

Childhood abuse

Significant proportions of patients with schizophrenia-spectrum disorders report histories of childhood abuse. For instance, Morgan and Fisher (2007), in their comprehensive review, reported average rates of childhood sexual abuse for female and male patients with a psychotic disorder of 42% and 28%, respectively, and rates of childhood physical abuse of 35% and 38%, respectively. This compares with general population figures of 11% for sexual abuse and 7% for physical abuse (May-Chahal and Cawson, 2005). In patients with other disorders, such as bipolar affective disorder (Hammersley *et al.*, 2003), post-traumatic stress disorder (Butler *et al.*, 1996) and dissociative identity disorder (Ross, 1989), experience of early maltreatment is also positively correlated with increased levels of auditory hallucinations and delusions. More recent studies using community samples have found that schizotypal features are more common in those who report adverse childhood experiences (e.g., Startup, 1999). Some research has also suggested that parental neglect during childhood is associated with higher rates of schizophrenia during adulthood (e.g., Jones *et al.*, 1994).

Furthermore, several large general population studies have found childhood maltreatment to be a significant predictor of later development of psychotic symptoms (Bebbington *et al.*, 2004; Janssen *et al.*, 2004; Spauwen *et al.*, 2006; Whitfield *et al.*, 2005). The Janssen *et al.* (2004) study is particularly noteworthy. The study was a prospective investigation of 4045 people in the Netherlands. Information on the experience, frequency and severity of various forms of abuse (physical, sexual, psychological and emotional) was collected at the beginning of the study and the sample was followed up over the subsequent two years to record all new cases of psychosis. Those who reported having been abused were seven times more likely than those without an abuse history to develop a psychotic disorder warranting treatment, after controlling for a range of possible confounding variables, including the presence of psychiatric problems at baseline and lifetime illicit drug use. However, the number of individuals with psychotic symptoms of a severity requiring care was small ($n=7$). The other population-based studies are also limited as they failed to take account of the timing, severity or duration of abuse (e.g., Bebbington *et al.*, 2004; Spauwen *et al.*, 2006), or because they used a single question to measure psychotic symptoms (e.g., Whitfield *et al.*, 2005). Moreover, the only study using contemporaneous records found no association between officially reported childhood sexual abuse and later hospital admission for schizophrenia (Spataro *et al.*, 2004). This non-significant finding could be due to a large number of sexual abuse cases going unreported in the general population or the possibility that intervention by state services provides a protective effect. These inconsistencies point to a need for more methodologically robust research.

Bullying

Bullying can be either direct (e.g., kicking, hitting) or relational (e.g., social exclusion, name-calling) and is considered to occur within the context of a real or perceived physical or psychological imbalance of power in which an individual is chronically exposed to deliberate harm or suffering by at least one other person (Olweus, 1993). Although psychiatric problems and utilisation of mental health services have been found amongst both bullies and their victims (Kumpulainen *et al.*, 1998), relatively few studies have considered these roles in terms of increased susceptibility to psychosis in adulthood. To date, there do not appear to be any studies exploring the rate of childhood bullying amongst psychotic patients, but two general population studies have demonstrated that this adverse experience significantly increases the risk of psychosis-like experiences in adolescence (Lataster *et al.*, 2006) and probable psychotic disorder in adulthood (Bebbington *et al.*, 2004). In the latter survey, those with a history of bullying victimisation were four times more likely to self-report psychotic symptoms, although this was reduced to less than twice after other types of victimisation were taken into account (Bebbington *et al.*, 2004). Moreover, bullying seems to have a persistent effect on individuals' subjective wellbeing after the development of non-affective psychosis (Hardy *et al.*, 2005), thus also potentially having an impact upon recovery.

Parental mental illness

Rutter and Quinton (1984) studied the offspring of consecutive new psychiatric cases and found that around a third exhibited some form of persistent disorder. However, few had a psychotic disorder. Moreover, this association is potentially confounded by other factors prevalent in such families, including marital discord, parental separation, emotional deprivation and low socioeconomic status (Harris *et al.*, 1987; Rutter and Quinton, 1984). High rates of parental psychosis have been found amongst severely abused children who came into contact with the judicial system in Boston (Taylor *et al.*, 1991). Consequently, having a parent with a psychotic disorder may increase exposure to the types of early adversity that have been linked to the subsequent development of psychosis. Disentangling the impact of these environmental factors and genetic risk is a major challenge for future research.

Methodological issues

Defining adversity

A problematic aspect of the studies reviewed above concerns the definition and assessment of the various forms of adversity. The concept of childhood adversity encompasses a diverse range of experiences, including sexual abuse, physical abuse, emotional or psychological abuse, neglect, bullying by peers, parental loss through separation or death, domestic violence and parental mental illness. Within each of these broad categories there are considerable variations in quantitative and qualitative aspects of the experiences that need to be taken into account. These include the frequency and severity of exposure, contextual factors, such as the age at which the exposure occurred, whether the perpetrator was a family member or outsider, and the presence of other aspects of adversity that might mitigate the likely impact. Some of these may include experiences, such as antipathy or neglect, that would not qualify as abuse in their own right but might nonetheless be important contributors to the overall impact. Different forms of abuse tend to overlap. Parents who physically abuse their children also tend to neglect them, and these different forms of adversity may have complex cumulative effects (Mullen *et al.*, 1993).

Measuring adversity

Most studies of early adversity and psychosis have relied on three sources of information – clinical case notes or other official records (e.g., Read, 1998; Read and Argyle, 1999; Read *et al.*, 2003), self-report questionnaires (e.g., Whitfield *et al.*, 2005) or one or two questions within a larger interview (Bebbington *et al.*, 2004; Darves-Bornoz *et al.*, 1995; Janssen *et al.*, 2004). Each approach has serious limitations. For example, abuse histories extracted from the records of psychiatric patients suffer from all the definitional weaknesses mentioned above, are unreliably recorded and consistently underestimate the prevalence of abuse (e.g., Read, 1998; Read and Argyle, 1999), particularly where reliance is solely on case notes (Wurr and Partridge, 1996). Moreover, Dill *et al.* (1991) demonstrated that confidential self-report questionnaires elicited twice as many reports of childhood abuse as routine psychiatric intake interviews. Reports based on official court and social service records of maltreatment are likely to be more carefully recorded and accurate, but these legal samples are restricted to the more extreme end of the spectrum. These samples may well exaggerate the importance of an association between abuse and psychosis both because of the extreme nature of the abuse and because these families may be dysfunctional in many other ways.

By far the most common measurement approach is one that relies on standardised questions. Typically, whether self-completed or by interview, standard questions are asked that require 'yes' or 'no' responses and the number of positive replies is used as the final measure. There are many problems with this approach. What threshold of experience to include is left to the respondent and what might be qualitatively quite different experiences are given the same score. Such checklist measures often fail to deal with time order and do not always distinguish childhood and adult trauma. For example, one of the more commonly cited studies that found a link between sexual abuse and psychosis (Bebbington *et al.*, 2004) did not determine the timing of the experience and probably includes adult sexual assault, which is considered by some authors to be more common than childhood sexual abuse (Coverdale and Turbott, 2000).

Detailed questioning in semi-structured interviews has produced more accurate recollections of adverse childhood experiences (Maughan and Rutter, 1997), especially when given together with assurances about the confidential treatment of disclosures (Dill *et al.*, 1991). Additionally, the availability of a manual and the need for training to be completed before administering the measure enhances inter-rater consistency in administration and interpretation (Roy and Perry, 2004). Very few of the existing studies have employed tools with published psychometric properties that meet such criteria (e.g., Fisher *et al.*, 2006). However, a few studies have attempted to rectify assessment problems and enhance validity by assigning high cut-offs to their definitions of adversity to capture only severe and persistent cases of childhood maltreatment (e.g., Janssen *et al.*, 2004). Similarly, in studies that have not employed specific tools to assess childhood abuse, such as Read *et al.* (2003), in which medical notes were screened, inter-rater reliability has occasionally been determined to check the consistency with which definitions of abuse have been applied (e.g., Read, 1998).

Of course it is not only the adversity that needs careful consideration. Psychosis and schizophrenia are broad, heterogeneous constructs and it may be too limiting merely to consider correlations involving patients who have received such diagnoses. Greater understanding may be reached by focusing on specific psychotic symptoms or 'complaints' (see Chapter 14). However, some studies have employed inadequate measures of such symptoms. For example, Whitfield *et al.* (2005) used a single question to determine the presence of hallucinations in their participants. Moreover, many studies have not specified which psychotic symptoms or types of trauma are being measured. Those that do often have sample sizes that are too small to detect associations between the different forms of adversity and psychosis (e.g., Bak *et al.*, 2005). Others have focused on just a single type of adversity (e.g., Darves-Bornoz *et al.*, 1995), preventing the potentially confounding effects of other types of abuse from being controlled.

Validity and retrospective assessment

The accuracy of recall of childhood maltreatment is contentious. In addition to the normal processes of forgetting over time, the traumatic nature of adversity may result in amnesia for such experiences (Feldman-Summers and Pope, 1994). Unfortunately, there is no easy way of removing the need for retrospective assessment for anything other than the most severe forms of neglect and abuse that come to the attention of social services.

Consequently, assessment tools have employed devices to minimise potential problems with recall. For instance, the Childhood Experiences of Care and Abuse interview (CECA: Bifulco et al., 1994) and a shorter investigator-administered screening questionnaire (CECA-Q: Bifulco et al., 2005) were developed to focus on factual aspects of behaviours, and require the respondents to give concrete examples of abuses that they have experienced. The interview starts with mapping the household arrangements from early childhood to the age of 17 and covers the care received from both parents and other carers. These, together with key dates (birthdays, major events), are then used to frame questions and trigger the individual's memory of past events. However, only two studies involving patients with psychotic conditions have employed these approaches (Fisher et al., 2006; Friedman et al., 2002).

Additional concerns about the reliability of patients' recall of abuse histories have been raised based on the cognitive impairments associated with psychotic disorders (Saykin et al., 1991) or the perception that such patients are more likely to report delusional accounts of abuse (Young et al., 2001). Although there is a large body of literature indicating that individuals with psychosis experience difficulties in acquiring, retaining and retrieving new information (Goldman-Rakic, 1994), there is no clear evidence of similar deficits with regard to information stored in the long-term memory (Gur et al., 2000). Several reviews have concluded that current psychopathology does not result in biased memories of childhood abuse (e.g., Maughan and Rutter, 1997). Reports of abuse by adult psychiatric patients have been shown to be reasonably reliable over time (Goodman et al., 1999) and reports by those with schizophrenia have been found to be as reliable as those made by the general population (Darves-Bornoz et al., 1995). Indeed, patients may be more likely to under-report instances of abuse (Dill et al., 1991).

Sample characteristics

Reasonably large numbers of participants are required to test statistically for effects, control for confounders and explore the differential influence of various types of abuse on risk of psychosis (Read et al., 2005). However, even the large general population studies only identified a small number of people with probable psychosis ($n = 60$: Bebbington et al., 2004; $n = 7$: Janssen et al., 2004). Moreover, many studies have been based on samples of inpatients suffering from chronic disorders, which are not representative of the broader population of individuals with psychosis (Saleptsi et al., 2004), let alone the many people who experience transient conditions or those who experience psychosis but do not seek treatment. It is consequently not clear from such studies whether the childhood trauma is associated with the onset or the course of the disorder.

The majority of studies in this area also lack a comparison group to compare findings against, thereby hindering attempts to determine whether the relationship between childhood adversity and psychosis is causal. Ideally, comparisons should be made with a randomly selected general population sample drawn from the same geographical area as patients and matched for sociodemographic characteristics (e.g., age, ethnicity, social class and educational level). The control group would also need to be of sufficient size to allow adjustments for potentially confounding factors to be made. It is only through investigations utilising different samples of patients and healthy control comparisons with an appropriate range of social conditions that causal relationships will emerge with any clarity (Rutter *et al.*, 2001).

Theoretical models

While the nature and strength of any association between childhood adversity and psychosis needs further clarification, models have nonetheless been proposed that identify potential mechanisms through which early trauma may increase the risk of later psychosis. It makes sense for these two strands of research (epidemiology and studies of biological, psychological and social mechanisms) to proceed simultaneously. Here we review some of the hypothesised models.

Biological

The most popular biological-level theory currently postulated to account for the correlation between childhood abuse and psychosis concerns the role of the hypothalamic-pituitary-adrenal (HPA) axis. It has been suggested that persistent exposure to stress during childhood may lead to prolonged periods of high glucocorticoid levels and subsequent impairment of the negative feedback system that dampens HPA activation (Walker and DiForio, 1997). This, in turn, may result in heightened sensitivity to future stress. This theory is supported by studies that have demonstrated HPA axis dysregulation in abused girls (Putnam *et al.*, 1991). Such over-sensitivity to stress is also considered to be a central feature of schizophrenia (Walker and DiForio, 1997). Further links between the HPA axis and schizophrenia are provided by the interdependency of HPA activation and dopamine release and synthesis following exposure to stressors (Depue and Collins, 1999). Dopamine is consistently linked to schizophrenia, and particularly the formation of persecutory delusions, owing to its perceived role in the interpretation of threat-related stimuli (Spitzer, 1995). Moreover, elevated dopamine metabolism has been found in girls who have been sexually abused compared with non-abused controls (De Bellis *et al.*, 1994). Of course, this proposed pathway from adverse childhood experiences to dysfunction in the HPA axis and dopamine system, and the subsequent development of psychosis, is very much speculative at this stage.

Alterations to brain structure and function present another biological-level explanation for the role of childhood adversity in the later development of psychosis. Teicher *et al.* (2003) have proposed that high levels of stress early in life resulting from maltreatment can produce major and enduring changes in brain development. They cite evidence that those who experience childhood trauma have stunted development of the hippocampus (e.g., Stein, 1997), amygdala (Driessen *et al.*, 2000) and corpus callosum (De Bellis *et al.*, 1999), although some studies have not found any reductions in these areas for abuse survivors compared with controls (Carrion *et al.*, 2001). Of particular relevance is their suggestion that the stress exerted on the limbic system during maltreatment may produce the same psychosis-type symptoms (e.g., perceptual distortions, brief hallucinations) that occur during temporal lobe seizures (Teicher *et al.*, 1993), which can be caused by abnormal development of the hippocampus or amygdala under the right neurochemical conditions (Gale, 1992). Indeed, Teicher *et al.* (1993) found that adults who had been physically or sexually abused as children exhibited high scores on a checklist of limbic symptoms. However, these are likely to be attenuated or sub-clinical psychotic symptoms and this theory does not clarify how a clinically relevant psychotic disorder develops. Once again, the hypothesis that early traumatic experiences result in structural and functional changes in the brain that subsequently lead to the emergence of psychosis is still tentative.

Psychological

A further appealing theory suggests that psychotic symptoms might emerge via over-sensitive threat-appraisal mechanisms resulting from childhood maltreatment (see Chapter 14). Crittendon and Ainsworth (1989) posited that children who are abused, particularly those who suffer physical abuse or bullying, have a strong tendency to be hyper-vigilant to hostile cues in their environment, which could initially be an adaptive response to unpredictable and threatening surroundings (Pollak *et al.*, 2005). This has been supported by research indicating that children who have experienced abuse attend to and remember negative and aggressive stimuli to a greater extent than non-abused children (Dodge *et al.*, 1995). If this coping mechanism persists, then it might become integrated into the individual's general social information processing model, leading to overly hostile attributions about the intentions of others (Dodge *et al.*, 1986). Consequently, such individuals may display inappropriate or maladaptive behaviours, such as aggression (Eisenberg *et al.*, 1994), leaving them vulnerable to developing conduct disorders. Equally, abused or bullied children may distance themselves from others and become overly suspicious of others' intentions and behaviour, leaving them predisposed to psychotic symptoms, such as paranoid delusional beliefs or ideas of reference (Frith, 1992).

This theoretical model, however, is only really valid in relation to adverse experiences involving perceived threat or actual harm (e.g., emotional, physical or potentially sexual abuse and bullying). By drawing on attachment theory, it is possible to extend this model to children who have experienced other types of adversity, including aberrant separation from the primary caregiver and severe maternal antipathy. Attachment involves the development of strong affectional bonds initially between an infant and his or her primary caregiver (Bowlby, 1969). This early attachment experience is thought to influence the individual in his or her future relationships and interactions throughout life (Ainsworth, 1989). More specifically, a secure attachment in childhood is thought to foster basic trust in both the self and others (Bowlby, 1973). Children who have been maltreated are at increased risk of forming insecure (Cole and Putnam, 1992) or disorganised attachments (O'Connor and Rutter, 2000) and such patterns of attachment may subsequently instil a general suspiciousness of other people. Indeed, Chadwick (1995) suggests that paranoid attitudes are more likely to develop when individuals lack mutually trusting relationships. Therefore, abuse during childhood or an extremely difficult relationship with the mother may increase an individual's vulnerability to developing beliefs with a delusional quality. However, these routes to misinterpretation of the intentions of others can only be utilised as a partial hypothesis to explain the development of psychosis. The focus is solely on paranoid delusions at the expense of hallucinations, which have been shown to be highly correlated with childhood abuse, and indeed other psychotic symptoms, such as forms of thought disorder (Read and Argyle, 1999).

Broader theories concerning faulty source monitoring may be able to account for the development of hallucinations given childhood experiences of adversity. Bentall (1990) has suggested that hallucinations are a form of bias in which internally generated items are attributed to external sources. In terms of childhood abuse and bullying, it is possible that intrusive, flashback memories of these traumatic events occur in adolescence and adulthood (Ehlers and Clark, 2000) and develop directly into hallucinations, particularly around relevant themes such as humiliation (Hardy et al., 2005). Alternatively, it may be that, to reduce the anxiety provoked by such intrusions, the individual appraises them as external events (Morrison et al., 1995). Potential evidence for the presence of such faulty source monitoring in people with histories of abuse comes from studies assessing locus of control. Children who have experienced adverse and unpredictable environments have been shown to experience a perceived lack of control over subsequent events (Chorpita and Barlow, 1998), and, therefore, may be more likely to assume that their behaviour is under external control (Rotter, 1966). Such an external locus of control in adolescents has been found to be a strong predictor of adult psychotic disorder (Frenkel *et al.*, 1995). However, this argument depends on the child appraising the maltreatment as extremely traumatic; some children clearly maintain a sense of internal control and are able to cope well with adversity (Luthar, 1991).

Behavioural

Social withdrawal is a common antecedent to a psychotic illness. While usually seen as an early manifestation of the illness itself, it is possible that it is one component of a complex causal chain. Animal models have demonstrated that severely aberrant parenting produces socially pathological behaviours in offspring, including social avoidance (e.g., Harlow and Suomi, 1971). A tendency to withdraw from social interactions is also a behavioural consequence of childhood maltreatment in human beings. This may reflect the belief that it is best to avoid social contact in order to be protected from potential sources of harm (Kaufman and Cicchetti, 1989), or it may be a behavioural manifestation of the distorted cognitive schema described above (e.g., Frith, 1992). Additionally, abused children are often less well liked by their peers and experience higher rates of rejection even by those they consider to be their best friends (Salzinger *et al.*, 1993). Impoverished social adjustment in infancy and adolescence is associated with later development of psychosis (e.g., Davidson *et al.*, 1999), and it has been suggested that individuals who are predominantly exposed to solitary environments, either self-imposed or through difficulties in developing friendships, are more prone to develop psychosis, possibly because they are not exposed to alternative and normalising explanations for anomalous psychotic experiences (White *et al.*, 2000). Therefore, childhood abuse may increase the risk for onset of psychotic disorders through its detrimental impact on social functioning. However, social withdrawal is unlikely to be either sufficient or necessary, as individuals with psychosis vary greatly in the nature and severity of their pre-morbid behavioural deficits, ranging from being highly functioning in the prodromal period to having marked impairments (Offord and Cross, 1969).

Another potential behavioural route through which adverse childhood experiences could influence later psychosis onset is by increasing the likelihood of substance misuse. Severe substance abuse problems occur more commonly in those who have a history of childhood maltreatment (Zlotnick *et al.*, 2004) and substance misuse is increasingly considered a major risk factor for psychosis (McGuire *et al.*, 1995). The use of cannabis, particularly heavy use, may be moderated by genetic factors (Caspi *et al.*, 2005) suggesting that it could be an individual's genetic make-up rather than experiences of childhood maltreatment that leads to substance misuse and the subsequent onset of psychosis. However, a recent general population study of 17 337 individuals revealed that those who had experienced the greatest number of types of childhood maltreatment had markedly increased rates of hallucinations compared with those without a history of abuse, even when controlling for substance misuse (Whitfield *et al.*, 2005).

Integrative theories

Is it possible to pull the various theories outlined above together into an integrated model that can provide a framework for continuing research in this area? The classic theory of schizophrenia that has attempted to incorporate these different levels of analysis is the 'diathesis–stress' model. This proposes that an individual who has a genetic predisposition ('diathesis') only becomes unwell when exposed to an environmental pathogen ('stress') that triggers the onset of the disorder (Zubin and Spring, 1977). However, Read *et al.* (2005) argue that this 'biopsychosocial' model is not a truly integrative model; rather it focuses too heavily on biological factors and assumes that the diathesis of the diathesis–stress model must be biological. In response to the perceived rigidity of this model, Read *et al.* (2001) advocate a traumagenic neurodevelopmental model, in which they propose that childhood maltreatment initiates abnormal neurodevelopmental processes (e.g., overreactivity of the HPA axis, structural neuroanatomical changes) and that this creates the vulnerability for later schizophrenia. Although this model makes some attempt to link these biochemical and structural aspects to the actual formation of psychotic symptoms, it does so only tentatively and without utilising other levels of analysis.

A framework that integrates both the biological and psychological levels to model the hypothetical link between childhood adversity and psychosis could be developed by unifying two integrative theories. Kapur (2003) has postulated that dysregulation of the dopaminergic system produces negative appraisals of external events (potentially leading to persecutory delusions) and aberrant salience of internal representations of perceptions and memories (potentially leading to hallucinations and, indirectly, to delusions through attempts to impose meaning on such experiences). Therefore, if the traumagenic neurodevelopmental model and Kapur's theory are combined (as suggested by Read *et al.*, 2005) then a hypothetical causal model of psychosis could be developed in which the stress of childhood maltreatment leads to impaired dopamine transmission, which results in faulty source monitoring and hostile attribution bias, and the subsequent formation of delusions and hallucinations.

The above strands are brought together in Figure 7.1. In this model, childhood trauma produces biological and psychological effects that endure into adulthood. The psychological response to trauma is the development of a view of the world as an essentially hostile source of threatening experiences over which the individual

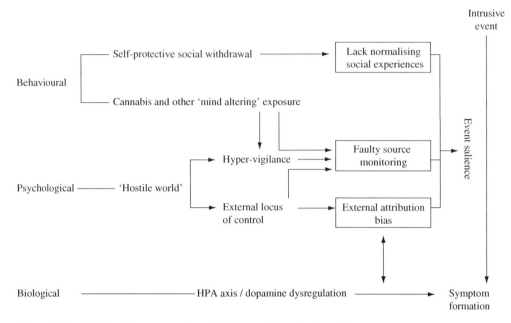

Figure 7.1 Childhood trauma and psychosis – an integrated model

has little personal control (i.e., an externalising locus of control) and for which he or she has to remain on perpetual alert (hyper-vigilance). Social withdrawal is one way of reducing exposure to this hostile environment. Childhood trauma and the subsequent life experiences that confirm the world as hostile interact with biological vulnerability, perhaps causing, but more likely heightening, an underlying dysregulation of the dopaminergic system, which, in turn, governs the salience of later stressors for the individual.

Conclusions

In conclusion, although the amount of research literature investigating a link between childhood adversity and the subsequent development of psychosis has increased in recent years, a corresponding increase in the methodological quality of studies is not yet evident. The definition and measurement of childhood maltreatment varies widely between studies and few have utilised standardised instruments with published psychometric properties. The samples employed tend to be small (at least in terms of the number of individuals with psychosis), heterogeneous with regard to psychiatric diagnosis and mainly composed of inpatients with chronic forms of the disorder. The retrospective and self-report nature of assessments of childhood adversity used by the majority of studies limits the reliability and validity of the data obtained, although attempts have been made to minimise potential biases. Therefore, present claims that a causal relationship between childhood adversity and onset of psychosis has been established (Read *et al.*, 2005) are premature. Nevertheless, the plausibility of the proposition that childhood adversity is aetiologically important in psychosis is bolstered by the fact that there are a number of theoretically coherent mechanisms that could account for a link between the two factors. Future research needs to be more methodologically rigorous and incorporate detailed, standardised instruments to measure adversity. Only then can causal assumptions be adequately tested (Rutter *et al.*, 2001).

REFERENCES

Ainsworth, M. D. S. (1989). Attachment beyond infancy. *American Psychologist*, **44**, 709–16.

Bak, M., Krabbendam, L., Janssen, I. *et al.* (2005). Early trauma may increase the risk for psychotic experiences by impacting on emotional response and perception of control. *Acta Psychiatrica Scandinavica*, **112**, 360–6.

Bebbington, P., Bhugra, D., Singleton, N. *et al.* (2004). Psychosis, victimisation and childhood disadvantage. *British Journal of Psychiatry*, **185**, 220–6.

Bentall, R. P. (1990). The syndromes and symptoms of psychosis: or why you can't play twenty questions with the concept of schizophrenia and hope to win. In *Reconstructing Schizophrenia*, ed. R. P. Bentall. London: Routledge, pp. 3–22.

Bifulco, A., Brown, G. W. and Harris, T. O. (1994). Childhood experience of care and abuse (CECA): a retrospective interview measure. *Journal of Child Psychology and Psychiatry*, **35**, 1419–35.

Bifulco, A., Bernazzani, O., Moran, P. M. *et al.* (2005). The Childhood Experiences of Care and Abuse Questionnaire (CECA.Q) – validation in a community series. *British Journal of Clinical Psychology*, **44**, 563–81.

Bowlby, J. (1969). *Attachment*. Vol. 1 of *Attachment and Loss*. New York: Basic Books.

Bowlby, J. (1973). *Separation*. Vol. 2 of *Attachment and Loss*. New York: Basic Books.

Butler, R. W., Mueser, K. T., Sprock, J. *et al.* (1996). Positive symptoms of psychosis in post-traumatic stress disorder. *Biological Psychiatry*, **39**, 839–44.

Carrion, V. G., Weems, C. F., Eliez, S. *et al.* (2001). Attenuation of frontal asymmetry in pediatric post-traumatic stress disorder. *Biological Psychiatry*, **50** (12), 943–51.

Caspi, A., Moffitt, T. E., Cannon, M. *et al.* (2005). Moderation of the effect of adolescent-onset cannabis use on adult psychosis by a functional polymorphism in the catechol-O methyl-transferase gene: longitudinal evidence of a gene X environment interaction. *Biological Psychiatry*, **57** (10), 1117–27.

Chadwick, P. (1995). *Understanding Paranoia*. London: Thorsons.

Chorpita, B. F. and Barlow, D. H. (1998). The development of anxiety: the role of control in the early environment. *Psychological Bulletin*, **124**, 3–21.

Cole, P. M. and Putnam, F. W. (1992). Effect of incest on self and social functioning: a developmental psychopathology perspective. *Journal of Consulting and Clinical Psychology*, **60**, 174–84.

Coverdale, J. H. and Turbott, S. H. (2000). Sexual and physical abuse of chronically ill psychiatric outpatients compared with a matched sample of medical outpatients. *Journal of Nervous and Mental Disease*, **188**, 440–5.

Crittendon, P. M. and Ainsworth, M. D. S. (1989). Child maltreatment and attachment theory. In *Childhood Maltreatment: Theory and Research on the Causes and Consequences of Child Abuse and Neglect*, ed. D. Cicchetti and V. Carlson. Cambridge: Cambridge University Press, pp. 432–63.

Darves-Bornoz, J. M., Lemperiere, T., Degiovanni, A. *et al.* (1995). Sexual victimisation in women with schizophrenia and bipolar disorder. *Social Psychiatry and Psychiatric Epidemiology*, **30**, 78–84.

Davidson, M., Reichenberg, A., Rabinowitz, J. *et al.* (1999). Behavioural and intellectual markers for schizophrenia in apparently healthy male adolescents. *American Journal of Psychiatry*, **156**, 1328–35.

De Bellis, M., Chrousos, G., Dorn, L. *et al.* (1994). Hypothalamic-pituitary-adrenal axis dysregulation in sexually abused girls. *Journal of Clinical Endocrinology and Metabolism*, **78**, 249–55.

De Bellis, M. D., Keshavan, M. S., Clark, D. B. *et al.* (1999). Developmental traumatology. Part II: brain development. *Biological Psychiatry*, **45** (10), 1271–84.

Depue, R. and Collins, P. (1999). Neurobiology of the structure of personality: dopamine, facilitation of incentive motivation, and extraversion. *Behavioural and Brain Sciences*, **22**, 491–569.

Dill, D. L., Chu, J. A., Grob, M. C. *et al.* (1991). The reliability of abuse history report: a comparison of two inquiry formats. *Comprehensive Psychiatry*, **32**, 166–9.

Dodge, K. A., Pettit, G. S., McClaskey, C. L. *et al.* (1986). Social competence in children. *Monographs of the Society for Research in Child Development*, **51**, (2, serial no 213).

Dodge, K. A., Pettit, G. S., Bates, J. E. *et al.* (1995). Social information processing patterns partially mediate the effects of early physical abuse on later conduct problems. *Journal of Abnormal Psychology*, **104**, 632–43.

Driessen, M., Herrmann, J., Stahl, K. *et al.* (2000). Magnetic resonance imaging volumes of the hippocampus and the amygdala in women with borderline personality disorder and early traumatization. *Archives of General Psychiatry*, **57** (12), 1115–22.

Ehlers, A. and Clark, D. M. (2000). A cognitive model of post-traumatic stress disorder. *Behaviour, Research and Therapy*, **38**, 319–45.

Eisenberg, N., Fabes, R. A., Nyman, M. *et al.* (1994). The relations of emotionality and regulation to children's anger-related reactions. *Child Development*, **65**, 109–28.

Feldman-Summers, S. and Pope, K. S. (1994). The experience of 'forgetting' childhood abuse: a national survey of psychologists. *Journal of Consulting and Clinical Psychology*, **62** (3), 636–9.

Fisher, H., Morgan, C., Fearon, P. *et al.* (2006). Childhood maltreatment as a risk factor for psychosis. *Schizophrenia Research*, **81** (suppl. 1), 235.

Frenkel, E., Kugelmass, M. N. and Ingraham, L. J. (1995). Locus of control and mental health in adolescence and adulthood. *Schizophrenia Bulletin*, **21**, 219–26.

Friedman, S., Smith, L., Fogel, D. *et al.* (2002). The incidence and influence of early traumatic life events in patients with panic disorder: a comparison with other psychiatric outpatients. *Journal of Anxiety Disorders*, **16**, 259–72.

Frith, C. D. (1992). *The Cognitive Neuropsychology of Schizophrenia*. Hove: Psychology Press.

Gale, K. (1992). Role of GABA in the genesis of chemoconvulsant seizures. *Toxicology Letters*, **64–65**, 417–28.

Goldman-Rakic, P. S. (1994). Working memory dysfunction in schizophrenia. *Journal of Neuropsychiatry and Clinical Neurosciences*, **6**, 348–57.

Goodman, L., Thompson, K., Weinfurt, K. *et al.* (1999). Reliability of reports of violent victimisation and post-traumatic stress disorder among men and women with serious mental illness. *Journal of Traumatic Stress*, **12**, 587–99.

Gur, R. C., Moelter, S. T. and Ragland, J. D. (2000). Learning and memory in schizophrenia. In *Cognition in Schizophrenia: Impairments, Importance and Treatment Strategies*, ed. T. Sharma and P. Harvey. Oxford: Oxford University Press, pp. 73–91.

Hammersley, P., Dias, A., Todd, G. *et al.* (2003). Childhood trauma and hallucinations in bipolar affective disorder: a preliminary investigation. *British Journal of Psychiatry*, **182**, 543–7.

Hardy, A., Fowler, D., Freeman, D. *et al.* (2005). Trauma and hallucinatory experience in psychosis. *Journal of Nervous and Mental Disease*, **193**, 501–7.

Harlow, H. F. and Suomi, S. J. (1971). Production of depressive behaviors in young monkeys. *Journal of Autism and Childhood Schizophrenia*, **13**, 246–55.

Harris, T., Brown, G. W. and Bifulco, A. (1987). Loss of parent in childhood and adult psychiatric disorder: the role of social class position and premarital pregnancy. *Psychological Medicine*, **16**, 641–59.

Janssen, I., Krabbendam, L., Bak, M. *et al.* (2004). Childhood abuse as a risk factor for psychosis. *Acta Psychiatrica Scandinavica*, **109**, 38–45.

Jones, P., Rodgers, B., Murray, R. *et al.* (1994). Child developmental risk factors for adult schizophrenia in the British 1946 birth cohort. *Lancet*, **344**, 1398–402.

Kapur, S. (2003). Psychosis as a state of aberrant salience: a framework linking biology, phenomenology, and pharmacology. *American Journal of Psychiatry*, **160**, 13–23.

Kaufman, J. and Cicchetti, D. (1989). Effects of maltreatment on school-aged children's socio-emotional development: assessment in a day camp setting. *Developmental Psychology*, **25**, 516–24.

Kumpulainen, K., Räsänen, E., Henttonen, I. *et al.* (1998). Bullying and psychiatric symptoms among elementary school-age children. *Child Abuse and Neglect*, **22**, 705–17.

Lataster, T., van Os, J., Drukker, M. *et al.* (2006). Childhood victimisation and developmental expression of non-clinical delusional ideation and hallucinatory experiences: victimisation and non-clinical psychotic experiences. *Social Psychiatry and Psychiatric Epidemiology*, **41** (6), 423–8.

Luthar, S. S. (1991). Vulnerability and resilience: a study of high-risk adolescents. *Child Development*, **62**, 600–16.

Maughan, B. and Rutter, M. (1997). Retrospective reporting of childhood adversity: issues in assessing long-term recall. *Journal of Personality Disorders*, **11**, 19–33.

May-Chahal, C. and Cawson, P. (2005). Measuring child maltreatment in the United Kingdom: a study of the prevalence of child abuse and neglect. *Child Abuse and Neglect*, **29**, 969–84.

McGuire, P., Jones, P. and Harvey, I. (1995). Cannabis and acute psychosis. *Schizophrenia Research*, **13**, 161–8.

Morgan, C. and Fisher, H. (2007). Environmental factors in schizophrenia: childhood trauma – a critical review. *Schizophrenia Bulletin*, **33**, 3–10.

Morgan, C., Kirkbride, J., Leff, J. *et al.* (2007). Parental separation, loss and psychosis in different ethnic groups: a case-control study. *Psychological Medicine*, **37** (4), 495–505.

Morrison, A. P., Haddock, G. and Tarrier, N. (1995). Intrusive thoughts and auditory hallucinations. *Psychological Medicine*, **26**, 669–79.

Mullen, P. E., Martin, J. L., Anderson, J. C. *et al.* (1993). Childhood sexual abuse and mental health in adult life. *British Journal of Psychiatry*, **163**, 721–32.

O'Connor, T. G. and Rutter, M. (2000). Attachment disorder behavior following early severe deprivation: extension and longitudinal follow-up. English and Romanian Adoptees Study Team. *Journal of the American Academy of Child and Adolescent Psychiatry*, **39** (6), 703–12.

Offord, D. and Cross, L. (1969). Behavioural antecedents of adult schizophrenia. *Archives of General Psychiatry*, **21**, 267–83.

Olweus, D. (1993). *Bullying at School: What We Know and What We Can Do*. Oxford: Blackwell.

Pollak, S. D., Vardi, S., Putzner Bechner, A. M. *et al.* (2005). Physically abused children's regulation of attention in response to hostility. *Child Development*, **76** (5), 968–77.

Putnam, F. W., Trickett, P., Helmers, K. *et al.* (1991). Cortisol abnormalities in sexually abused girls. In *New Research Abstracts. Proceedings of the 144th Annual Meeting of the American Psychiatric Association*, ed. S. J. Fiester, Washington, DC, p. 107.

Read, J. (1998). Child abuse and severity of disturbance among adult psychiatric inpatients. *Child Abuse and Neglect*, **22**, 359–68.

Read, J. and Argyle, N. (1999). Hallucinations, delusions, and thought disorder among adult psychiatric inpatients with a history of child abuse. *Psychiatric Services*, **50**, 1467–72.

Read, J., Perry, B. D., Moskowitz, A. *et al.* (2001). The contribution of early traumatic events to schizophrenia in some patients: a traumagenic neurodevelopmental model. *Psychiatry*, **64** (4), 319–45.

Read, J., Agar, K., Argyle, N. *et al.* (2003). Sexual and physical abuse during childhood and adulthood as predictors of hallucinations, delusions and thought disorder. *Psychology and Psychotherapy: Theory, Research and Practice*, **76**, 1–22.

Read, J., van Os, J., Morrison, A. P. *et al.* (2005). Childhood trauma, psychosis and schizophrenia: a literature review with theoretical and clinical implications. *Acta Psychiatrica Scandinavica*, **112**, 330–50.

Ross, C. (1989). *Multiple Personality Disorder: Diagnosis, Clinical Features, and Treatment*. London: John Wiley and Sons.

Rotter, J. B. (1966). Generalised expectancies for internal control of reinforcement. *Psychological Monographs*, **80**, 1–28.

Roy, C. A. and Perry, J. C. (2004). Instruments for the assessment of childhood trauma in adults. *The Journal of Nervous and Mental Disease*, **192** (5), 343–51.

Rutter, M., Pickles, A., Murray, R. *et al.* (2001). Testing hypotheses on specific environmental causal effects on behaviour. *Psychological Bulletin*, **127** (3), 291–324.

Rutter, M. and Quinton, D. (1984). Parental psychiatric disorder: effects on children. *Psychological Medicine*, **14** (4), 853–80.

Saleptsi, E., Bichescu, D., Rockstroh, B. *et al.* (2004). Negative and positive childhood experiences across developmental periods in psychiatric patients with different diagnoses – an exploratory study. *BMC Psychiatry*, **4**, 40–54.

Salzinger, S., Feldman, R. S., Hammer, M. *et al.* (1993). The effects of physical abuse on children's social relationships. *Child Development*, **64**, 169–87.

Saykin, A. J., Gur, R. C., Gur, R. E. *et al.* (1991). Neuropsychological functioning in schizophrenia: selective impairment in memory and learning. *Archives of General Psychiatry*, **48**, 618–24.

Spataro, J., Mullen, P. E., Burgess, P. M. *et al.* (2004). Impact of child sexual abuse on mental health. *British Journal of Psychiatry*, **184**, 416–21.

Spauwen, J., Krabbendam, L., Lieb, R. *et al.* (2006). Impact of psychological trauma on the development of psychotic symptoms: relationship with psychosis proneness. *British Journal of Psychiatry*, **188**, 527–33.

Spitzer, M. (1995). A neurocomputational approach to delusions. *Comprehensive Psychiatry*, **36**, 83–105.

Startup, M. (1999). Schizotypy, dissociative experiences and childhood abuse: relationships among self-report measures. *British Journal of Clinical Psychology*, **38**, 333–44.

Stein, M. B. (1997). Hippocampal volume in women victimised by childhood sexual abuse. *Psychological Medicine*, **27** (4), 951–9.

Taylor, C. G., Norman, J., Murphy, M. *et al.* (1991). Diagnosed intellectual and emotional impairment among parents who seriously mistreat their children: prevalence, type and outcome in a court sample. *Child Abuse and Neglect*, **15**, 389–401.

Teicher, M. H., Glod, C. A., Surrey, J. *et al.* (1993). Early childhood abuse and limbic system ratings in adult psychiatric outpatients. *Journal of Neuropsychiatry and Clinical Neuroscience*, **5** (3), 301–6.

Teicher, M. H., Andersen, S. L., Polcari, A. *et al.* (2003). The neurobiological consequences of early stress and childhood maltreatment. *Neuroscience and Behavioral Reviews*, **27**, 33–44.

Walker, E. and DiForio, D. (1997). Schizophrenia: a neural diathesis–stress model. *Psychological Review*, **104**, 667–85.

Wicks, S., Hjern, A., Gunnell, D. *et al.* (2005). Social adversity in childhood and the risk of developing psychosis: a national cohort study. *American Journal of Psychiatry*, **162**, 1652–7.

White, R., Bebbington, P., Pearon, J. *et al.* (2000). The social context of insight in schizophrenia. *Social Psychiatry and Psychiatric Epidemiology*, **35** (11), 500–7.

Whitfield, C., Dube, S., Felitti, V. *et al.* (2005). Adverse childhood experiences and hallucinations. *Child Abuse and Neglect*, **29**, 797–810.

Wurr, J. C. and Partridge, I. M. (1996). The prevalence of a history of childhood sexual abuse in an acute adult inpatient population. *Child Abuse and Neglect*, **20**, 867–72.

Young, M., Read, J., Barker-Collo, S. *et al.* (2001). Evaluating and overcoming barriers to taking abuse histories. *Professional Psychology: Research and Practice*, **32**, 407–14.

Zlotnick, C., Tam, T. and Robertson, M. J. (2004). Adverse childhood events, substance abuse, and measures of affiliation. *Addictive Behaviors*, **29**, 1177–81.

Zubin, J. and Spring, B. (1977). Vulnerability – a new view of schizophrenia. *Journal of Abnormal Psychology*, **86** (2), 103–26.

8

Family environment and psychosis

Pekka Tienari and Karl-Erik Wahlberg

Introduction

As with all forms of illness and disability, the primary burden of care for those with an enduring mental illness frequently falls on the family. Undoubtedly, without the ongoing support provided by close family, the impact of schizophrenia and other psychoses on the lives of many sufferers would be greatly increased. Families can provide emotional and practical support, continuity of care, and much needed help in negotiating interactions with professional mental health services. It is no surprise, then, that suggestions that families cause schizophrenia, as some asserted in the 1960s and 1970s (see Hirsch and Leff, 1975), were met with disbelief and anger. Singer and Wynne (1965) stated in their paper concerning the family relationships of patients with schizophrenia that biological and hereditary factors do contribute to disturbed transactions in some families. The majority of pioneers of family dynamic research did not, in fact, assert that parents were responsible for the psychosis in their children. Instead, they thought that many parents themselves were in need of help. However, many relatives felt that they were being blamed; they felt hurt, alienated and negatively labelled (Hatfield et al., 1987).

It is important, therefore, that any discussion of families, the family environment and psychosis begin with three important disclaimers. First, as noted above, families frequently provide invaluable support and shoulder a large burden of care. Second, families (and specifically mothers) do not cause schizophrenia or any other psychosis. Third, the overwhelming majority of families provide positive, nurturing environments. However, this should not, and does not, lead to the conclusion that family environment is irrelevant in understanding the onset and course of psychosis. Hirsch and Leff (1975), in their early review, concluded that there was a need for further research to test the more modest propositions that difficult and problematic family environments may increase the risk of schizophrenia and other psychoses, and worsen the course of these disorders.

Society and Psychosis, ed. Craig Morgan, Kwame McKenzie and Paul Fearon. Published by Cambridge University Press. © Cambridge University Press 2008.

In this chapter, we aim to provide an overview of research relating to family environment and schizophrenia and other psychoses. The most frequently studied intrafamilial factors are family communication and 'expressed emotion' (EE), and we will focus specifically on these in assessing the evidence for the role of family environment in the aetiology and course of psychosis. Within the scope of this chapter, it is not possible to discuss fully the methodological issues in the study of family environment and psychosis. A thorough book is available on this topic (Jacob, 1987).

History: early studies

Apart from the question of the aetiology of schizophrenia, early studies of the families of patients with schizophrenia made two major contributions to our understanding of family dynamics: first, their focus on the family group was an important advance over traditional, individual-focused approaches; second, through the development of specific concepts, such as 'double bind', 'fragmentation' and 'pseudo-mutuality', they alerted us to certain potentially important phenomena in family life (Mishler and Waxler, 1965).

Goldstein and Strachan (1987) reviewed in detail the different aspects of earlier family research in relation to schizophrenia. They concluded that the large number of cross-sectional family studies has shown one consistent finding: the parents of patients with schizophrenia tend to show a deficit in their ability to share a focus of attention, to adopt the perspective of another person, and to communicate meaning clearly and accurately. But only in the area of communication accuracy have cross-sectional comparison studies revealed consistent differences between families of patients with schizophrenia and other families. They further concluded that disturbed communication and negative affect in families precede the development of schizophrenia spectrum disorders. It is, however, doubtful whether these findings are specific to schizophrenia. Further, their review suggested that family factors affect the course of schizophrenia, and that there is considerable continuity between the negative affective factors that precede the onset of the disorder and those that are predictive of course and outcome. To disentangle these issues further, they emphasised the value of high-risk longitudinal designs.

After the initial enthusiasm in the 1950s and 1960s, research on family dynamics declined, partly for the reasons outlined above. However, investigations on intrafamilial communication, EE and the efficacy of family interventions have been actively continued. In addition, interest in the interplay of genetic and environmental factors has been maintained. It is to this more recent research that we now turn.

Familial communication in schizophrenia

Early research, as noted above, hinted at there being unclear and ambiguous communication patterns in the families of patients with schizophrenia. Research findings appear to confirm a greater prevalence of communication disturbance in the parents of schizophrenic patients than in other parents (e.g., Docherty *et al.*, 1998; Goldstein, 1987a). There is further evidence that siblings of those with schizophrenia have more communication problems than other children (Docherty *et al.*, 2004). These findings have been interpreted as suggesting that communication disturbances are indicators of genetic vulnerability in parents (e.g., Subotnik *et al.*, 2002). However, this seems to be too simplified an explanation of the origin of disturbed communication patterns.

The 'communication deviance' (CD) construct and scale were developed by Wynne and Singer (Singer *et al.*, 1978) to describe the disturbed communication styles found in the families of patients diagnosed with schizophrenia. Communication deviance is a scale that measures the degree to which a person does not share and maintain a focus of attention when communicating with other persons (Singer and Wynne, 1966), and to which meanings are not consensually or visibly validated. The scale consists of 42 categories adapted from the Singer–Wynne Rorschach scoring manual (Singer and Wynne, 1966, unpublished 1986 version, by M. T. Singer and L. C. Wynne). The most frequent and influential items of the CD scale are 'abandoned, abruptly ceased, uncorrected remarks', 'inability or failure to verify own responses', 'odd sentence construction' and 'reiteration'. Communication deviance has most often been measured from standardised, verbatim Rorschach test records, and the essential issue is not the intrapsychic phenomena as traditionally interpreted, but more the pattern of reciprocal shared perceptions, focusing on attention and meaning in the communication process. In one study using this construct, in a subsample of the Finnish Adoptive Family Study of Schizophrenia, Wahlberg *et al.* (1997) found that adoptees at a high genetic risk, and with high-CD adoptive parents, had more sub-syndromal thought disorder than low-risk adoptees with high-CD adoptive parents. The high-risk adoptees with low-CD adoptive parents had slightly lower levels of sub-syndromal thought disorder than the low-risk adoptees of low-CD adoptive parents, findings which are suggestive of a gene–environment interaction and sensitivity of the genetic high-risk adoptees to the family environment (see below). Further, Wahlberg *et al.* (2004) provide more evidence of gene–environment interaction in schizophrenia. They found that high-risk adoptees with high-CD adoptive parents had more mental disorders than low-risk adoptees with high-CD adoptive parents. Again, high-risk adoptees with low-CD adoptive parents had the same incidence of mental disorders as low-risk adoptees with low-CD adoptive parents. These findings support the biopsychosocial concept of an interaction between genetic vulnerability or sensitivity and risk factors in the family rearing environment. The form of communication style considered here is likely to hinder a child's cognitive development (especially in logical thinking and problem solving). These findings further suggest that more common communication styles support the cognitive development of high-risk children, perhaps protecting the vulnerable from schizophrenia. These results suggest that schizophrenia has both a genetic and an environmental base, and that neither alone can fully account for the illness.

Origins of communication deviance

It has been proposed that some children, exhibiting strange and incomprehensible behaviour indicative of an increased genetic risk for schizophrenia, evoke in their parents more negative and inconsistent ways of communicating (Bell, 1968). This may well be true in some cases, but it is questionable whether a child's behaviour can evoke such changes in parents in the long term. For example, levels of CD have been found to be stable during adulthood over an 11 year time span (Wahlberg et al., 2001). Communication deviance also remains stable when a person is tested either alone or with his or her spouse and child (Keskitalo, 2000). Wahlberg et al. (1997) have further found that levels of CD in parents of adoptees at high genetic risk are similar to those of parents of adoptees at low genetic risk. This suggests that behavioural manifestations of genetic vulnerability for schizophrenia in adopted children do not provoke communication disturbances in parents. In the Wahlberg et al. (2004) study, all adoptees were mentally healthy at the time the CD of the adoptive parents was measured. The presence of mental disorder in the adoptees was measured 11 years later. Putting these findings together, we can assume that CD is a stable trait and not simply a reflective product of a disturbed child. The stability of CD indicates that high parental CD scores contribute to an enduring atmosphere in the family, which may shape cognitive function, especially the thought processes of a developing child.

Expressed emotion

Expressed emotion is a measure of family environment that is based on how the parents or other carers talk about their ill relative. Based on the Camberwell Family Interview (CFI) (Vaughn and Leff, 1976), a long and detailed tape-recorded semi-structured interview, parents or other carers are classified as being high in EE if they make more than a specified number of critical comments or show any signs of hostility or marked emotional over-involvement. Positive aspects of the relationship may also be measured in the form of positive comments – a frequency count – and warmth, a scaled score taking into account attitudes and comments evidenced throughout the interview. However, it is the dimensions of criticism, hostility and emotional over-involvement that are used to determine high and low levels of EE (Barrowclough and Hooley, 2003). In some studies, scoring has been based on a five-minute speech sample (Magana, 1990; Marom *et al.*, 2005). Kavanagh *et al.* (1997) have developed a 30-item self-completed questionnaire for relatives, called the Family Attitude Scale. However, the CFI remains the gold standard.

Expressed emotion has been found to be a reliable psychosocial predictor of relapse in schizophrenia (e.g., Butzlaff and Hooley, 1998). Marom *et al.* (2005) demonstrated the prolonged (up to seven years) predictive validity of EE in respect to psychiatric hospitalisation. There is also a growing literature concerning the role of EE in unipolar depression, bipolar disorder and eating disorders. Indeed, rather than being a construct of interest solely with respect to schizophrenia, EE is a more general predictor of poor outcome across a range of conditions. Furthermore, EE is a construct that is modifiable (Butzlaff and Hooley, 1998). In the University of California at Los Angeles (UCLA) High Risk Project (Goldstein, 1987b), EE preceded and predicted the development of schizophrenia spectrum disorders (communication deviance and affective style were even stronger predictors). It seems that EE may have some role in the aetiology of psychosis, even though its ability to predict relapse has been more strongly confirmed.

Evidence is accumulating to show that high-EE and low-EE relatives may differ in the beliefs they hold about the patient and the problem behaviours associated with the patient's illness. In particular, several studies have shown that critical relatives are more likely to hold patients responsible for their difficulties (Barrowclough and Hooley, 2003). Compared with low-EE relatives, high-EE relatives appear more conventional in their behaviour (higher norm favouring) and less satisfied with themselves and their lives (lower self-realisation). High-EE relatives may also be less flexible and tolerant and rate lower on empathy and achievement through independence than low-EE relatives. In a study by Hooley and Hiller (2000), even after potential demographic confounders were controlled, inflexibility remained a significant predictor of high-EE. Heikkilä *et al.* (2006), in a study of consecutive first-episode patients from a defined geographic area, found evidence that good cognitive functioning in patients may be associated with higher EE scores in relatives, a finding that may reflect the higher expectations (and consequent disappointments) of relatives of intellectually more able children. In another study, Patterson *et al.* (2005) found that a high-EE relationship involving high emotional over-involvement and critical comments may have adaptive functions, for example, in enabling the relative to respond to the crisis of a family member developing a psychosis.

Kuipers *et al.* (2006) found that patients whose carers showed high EE had significantly higher levels of anxiety and depression, but not more psychotic symptoms or lower self-esteem. Thus, their research hypothesis suggesting that the effect of high EE is mediated through affective changes in patients was partially supported. Even at the time of the first episode, the carers' psychological appraisal, rather than the patient's illness, appears to be influential in determining high EE (Raune *et al.*, 2004).

Family interventions

Studies of the efficacy of family interventions for those with psychosis provide further relevant evidence. The Schizophrenia Patient Outcome Research Team, funded by the US National Institute of Mental Health (NIMH) (Lehman *et al.*, 1998), suggested that individual and group psychotherapies adhering to a psychodynamic model and family therapies based on the premise that family dysfunction is of primary importance in the aetiology of the schizophrenia should be avoided. Psychotherapists and family therapists did not accept this view. Many felt that the recommendations were not based on a full exploration of the field of psychological therapies (Silver and Larsen, 2003). They have since been modified. The Schizophrenia Patient Outcome Research Team, in their updated treatment recommendations, stated that: 'Persons with schizophrenia and their families who have ongoing contact with each other should be offered a family intervention, the key elements of which include a duration of at least nine months, illness education, crisis intervention, emotional support, and training in how to cope with illness symptoms and related problems.' (Lehman *et al.*, 2004, p. 202.)

Pitschel-Walz *et al.* (2001) and Pilling *et al.* (2002) have both published meta-analyses of family intervention studies. Both included randomised controlled trials only. Pilling and colleagues, basing their review on 'intention to treat' analyses, found that family intervention reduced relapse rates and re-hospitalisations, and improved compliance with medication.

Alanen (2004) has described the implementation of family interventions for patients with schizophrenia in Finland. Correspondingly, family interventions in bipolar disorders have been described in detail by Miklowitz and Goldstein (1997) and Callahan and Bauer (1999). The cause-and-effect relationships between mood disorder symptoms and family environmental factors are bidirectional; families are affected by the bipolar disorder as much as they affect it. There is no convincing evidence that disturbed family relationships cause the onset of bipolar disorder. In the absence of longitudinal high risk research, it is not possible to establish, with any certainty, causal connections between features of the childhood family environment and the eventual onset of bipolar disorder (or schizophrenia or other psychoses) in adulthood. Stierlin *et al.* (1986) reported their observations from a study of families, each with a young adult member who had been diagnosed as manic-depressive (and, in a separate sample, with schizoaffective disorder). All families could be described as extremely rigid and bound-up systems. Many of them were characterised by a 'restrictive parental complementarity' and by reciprocal delegation. Families with a relative with manic-depression showed both similarities and differences when compared with those with a relative with schizophrenia or a serious psychosomatic disorder. The authors also describe the therapeutic problems and the typical phases of the family therapeutic process (Weber et al., 1988), and report on a follow-up study in which they found a reduced relapse rate compared with the earlier histories of these patients with bipolar or schizoaffective psychoses (Retzer et al., 1991). Lindelöw (1999) showed that indicators of a lack of positive parent–child interactions, based on maternal reports for children at 10 years old, were significantly associated with (non-psychotic) depression in the children some 20 years later.

Interplay of genes and the family environment

Rutter (2005a) has recently reviewed research on environmental risks for mental health and psychopathology. He underlined the need to differentiate between risk indicators and risk mediators, and the need to better understand the kinds of environmental influences that have major risk effects. Another challenge is to identify the origins of environmental risk factors and to find out whether they lie in gene–environment correlations (see Chapter 5), societal elements or personal experiences. It is also a challenge to determine the changes in the organism that provide the basis for the persistence of environmental effects on psychological functioning or psychopathology. Rutter (2005b), in summarising the main findings, emphasised the point that environmentally mediated risk effects are both real and important. Some effects operate predominantly on individual differences in liability, but some mainly affect the level of a trait or the rate of a disorder. The effects operate within a wide range of environments (and not just at the very extremes). They derive from influences in the family, school, peer group and community, as well as in the prenatal environment. The effects are often dependent on genetic susceptibility, i.e., they operate through gene–environment interactions.

In an editorial, Arrindell and Perris (1999) underlined the importance of parental rearing behaviour because of its relevance for attachment and its later influence on personality development and mental health. In the Northern Finland 1966 Birth Cohort, unwanted pregnancy was found to be associated with an increased risk of schizophrenia. This factor may operate directly or may be a marker for other risk factors. Furthermore, first-born sons had an increased risk of schizophrenia in this cohort. However, some factors that have been found to be associated with schizophrenia in other studies were not replicated in this cohort:

living in a single-parent family, size of the family of origin and antenatal depression in the mother (Isohanni *et al.*, 2005). These results cannot be easily dismissed because they come from the study of a birth cohort, and thus are not as prone to the problems of bias and reverse causality common to case-control and other retrospective studies.

To an important degree, genetic effects on behaviour arise either because they influence the extent to which the individual is likely to be exposed to environmental risk or because they affect the individual's susceptibility to environmental adversities (Rutter, 2002; van Os and Sham, 2003). Gene–environment interaction can be defined as genetic control of sensitivity to environmental factors, or environmental control of gene expression (Kendler and Eaves, 1986). Thus, individuals with some genotypes are more likely than others to develop a disorder in the event of exposure to certain environmental factors. Given the existence of gene–environment interactions, it is possible that disorders cluster in families not just because of direct genetic effects, but also because relatives are more vulnerable to the risk-increasing effect of a prevalent environmental risk factor (van Os and Marcelis, 1998). A moderator (genotype) specifies on whom or under what conditions a mediator, such as rearing environment, will produce a certain outcome (Kraemer *et al.*, 2001).

Adoption studies of schizophrenia

In adoption studies, genetic and rearing factors can be differentiated because, simply, the biological parents are not the rearing parents. Earlier adoption studies have convincingly confirmed the importance of a genetic contribution to schizophrenia (Kendler *et al.*, 1994; Kety *et al.*, 1994; Rosenthal *et al.*, 1971, 1975). They have not, however, adequately examined the environmental contribution; they did not, for example, incorporate observations on rearing family environments. Rosenthal *et al.* (1975) conducted retrospective interviews with a group of adoptees about how they recalled their parent–child relationships. Wynne *et al.* (1976) pointed out that parental psychopathology has often been used as a rearing variable, although parental psychopathology is not necessarily relevant to the quality of their parenting.

One aim of the Finnish Adoption Study was to investigate whether genetic risk for schizophrenia moderates the effects of adoptive rearing families (Tienari *et al.*, 2003, 2004; Wahlberg *et al.*, 1997, 2004). A national sample of adopted-away offspring of biological mothers with schizophrenia spectrum disorders was blindly compared with control adoptees of biological mothers with no diagnosis or non-schizophrenia spectrum diagnosis. The biological parents were diagnosed using personal structured interviews or hospital records. Adoptive families were assessed at initial phase with joint and individual interviews and psychological tests. High-risk adoptees ($n = 190$) had a biological mother with a schizophrenia spectrum disorder. Low-risk adoptees ($n = 192$) had a biological mother with a non-spectrum or no disorder. Adoptees were personally interviewed a median of 12 years after the initial interview by a new psychiatrist blind to initial evaluations. All subjects ($n = 1741$) were followed up 21 years later using national registers.

The age-corrected morbid risk for (narrowly defined) definite DSM-III-R schizophrenia in low-genetic-risk adoptees reared in 'healthy' families was 0% (no genetic risk and no environmental risk), while that in high-genetic-risk adoptees (indexed by having a biological mother with a schizophrenia spectrum disorder) reared in 'healthy' families was 1.49% (genetic risk in the absence of environmental risk). The morbid risk for schizophrenia was 4.84% in low-genetic-risk adoptees reared in 'dysfunctional' families (environmental risk in the absence of genetic risk), but 13.04% in high-genetic-risk adoptees reared in 'dysfunctional' families (families with both a genetic risk and an 'environmental risk' present) (Tienari et al., 2002). The family's overall health was rated by the interviewing psychiatrist using the Global Health Pathology Scale ranging from healthy (01) to pathological (99) (see Tienari et al., 2005).

Disordered rearing in adoptive families predicted schizophrenia spectrum disorders in adoptees in a 21-year follow-up. However, it was only for adoptees at genetic high risk that a significant association between the measure of adoptive family functioning and the adoptee's spectrum diagnosis was found. A similar result was obtained when the subgroup of adoptees with schizophrenia spectrum diagnoses at initial assessment was excluded. These findings indicate that adoptees at high genetic risk are more sensitive than adoptees at low genetic risk to both adverse and protective environmental effects in their rearing environments. This supports the hypothesis of interaction between the genotype and the environment (Tienari et al., 2004).

In the same study, family ratings were made, based on joint family interviews in their homes using the Oulu Family Rating Scale. In the Oulu Family Rating Scale, 33 scales from a variety of sources were selected for ratings of specific aspects of adoptive family functioning (Tienari et al., 2004, 2005), each defined operationally at five levels from 'healthy' to 'severely dysfunctional'. Some of the scales, borrowed from family researchers, had generalised applicability for the study of family relationships, for example, 'non-acknowledgement' and 'manifest anxiety'. Other scales were constructed to tap concepts that have been hypothesised as especially relevant to families with schizophrenic members, for example, 'narrow range of affect' and 'disrupted communication'. Extensive pilot testing and statistical evaluations of the ratings were carried out to examine inter-rater reliability and raters' consensual understanding of the items. The family interviewers rated families both from personal observation and from tape recordings of one another's interviews. Finally, nine scales were deleted as psychometrically unsatisfactory and the remaining 24 were factor analysed into three groups, labelled as 'critical or conflictual', 'constricted' and 'boundary problems'. These ratings were then used to assess the putative family rearing environments separately and jointly with the diagnoses of the proband birth mothers.

The results showed that adoptees at high genetic risk were more sensitive to problems in the rearing adoptive family, in terms of *both* the three domains (factor groups) indicative of problematic adoptive rearing, i.e., 'critical or conflictual', 'constricted' and 'boundary problems', *and* the total score of the three domains (Tienari *et al.*, 2004). An alternative way to view the findings is that there appears to be a protective effect of having been reared in a 'healthy' adoptive family with a low Oulu Family Rating Scale rating. High-genetic-risk adoptees reared in families with low Oulu Family Rating Scale scores had significantly fewer schizophrenia spectrum outcomes than high-genetic-risk adoptees with high Oulu Family Rating Scale scores. The joint effect of high genetic risk and a 'dysfunctional' rearing family environment is essentially equal for each of the three groups that were differentiated in the factor analysis. This finding suggests that there is no specific, sharply delimited form of family environmental problem, and that the psychosocial environment has multiple components, perhaps similar to multifactorial genetics.

Conceptually, the findings support the hypothesis of significant genotype by environment interaction, as defined by Kendler and Eaves (1986), implying genetic control of sensitivity to the environment or environmental control of genetic expression. In other words, a moderator (genotype) specifies on whom or under what conditions a rearing environment is associated with outcome (schizophrenia spectrum disorder in adoptees). Carter *et al.* (2002) demonstrated that gene–environment interaction was the most powerful predictor of schizophrenia in their multivariate analyses. The results are also in accordance with the hypothesis of Gottesman and Bertelsen (1989), which proposes that discordance in monozygotic twins may primarily be explained by the capacity of the schizophrenic genotype or diathesis to be unexpressed, unless released by some kind of environmental, including non-familial, stressors.

The results support the popular diathesis–stress model of the aetiology of psychopathology. In this model, environmental stressors are hypothesised to have a particularly deleterious effect only on the individuals with a genetic diathesis, or a predisposition to a particular psychopathology (Rosenthal, 1963). Theoretically, one can hypothesise the possibility of an evocative gene–environment correlation if the child's genetically influenced characteristics play a role in shaping his or her environment. Reciprocal bi-directional effects between rearing parents and their children almost certainly take place. One would then expect adoptive families with genetically high-risk adoptees to differ from those with genetically low-risk adoptees. However, high versus low genetic risk adoptees did not generate any such difference between 'healthy' and 'dysfunctional' families, at least when assessed using the Oulu Family Rating Scale ratings of the adoptive families. This is consistent with the finding that there was no difference in 'communication deviance' (CD) between the adoptive parents of the high genetic-risk and low genetic-risk groups (Wahlberg *et al.*, 1997, 2004). These results indicate that the adoptees at genetic risk did not have a special measurable impact in producing increased CD in their rearing parents or generating other observable problems in their adoptive families. It should also be emphasised that, when the adoptees with serious mental disorders at initial assessment (when the family assessments were made) were excluded, family variables (Oulu Family Rating Scale, CD) still had a statistically significant association with the diagnoses of the adoptees at follow-up. These findings are important when considering the direction of observed effects.

Goldstein (1987a) found that CD in the parents of troubled adolescents predicted schizophrenia spectrum diagnoses in children 15 years later. In the Finnish adoption study, Wahlberg *et al.* (2004) found that, in a group of adoptees without a psychiatric diagnosis at initial assessment, CD in adoptive parents predicted adoptee diagnoses at a 19-year follow-up. When genetic high risk is combined with rearing by high-CD parents, the risk for a psychiatric diagnosis is significantly increased compared with genetic low risk combined with low-CD rearing (as well as in high-genetic risk adoptees in adoptive families with low-CD parents). Johnson *et al.* (2001) showed that, in a large population cohort interviewed repeatedly, disordered parenting was a more important predictor of the child's psychiatric diagnosis than parental psychiatric diagnosis.

Conclusions and future directions

There is clear and accumulating evidence that the early family environment is of aetiological importance in schizophrenia and, perhaps, other psychoses. This is not a return to the simplistic and unthinking family blaming of the past. It acknowledges that the emotional environment of childhood can have lasting effects on development (as can more severe childhood experiences; see Chapter 7). In the presence of a pre-existing vulnerability, be it genetic or other, this may increase the risk of later schizophrenia. The potential implications for prevention and intervention are clear.

There is still a need, however, to confirm and extend the findings reviewed here through further research. In future, it would be useful to simplify methods of communication measurements. If they could be used in child guidance clinics, for example, measurements could be made before disorders become manifest. The identification of at-risk children would provide possibilities for more attention to be paid to potential preventive measures. In terms of educating health personnel, increasing knowledge about family functioning and the provision of supervision for working with whole families would help with the earlier identification of problems. Screening problem families from a birth cohort, and careful evaluation of their functioning, would help develop methods that are useful in identifying factors related to dysfunction. Of course, longitudinal studies would be ideal – but these remain logistically challenging and expensive.

REFERENCES

Alanen, Y. O. (2004). The need-adapted approach – developing an integrated and individualized psychotherapeutically oriented treatment of schizophrenic patients. *Archives of Psychiatry and Psychotherapy*, **6**, 5–21.

Arrindell, W. A. and Perris, C. (1999). Parental influences do matter! *Acta Psychiatrica Scandinavica*, **100**, 249–51.

Barrowclough, C. and Hooley, J. M. (2003). Attributions and expressed emotion: a review. *Clinical Psychology Review*, **23**, 849–80.

Bell, R. Q. (1968). A reinterpretation of the direction of effects in studies of socialization. *Psychological Review*, **75**, 81–95.

Butzlaff, R. L. and Hooley, J. M. (1998). Expressed emotion and psychiatric relapse: a meta-analysis. *Archives of General Psychiatry*, **55**, 547–52.

Callahan, A. M. and Bauer, M. S. (1999). Psychosocial interventions for bipolar disorders. In *Bipolarity: Beyond Classic Mania*, ed. H. S. Akiskal. Philadelphia: W. B. Saunders Company, pp. 675–88.

Carter, J. W., Schulsinger, F., Parnas, J. *et al.* (2002). A multivariate prediction model of schizophrenia. *Schizophrenia Bulletin*, **28**, 649–82.

Docherty, N. M., Rhinewine, J. P., Labhart, R. P. *et al.* (1998). Communication disturbances and family psychiatric history in parents of schizophrenic patients. *Journal of Nervous and Mental Disease*, **186**, 761–8.

Docherty, N. M., Gordinie, S. W., Hall, M. J. *et al.* (2004). Referential communication disturbances in the speech of non-schizophrenic siblings of schizophrenia patients. *Journal of Abnormal Psychology*, **113**, 399–405.

Goldstein, M. J. (1987a). Family interaction patterns that antedate the onset of schizophrenia and related disorders: a further analysis of data from a longitudinal, prospective study. In *Understanding Major Mental Disorder: The Contribution of Family Interaction Research*, ed. K. Hahlweg and M. J. Goldstein. New York: Family Process Press, pp. 11–32.

Goldstein, M. J. (1987b). The UCLA High-Risk Project. *Schizophrenia Bulletin*, **13**, 505–14.

Goldstein, M. J. and Strachan, A. M. (1987). The family and schizophrenia. In *Family Interaction and Psychopathology: Theories, Methods and Findings*, ed. T. Jacob. New York: Plenum Press, pp. 481–508.

Gottesman, I. I. and Bertelsen, A. (1989). Confirming unexpressed genotypes for schizophrenia. Risks in the offspring of Fischer's Danish identical and fraternal discordant twins. *Archives of General Psychiatry*, **46**, 867–72.

Hatfield, A. B., Spaniol, L. and Zipple, A. M. (1987). Expressed emotion: a family perspective. *Schizophrenia Bulletin*, **13**, 221–6.

Heikkilä, J., Ilonen, T., Karlsson, H. *et al.* (2006). Cognitive functioning and expressed emotion among patients with first-episode severe psychiatric disorders. *Comprehensive Psychiatry*, **47**, 152–8.

Hirsch, S. R. and Leff, J. P. (1975). *Abnormalities in Parents of Schizophrenics*. London: Oxford University Press.

Hooley, J. M. and Hiller, J. B. (2000). Personality and expressed emotion. *Journal of Abnormal Psychology*, **109**, 40–4.

Isohanni, M., Lauronen, E., Moilanen, K. *et al.* (2005). Predictors of schizophrenia. Evidence from the Northern Finland 1966 birth cohort and other sources. *The British Journal of Psychiatry*, **187**, 4–7.

Jacob, T. (ed.) (1987). *Family Interaction and Psychopathology: Theories, Methods and Findings*. New York: Plenum Press.

Johnson, J. G., Cohen, P., Kasen, S. *et al.* (2001). Association of maladaptive parental behavior with psychiatric disorder among parents and their offspring. *Archives of General Psychiatry*, **58**, 453–60.

Kavanagh, D. J., O'Halloran, P., Manicavasagar, V. *et al.* (1997). The Family Attitude Scale: reliability and validity of a new scale for measuring the emotional climate of families. *Psychiatry Research*, **70**, 185–95.

Kendler, K. S. and Eaves, L. J. (1986). Models for the joint effect of genotype and environment on liability to psychiatric illness. *American Journal of Psychiatry*, **143**, 279–89.

Kendler, K. S., Gruenberg, A. and Kinney, D. (1994). Independent diagnoses of adoptees and relatives as defined by DSM-III in the provincial and national samples of the Danish Adoption Study of Schizophrenia. *Archives of General Psychiatry*, **51**, 456–68.

Keskitalo, P. (2000). Stability of parental communication deviance and the correlation with the development of thinking in adopted children predisposed to schizophrenia and controls. *Acta Universitatis Ouluensis, Medica D*, **599**.

Kety, S. S., Wender, P. H., Jacobsen, B. *et al.* (1994). Mental illness in the biological and adoptive relatives of schizophrenic adoptees. Replication of the Copenhagen study in the rest of Denmark. *Archives of General Psychiatry*, **51**, 442–55.

Kraemer, H. C., Stice, E., Kazdin, A. *et al.* (2001). How do risk factors work together? Mediators, moderators and independent, overlapping, and proxy risk factors. *American Journal of Psychiatry*, **158**, 848–56.

Kuipers, L., Bebbington, P., Dunn, G. *et al.* (2006). Influence of carer expressed emotion and affect on relapse in non-affective psychosis. *British Journal of Psychiatry*, **188**, 173–9.

Lehman, A. F., Steinwachs, D. M. and the co-investigators of the PORT-Projects (1998). At issue – translating research into practice: the Schizophrenia Patients' Outcomes Research Team (PORT) treatment recommendation. *Schizophrenia Bulletin*, **24**, 1–10.

Lehman, A. F., Kreyenbuhl, J., Buchanan, R. W. *et al.* (2004). The Schizophrenia Patient Outcomes Research Team (PORT): updated treatment recommendations 2003. *Schizophrenia Bulletin*, **30**, 193–217.

Lindelöw, M. (1999). Parent–child interaction and adult depression: a prospective study. *Acta Psychiatrica Scandinavica*, **100**, 270–8.

Magana, A. (1990). *Manual for Coding Expressed Emotions from the Five Minute Speech Sample*. Los Angeles, CA: UCLA Family Project.

Marom, S., Muniz, H., Jones, B. P. *et al.* (2005). Expressed emotion: relevance to re-hospitalization in schizophrenia over 7 years. *Schizophrenia Bulletin*, **31**, 751–8.

Miklowitz, D. J. and Goldstein, M. J. (1997). *Bipolar Disorder: A Family-Focused Treatment Approach*. New York: The Guilford Press.

Mishler, E. G. and Waxler, N. E. (1965). Family interaction processes and schizophrenia: a review of current theories. *The Merrill-Palmer Quarterly of Behavior and Development*, **11**, 375–415.

Patterson, P., Birchwood, M. and Cocrane, R. (2005). Expressed emotion as an adaptation to loss. Prospective study in first-episode psychosis. *British Journal of Psychiatry*, **187**, 59–64.

Pilling, S., Bebbington, P., Kuipers, E. *et al.* (2002). Psychological treatments in schizophrenia: I. Meta-analysis of family intervention and cognitive behavior therapy. *Psychological Medicine*, **32**, 763–82.

Pitschel-Walz, G., Leucht, S., Bäuml, J. *et al.* (2001). The effect of family intervention on relapse and re-hospitalization in schizophrenia – a meta-analysis. *Schizophrenia Bulletin*, **27**, 73–92.

Raune, D., Kuipers, E. and Bebbington, P. E. (2004). Expressed emotion at first-episode psychosis: investigating a carer appraisal model. *British Journal of Psychiatry*, **184**, 321–6.

Retzer, A., Simon, F., Weber, G. *et al.* (1991). A follow-up study of manic-depressive and schizoaffective psychoses after systemic family therapy. *Family Process*, **30**, 139–53.

Rosenthal, D. (1963). *The Genain Quadruplets: A Case Study and Theoretical Analysis of Heredity and Environment in Schizophrenia*. New York: Basic Books.

Rosenthal, D., Wender, P. H., Kety, S. S. *et al.* (1971). The adopted-away offspring of schizophrenics. *American Journal of Psychiatry*, **128**, 307–11.

Rosenthal, D., Wender, P. H., Kety, S. S. *et al.* (1975). Parent–child relationships and psychopathological disorder in the child. *Archives of General Psychiatry*, **32**, 466–76.

Rutter, M. (2002). The interplay of nature, nurture, and developmental influences. The challenge ahead for mental health. *Archives of General Psychiatry*, **59**, 996–1000.

Rutter, M. (2005a). How environment affects mental health. *British Journal of Psychiatry*, **186**, 4–6.

Rutter, M. (2005b). Environmentally mediated risks for psychopathology: research strategies and findings. *Journal of the American Academy of Child Adolescent Psychiatry*, **44**, 3–18.

Silver, A. L. and Larsen, T. K. (eds) (2003). The schizophrenic person and the benefits of the psychotherapies – seeking PORT in the storm. *The Journal of American Academy of Psychoanalysis and Academic Psychiatry*, **31** (1) (special issue), 1–268.

Singer, M. and Wynne, L. C. (1965). Thought disorder and family relations of schizophrenics. *Archives of General Psychiatry*, **12**, 210–12.

Singer, M. and Wynne, L. C. (1966). Principles for scoring communication defects and deviances in parents of schizophrenics: Rorschach and TAT scoring manuals. *Psychiatry*, **29**, 260–88.

Singer, M., Wynne, L. C. and Toohey, M. L. (1978). Communication disorders and the families of schizophrenics. In *The Nature of Schizophrenia: New Approaches to Research and Treatment*, ed. L. C. Wynne, R. L. Cromwell and S. Matthysse. New York: John Wiley and Sons, pp. 499–511.

Stierlin, H., Weber, G., Schmidt, G. *et al.* (1986). Some features of families with major affective disorders. *Family Process*, **25**, 325–36.

Subotnik, K. L., Goldstein, M. J., Nuechterlein, K. H. *et al.* (2002). Are communication deviance and expressed emotion related to family history of psychiatric disorders in schizophrenia? *Schizophrenia Bulletin*, **28**, 719–29.

Tienari, P., Wynne, L. C., Sorri, A. *et al.* (2002). Genotype-environment interaction in the Finnish adoptive family study – interplay between genes and environment? In *Risk and Protective Factors in Schizophrenia: Towards a Conceptual Model of the Disease Process*, ed. H. Häfner. Darmstadt: Springer-Verlag, pp. 29–38.

Tienari, P., Wynne, L. C., Läksy, K. *et al.* (2003). Genetic boundaries of the schizophrenia spectrum: evidence from the Finnish adoptive family study. *American Journal of Psychiatry*, **160**, 1587–94.

Tienari, P., Wynne, L., Sorri, A. *et al.* (2004). Genotype–environment interaction in schizophrenia spectrum disorder: long-term follow-up study of Finnish adoptees. *British Journal of Psychiatry*, **184**, 216–22.

Tienari, P., Wynne, L., Lahti, I. *et al.* (2005). Observing relationships in Finnish adoptive families: Oulu Family Rating Scale. *Nordic Journal of Psychiatry*, **59**, 253–63.

van Os, J. and Marcelis, M. (1998). The ecogenetics of schizophrenia. *Schizophrenia Research*, **32**, 127–35.

van Os, J. and Sham, P. C. (2003). Gene–environment correlation and interaction in schizophrenia. In *The Epidemiology of Schizophrenia*, ed. R. M. Murray, P. Jones, E. Susser, J. van Os and M. Cannon. Cambridge: Cambridge University Press, pp. 235–53.

Vaughn, C. E. and Leff, J. P. (1976). The measurement of expressed emotion in the families of psychiatric patients. *British Journal of Social and Clinical Psychology*, **129**, 125–37.

Wahlberg, K. E., Wynne, L. C., Oja, H. *et al.* (1997). Gene–environment interaction in vulnerability to schizophrenia: findings from the Finnish Adoptive Family Study of Schizophrenia. *American Journal of Psychiatry*, **154**, 355–62.

Wahlberg, K. E., Wynne, L. C., Keskitalo, P. *et al.* (2001). Long-term stability of communication deviance. *Journal of Abnormal Psychology*, **110**, 443–8.

Wahlberg, K. E., Wynne, L. C., Hakko, H. *et al.* (2004). Interaction of genetic risk and adoptive parent communication deviance: longitudinal prediction of adoptee psychiatric disorders. *Psychological Medicine*, **34**, 1531–41.

Weber, G., Simon, F., Stierlin, H. *et al.* (1988). Therapy for families manifesting manic-depressive behavior. *Family Process*, **27**, 33–49.

Wynne, L. C., Singer, M. T. and Toohey, M. L. (1976). Communication of the adoptive parents of schizophrenics. In *Schizophrenia 75. Psychotherapy, Family Studies, Research, Proceedings of the Vth International Symposium on the Psychotherapy of Schizophrenia, Oslo, Norway, August 13–17, 1975*, ed. J. J. Jorstad and E. Ugelstad. Oslo: Universitetsforlaget, pp. 413–52.

9

Adult adversity: do early environment and genotype create lasting vulnerabilities for adult social adversity in psychosis?

Inez Myin-Germeys and Jim van Os

Introduction

It has long been acknowledged that adult stress is an important factor in the development of psychosis. The vulnerability–stress model (Nuechterlein and Dawson, 1984) has been widely accepted as a heuristically useful framework for the study of the aetiology and clinical course of schizophrenia. According to this model, psychiatric symptoms emerge when a threshold of stressors exceeds the individual's vulnerability level, the latter being a stable within-person characteristic (Zubin *et al.*, 1983). However, despite the apparent agreement that adult stress is a component cause contributing to psychosis, only a limited amount of research is available addressing the question of how stressors impact on vulnerable individuals. The mechanisms underlying the association between life stress and psychosis thus remain unclear.

In this chapter, we will first give an overview of evidence concerning adult adversity and risk of psychosis. In the second part, two possible ways of approaching the question of how the adult environment interacts with the individual to increase the risk of psychosis will be discussed. First, we will ask whether the impact of the adult environment on the risk of psychosis reflects the expression of a lasting vulnerability for adult stress caused by adversity early in life (we will refer to this as behavioural sensitisation). We hypothesise that exposure to *early* developmental exposures, such as childhood trauma and growing up in an urban environment, increase vulnerability for psychosis by sensitising people to *later* adverse events. Second, we will ask whether early or later environmental exposures can cause psychotic disorder by interacting with pre-existing genetic vulnerability (i.e., a gene–environment interaction).

Society and Psychosis, ed. Craig Morgan, Kwame McKenzie and Paul Fearon. Published by Cambridge University Press. © Cambridge University Press 2008.

Adult social risk factors for psychosis

Adult life events

It has long been reported that patients suffering from schizophrenia are sensitive to life events (e.g., Bebbington *et al.*, 1993), defined as situations or occurrences that entail a positive or negative change in personal circumstances (Brown and Harris, 1978). Life events have consistently been found to influence the course and outcome of psychotic disorders, with a number of studies showing associations with higher levels of symptomatology and increased relapse rates (Bebbington *et al.*, 1993; Bebbington *et al.*, 1996; Carr *et al.*, 2000; Norman and Malla, 1993). However, both Bebbington *et al.* (1993, 1996) and Hirsch *et al.* (1996) have suggested that life events do not directly trigger relapse in psychosis, but rather contribute to a cumulatively increasing risk for psychosis with successive exposures. Furthermore, it has been suggested that the experience of recent life events might be particularly relevant in earlier episodes, as recurrent episodes (>3) appear less related to the experience of life events (Castine *et al.*, 1998).

Whereas most studies have relied on retrospective data, Ventura *et al.* (2000) conducted a prospective study investigating a sample of recent-onset patients diagnosed with schizophrenia over a period of 12 months. They found an increased risk for both psychotic and depressive exacerbation following a life event. Horan *et al.* (2005) compared this group of patients with a non-patient control sample, and while patients reported a lower frequency of life events than controls, they expressed diminished self-efficacy in their appraisals of the life events, i.e., they rated them as less controllable and more poorly handled compared with controls.

Two recent studies, based on data from the British National Psychiatric Morbidity Survey, have extended previous findings to sub-clinical psychotic experiences in the general population, which research suggests are on a phenomenological and aetiological continuum with clinical psychotic disorders (Johns *et al.*, 2004; Wiles *et al.*, 2006). These found that the experience of adverse life events during the preceding six months was associated, cross-sectionally and longitudinally, with psychotic experiences (Johns *et al.*, 2004; Wiles *et al.*, 2006). Finally, in a study of people at high risk for schizophrenia from the Edinburgh High Risk study, it was found that a lifetime experience of stress, and particularly upsetting life events, was associated with higher levels of psychotic symptoms at the time of assessment (Miller *et al.*, 2001). However, another study in individuals with 'at-risk mental states' found recent life events not to be highly predictive of transition to a psychotic disorder (Mason *et al.*, 2004). This latter finding fits with the notion of a cumulative rather than a triggering effect of life events on psychosis.

Discrimination and social defeat

Accumulating evidence suggests that migration is a putative risk factor for schizophrenia (van Os *et al.*, 2005; also see Chapter 10). Cantor-Graae and Selten (2005), in a meta-analysis of 18 studies, found a mean relative risk for psychosis of 2.7 (95% CI 2.3–3.2) in first-generation migrants and of 4.5 (95% CI 1.5–13.1) in second-generation migrants. Migrants from developing countries had a higher risk compared with migrants from developed countries (relative risk: 3.3, 95% CI 2.8–3.9) and migrants from countries where the majority of the population was black had an increased risk for schizophrenia that was almost twice as great as that for migrants from other countries.

It has been shown that the association between migrant status and psychosis is not solely due to selection (Cantor-Graae and Selten, 2005). An alternative explanation is that repeated experiences of discrimination and social defeat may increase risk in migrant groups. This would fit with the finding that black migrants are particularly at risk, since it is these groups who most often face discrimination in Western societies (Cantor-Graae and Selten, 2005). A prospective study in a general population sample reported that exposure to discrimination, be this due to age, sex, appearance, sexual orientation or handicap, was associated with an increased risk of psychosis (Janssen *et al.*, 2003). Boydell *et al.* (2001) found that the incidence of schizophrenia in non-white ethnic minorities increased in a dose–response fashion as they formed a decreasing proportion of the local population.

Mechanisms (1) Sensitisation to stress

One mechanism through which environmental exposures might impact on the risk for psychosis is sensitisation. Sensitisation indicates that a *previous* exposure to adversity or stress makes individuals more sensitive or responsive rather than more resistant to the *later* occurrence of stress. It is attractive to hypothesise that previous exposure to social adversity might sensitise people to later stressors, thus putting them at increased risk of psychosis.

Empirical evidence

To understand the mechanism of sensitisation it is pivotal to understand how stress impacts on individuals who are at risk of developing psychosis. In a series of studies by our group (for review see: Myin-Germeys and van Os, 2007), the effect of small stressors and disturbances in the natural flow of daily life was investigated in participants with different degrees of underlying vulnerability for psychosis. Previously, it had been suggested that the course of psychosis is influenced not so much by rare major life events but rather by the much more prevalent smaller events that occur in the flow of daily life. Thus, minor daily events have been reported to have an impact on psychological symptoms in general (Kanner *et al.*, 1981; Monroe, 1983), subjective distress (Norman and Malla, 1991) and relapse rates in schizophrenia (Malla *et al.*, 1990).

We used the Experience Sampling Method (ESM) – a structured diary technique – to investigate the impact of small stressors in the flow of daily life. The participants in these studies were signalled 10 times daily during a six day period to prompt completion of a questionnaire collecting reports of thoughts, current context (activity, persons present, location), appraisals of the current situation and mood after each signal (Myin-Germeys *et al.*, 2001).

In one study, the ESM was applied to investigate how small daily life stressors affected emotions in a sample of participants with differing degrees of vulnerability for psychosis: patients diagnosed with psychosis in a current state of remission; first-degree relatives of patients diagnosed with a psychotic disorder; and healthy controls. Emotional reactivity to stress was defined as an increase in negative affect (NA) and a decrease in positive affect (PA) associated with subjective appraisals of stress in daily life. Negative affect consisted of the mood items 'I feel anxious right now', 'I feel lonely right now', 'I feel insecure right now', 'I feel irritated right now', 'I feel down right now' and 'I feel guilty right now'. Positive affect was similarly defined as feeling happy, satisfied, cheerful and relaxed. Stress was conceptualised as the subjectively appraised stressfulness of distinctive events and minor disturbances in the natural flow of daily life.

We found that underlying vulnerability to psychotic disorder modified emotional responses to stress in daily life (see Myin-Germeys *et al.*, 2001). The two vulnerable groups (patients and relatives) reported a similarly significant decrease in positive affect associated with stress, compared with controls. For negative affect associated with stress, the relatives showed a significantly greater increase than the controls; the patients reported an even larger increase in negative affect compared with the controls. Thus, higher levels of familial risk for psychosis were associated with higher levels of emotional reactivity to daily life stress in a dose–response fashion. These data suggest that subtle alterations in the way persons interact with the environment may constitute part of the vulnerability for psychosis. Part of this vulnerability to daily life stress may be genetic, part may be environmental (see below).

In a further study, we investigated whether stress also has a direct impact on moment-to-moment fluctuations in the intensity of psychotic experiences in daily life (Myin-Germeys *et al.*, 2005a). Given that delusions and hallucinations vary in intensity, and that this variability may occur over weeks, days or even consecutive moments, it is attractive to investigate the effect of daily stress on such fluctuations. In the ESM booklets, symptom-relevant information is collected through self-report items enquiring about hallucinations and experiences related to the concept of delusions, such as 'I feel suspicious right now', 'I am preoccupied by my thoughts' and 'I feel controlled'. To investigate this, we recruited a sample of currently remitted patients at risk of relapse and first-degree relatives (Myin-Germeys et al., 2005a), this latter group being, on average, at increased risk of developing psychotic experiences, including subtle psychosis-like or schizotypal experiences (e.g., Bergman et al., 2000). The data showed a clear association between the occurrence of minor stresses and the intensity of psychotic experiences. This effect was interpreted as evidence of behavioural sensitisation, since it implies an enduring enhancement of the psychotic response to stress (Myin-Germeys et al., 2005a). It could be argued that these findings do not suggest a direct effect of stress on psychosis, but rather an artefact of increased negative mood, which is also associated with daily stress. However, the effect of stress on psychosis remained strong and significant after controlling for mood, suggesting a direct effect of daily stress on psychosis, independent of mood.

Mechanisms (2) Early adversity and behavioural sensitisation

The studies described above demonstrate that people who are vulnerable to developing psychosis are indeed sensitised to stress. They react with larger changes in mood and psychosis intensity in response to daily stress compared with healthy controls. Is this sensitised state, at least in part, the result of a sensitisation process caused by early environmental adversity or only the result of an inherited vulnerability for psychosis?

Empirical evidence

To demonstrate a process of sensitisation consisting of an enduring vulnerability caused by early environmental risk factors rather than genetic risk factors alone, evidence showing alterations in current stress as a function of previous stressful exposures is necessary. We investigated this in a sample of 42 patients in remission from psychosis. Life events were assessed with the Brown and Harris Life Events and Difficulties Schedule (Brown and Harris, 1978). We examined whether: (1) the occurrence of life events in the past year moderated the subjective stressfulness of daily hassles and (2) whether previous exposure to life events moderated emotional reactivity to daily hassles, assessed using the ESM (Myin-Germeys et al., 2003). We found that life events did not influence subjective appraisals of stress: life events did not change the stressfulness of daily events, nor did life events increase the appraised stressfulness of activities in which subjects were involved. Life events, however, did moderate the emotional reactivity to stress both in models predicting negative and positive affect (Figure 9.1).

Evidence suggests that recent life events also influence underlying biological mechanisms in newly admitted patients with psychosis; in particular pre-treatment cortisol may be increased after life events (Mazure et al., 1997). These results further

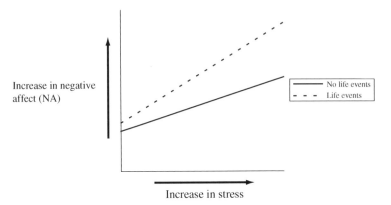

Increase in negative
affect (NA)

No life events
— — — Life events

Increase in stress

.**Figure 9.1**   The effect of stress negative affect, stratified for the experience of life events in the past year, in patients with psychosis

support the hypothesis that environmental effects sensitise people to smaller stresses encountered in daily life.

Another environmental risk factor associated with psychosis is the experience of trauma or victimisation, particularly in childhood (see Chapter 7). It is attractive to hypothesise that the relationship between childhood trauma and psychosis may in part be mediated by lasting alterations in adult stress-sensitivity. We thus investigated the effect of childhood trauma on stress sensitivity in adult life in a sample of 90 frequent general practice attendees, a sample selected because of the high prevalence of childhood trauma: 29 individuals had experienced serious trauma during childhood (Glaser *et al.*, 2006). The study examined whether childhood trauma moderated emotional reactivity to small, daily life stressors, which were again assessed using the Experience Sampling Method. The results showed that subjects with a history of childhood trauma did indeed report increased emotional reactivity to daily stress, reflected in an increase in negative affect. This effect was significantly stronger for the subjects who experienced trauma before the age of 10 (Glaser *et al.*, 2006). This provides some evidence for a long-lasting and enduring effect of childhood trauma on adult stress-sensitivity. However, these data were gathered in a normal population sample, and it is important to investigate these questions in samples of subjects who are vulnerable to developing psychosis. In this way, it may be possible to assess more fully the hypothesised causal chain from trauma through behavioural sensitisation to psychosis.

Mechanisms (3) Biology and behavioural sensitisation

We have presented evidence to suggest that behavioural sensitisation may be one mechanism linking the experience of previous larger stresses, such as significant life events or childhood trauma, and psychosis. The sensitised state, in these studies, was operationalised as increased emotional and psychotic responses to the small stresses of every day life. We now turn to the question of whether biological evidence for this sensitisation process can be found (see also: Myin-Germeys and van Os, 2007).

One obvious mechanism that may be involved in altered responses to stress in psychosis is the hypothalamic-pituitary-adrenal (HPA) axis, which is one of the major mediating systems involved in stress responsivity (Walker and Diforio, 1997). However, only a limited amount of research has been conducted investigating HPA axis activity in psychosis. Overall, the data suggest that patients with psychosis show evidence of overactivity of the HPA axis (Cotter and Pariante, 2002; Walker and Diforio, 1997), demonstrated by higher baseline cortisol levels (Ryan et al., 2004), increased pituitary volume (Pariante et al., 2004; Pariante et al., 2005) and higher cortisol levels after a dexamethasone suppression test (i.e., HPA axis challenge test) (for review, see Walker and Diforio, 1997). Similar findings were reported in subjects with schizotypal personality disorder and in individuals at ultra-high risk of developing psychosis (Garner et al., 2005; Walker and Diforio, 1997). However, studies using metabolic and psychosocial stress challenges have reported inconclusive results. Some studies suggest blunted cortisol responses in patients with schizophrenia and in patients with schizotypal personality disorder, and in first-degree relatives (albeit to a lesser degree) (Jansen et al., 1998; Marcelis et al., 2004; Mitropoulou et al., 2004). Others have found increased cortisol responses (Elman et al., 1998). However, all of the patients in these studies were receiving antipsychotic medication, which may have influenced the results. Thus, further examination of HPA axis functioning, especially in relation to stress challenges and possibly daily life stressors, is necessary to resolve this issue.

An alternative mechanism that may underlie sensitisation to stress in psychosis is dopamine sensitisation resulting in alterations in dopamine transmission. That is, prolonged or severe stress may lead to hyper-reactivity of dopamine (DA) neurons in response to further environmental stimuli, such that even exposure to moderate levels of stress become associated with an excessive dopamine response (Laruelle, 2000; Laruelle and Abi-Dargham, 1999). There are already relevant data. Neuroimaging techniques, such as positron emission tomography and single-photon emission tomography techniques, have demonstrated enhanced dopamine D2 receptor signalling in the striatum following acute amphetamine challenge in actively ill patients (Laruelle and Abi-Dargham, 1999). In addition, studies using metabolic perturbation have demonstrated increased plasma homovanillic acid (HVA) elevations in patients in a clinical state of remission (Breier et al., 1993; Marcelis et al., 2004), an effect that was also seen, albeit to a lesser degree, in first-degree relatives of patients (Marcelis et al., 2004). It has been suggested that a dysregulated, hyper-dopaminergic state may lead to stimulus-independent release of DA, which may take over the normal process of contextually driven salience attribution, resulting in aberrant, psychotic assignment of salience to external objects and internal representations (Kapur, 2003). Studies assessing dopamine transmission following acute amphetamine challenge have demonstrated that elevated DA response is associated with activation of psychotic symptomatology (Laruelle and Abi-Dargham, 1999).

Using the ESM, we investigated whether increased psychotic reactivity to stress assessed in daily life is associated with dopamine hyper-responsivity (Myin-Germeys et al., 2005b). We did this in a sample of 47 first-degree relatives, since they did not use antipsychotic medication and were at risk of psychotic experiences (e.g., Bergman et al., 2000). Altered dopamine reactivity was defined as plasma HVA elevation following metabolic perturbation (i.e., induction of the glucose analogue, 2-deoxyglucose, which inhibits intracellular glucose metabolism, thus inducing a mild, transient state of intracellular hypoglycemia – conforming to the paradigm developed by Breier et al. (1993)). The findings showed a large and significant interaction effect between psychotic reactivity to stress in daily life and HVA response to the metabolic perturbation in the relatives, indicating that the degree of underlying HVA reactivity moderated ESM psychotic experiences in response to daily life stress. No such effect was found in control subjects (Figure 9.2). These findings suggest that psychotic experiences may represent the functional state of underlying abnormal dopamine reactivity in subjects at risk of developing psychosis. Altered dopamine reactivity may be an essential mechanism underlying sensitisation to stress in psychosis. (Figure 9.2).

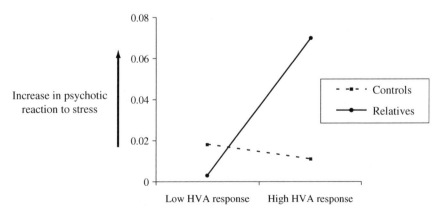

Figure 9.2   The effect of dopamine transmission expressed as low and high HVA response on psychotic reactivity to stress, stratified for underlying vulnerability for psychosis

Mechanisms (4) Gene–environment interactions

Another mechanism that is important in understanding the effect of adult adversities on the risk of psychosis is gene–environment interaction (see Chapter 5). Some recent studies have provided evidence for gene–environment interaction in the cause of psychiatric disorders (Caspi *et al.*, 2002; Caspi *et al.*, 2003). Some direct and indirect evidence for mechanisms of gene–environment interaction in psychosis will be provided next.

Empirical evidence (1) A developmental interactive model of psychosis

Recent research strongly points to a developmental interactive model of psychosis, in which gene–environment interactions are likely to play a role. First, the expression of psychosis, whether it be psychotic disorders (prevalence 1%), isolated psychotic symptoms (prevalence around 5%) and broadly defined psychotic experiences (prevalence around 15%), is much more common in young people and declines with age (Johns and van Os, 2001; Myin-Germeys *et al.*, 2004; Verdoux and Cougnard, 2006; Verdoux and van Os, 2002; Wittchen and Jacobi, 2005). Second, follow-up studies of young people with psychosis-like symptoms at the sub-clinical level reveal that the great majority do not experience such symptoms at any level at follow-up (Hanssen *et al.*, 2005). Third, the expression of psychosis at the sub-clinical or 'schizotypal'-level clusters in families and is influenced in part by genetic factors (Hanssen *et al.*, 2005). Finally, the generally good, because transitory, outcome of sub-clinical psychotic experiences may be altered negatively if subjects are exposed to additional (proxy) environmental risk factors. Examples of these are trauma (Spauwen *et al.*, 2006a), cannabis (Henquet *et al.*, 2005; van Os *et al.*, 2002) and urbanicity (Spauwen

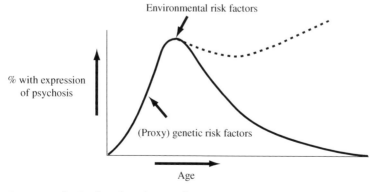

Figure 9.3 Onset psychotic disorder: abnormal persistence of developmentally normal expression of psychosis (dotted line)

et al., 2006b; van Os, 2004; van Os et al., 2003). In other words, the normal developmental expression of psychosis-like symptoms may become abnormally persistent and clinically relevant depending on the degree of environmental load the person is additionally exposed to (Figure 9.3). The relevant findings are discussed in more detail next.

Empirical evidence (2) Indirect evidence for gene–environment interaction

Growing up in an urban area is one of the most important environmental factors related to schizophrenia, explaining up to 30% of all schizophrenia incidence (Krabbendam and van Os, 2005; see Chapter 6). However, if gene–environment interaction is involved, one would expect that not everyone would be equally affected by this environmental risk factor.

A study by our group investigated this in a general population sample of 5618 subjects (van Os et al., 2003). We found that the level of urbanicity (defined in five levels based on the density of addresses in km^2) was associated both with sub-clinical and clinical psychosis outcomes. Genetic risk for psychosis was indirectly assessed based on family history. Participants with a first-degree relative who had ever experienced delusions or hallucinations or a first-degree relative who had ever received treatment from a psychiatrist for psychotic symptoms were considered to be genetically at risk. Three hundred and ten (5.6%) probands had a first-degree relative with delusions or hallucinations and 201 of these (3.6%) indicated that they had received treatment.

The results showed that the effect of urbanicity on psychosis risk was greatest in those with higher levels of familial liability for psychosis, independent of familial liability for other psychiatric disorders. Around 60–70% of the psychosis outcome in probands exposed to both familial liability and urbanicity was attributable to the synergistic action of these two factors, thus providing strong evidence for gene–environment interaction (van Os et al., 2003).

This result was replicated in a much larger sample of over one million Danish people (data from the Danish Civil Registration System) (van Os et al., 2004). In line with the previous study, it was found that a family history of psychosis, a proxy genetic risk factor, interacted synergistically with level of urbanicity, a proxy environmental risk factor, thus providing further support for gene–environment interaction. In this sample, a fifth to a third of individuals exposed to both the environmental and the genetic risk factors developed the disorder because of their coparticipation.

In a further study, the mechanism of gene–environment interaction was investigated using a more direct indicator of genetic liability at the level of the person, rather than at the level of the family (Spauwen et al., 2006b). In a sample of 3000 young adolescents from the Early Developmental Stages of Psychopathology study

(Lieb *et al.*, 2000), we examined whether the outcome of sub-clinical psychosis (as an indicator of psychosis-proneness) would be worse for those growing up in an urban environment. We found that the risk-increasing effect of urbanicity was only apparent in those with pre-existing psychotic experiences, thus providing more direct evidence for a synergistic interaction between a proxy genetic risk factor and a proxy environmental risk factor.

Empirical evidence (3) Direct evidence for gene–environment interaction

A more direct way to study gene–environment interaction is to investigate whether certain functional polymorphisms are related to the ways individuals respond to the environment. Moffit *et al.* (2005) have recently put forward criteria to ensure careful and deliberate gene–environment hypothesis testing. In terms of candidate environmental pathogens, it is necessary to find environmental risk factors (1) with variability in response, i.e., not everyone is equally affected, (2) that affect a neurobiological pathway to the disorder, and (3) that are true environmental pathogens having causal effects. Furthermore, it is better to investigate proximal rather than distal environmental pathogens, to take into account the cumulative nature of the environmental influence, and to exercise caution with retrospective measures of environmental pathogens since, for example, memories of events are under the influence of genes and these same genes influence personality and behaviour. In the previous part of this chapter, we described how daily hassles may have a direct effect on mood and psychosis. In addition, not all individuals were equally affected by these hassles; evidence was provided for a link with a neurobiological pathway (i.e., dopamine sensitisation), and there is evidence that such hassles constitute a true environmental pathogen (i.e., there is a direct effect on psychosis). Furthermore, it is a proximal measure, taking into account cumulative exposure, and prospectively measured. Daily hassles thus seem to provide a good candidate environmental pathogen in the study of gene–environment interactions. In terms of selecting the proper gene, Moffit *et al.* (2005) suggested focusing on common polymorphic variants, with a direct gene-to-disorder association and functional significance in relation to the environmental pathogen. A functional polymorphism on the catechol-O-methyltransferase gene (COMT) that results in a change from valine (*Val*) to methionine (*Met*) meets these criteria. First, the functional polymorphic variants are relatively common in the population (Palmatier *et al.*, 1999). Second, several studies have related the Val[158]Met COMT polymorphism to schizophrenia, although there is substantial inconsistency in the findings (Fan *et al.*, 2005; Glatt *et al.*, 2003; Munafo *et al.*, 2005). Third, the Val[158]Met COMT polymorphism has functional effects on dopamine neurotransmission (Bilder *et al.*, 2004); we have already shown that dopamine may mediate psychotic reactions to stress (Myin-Germeys *et al.*, 2005b).

In a recent ESM study, we examined whether variation in the Val[158]Met COMT polymorphism mediates the psychotic reaction to stress, in an attempt to provide more direct evidence for gene–environment interaction (van Winkel, R. *et al.*, in press). According to the tonic-phasic dopamine model (Bilder *et al.*, 2004; Grace, 1991), the enzyme containing *Val* favours reduction in tonic dopamine but increases in phasic dopamine, giving rise to decreased cognitive stability but increased cognitive flexibility. For the enzyme containing *Met*, the opposite would hold. We hypothesised that *Met* subjects would react more strongly to daily life events, on the basis that they would experience more difficulties in adapting to changes in the environment. The study sample consisted of 31 patients with a psychotic disorder, 7 first-degree and second-degree relatives and 25 healthy controls. The data showed that *Met/Met* subjects indeed reported significantly greater increases in psychotic experiences, especially delusional experiences, in reaction to daily stress than subjects with the *Val/Met* or *Val/Val* genotype. This effect was particularly evident in the patients. Furthermore, *Met/Met* subjects reported a larger increase in negative affect in reaction to stress than subjects of the other genotypes. This effect was apparent in both patients and controls.

This study, thus, provides direct evidence of a gene–environment interaction between the Val[158]Met COMT polymorphism and daily stress in terms of both psychotic and affective reactions. However, it involved a relatively small and select sample of subjects (all subjects were cannabis-users), thus limiting the generalisability of the findings.

Conclusion

There is evidence that adult adversity is a component cause of psychosis, in interaction with enduring liabilities created by both genetic and early environmental factors. The concepts of behavioural sensitisation and gene–environment interaction are useful in designing studies of the person-environment interactions that may cause continuous variation on the psychosis continuum.

REFERENCES

Bebbington, P., Wilkins, S., Jones, P. *et al.* (1993). Life events and psychosis. Initial results from the Camberwell Collaborative Psychosis study. *British Journal of Psychiatry*, **162**, 72–9.

Bebbington, P., Wilkins, S., Sham, P. *et al.* (1996). Life events before psychotic episodes: do clinical and social variables affect the relationship? *Social Psychiatry and Psychiatric Epidemiology*, **31** (3–4), 122–8.

Bergman, A. J., Silverman, J. M., Harvey, P. *et al.* (2000). Schizotypal symptoms in the relatives of schizophrenia patients: an empirical analysis of the factor structure. *Schizophrenia Bulletin*, **26** (3), 577–86.

Bilder, R. M., Volavka, J., Lachman, H. M. *et al.* (2004). The catechol-O-methyltransferase polymorphism: relations to the tonic-phasic dopamine hypothesis and neuropsychiatric phenotypes. *Neuropsychopharmacology*, **29** (11), 1943–61.

Boydell, J., van Os, J., McKenzie, K. *et al.* (2001). Incidence of schizophrenia in ethnic minorities in London: ecological study into interactions with environment. *British Medical Journal*, **323** (7325), 1336–8.

Breier, A., Davis, O. R., Buchanan, R. W. *et al.* (1993). Effects of metabolic perturbation on plasma homovanillic acid in schizophrenia. Relationship to prefrontal cortex volume. *Archives of General Psychiatry*, **50** (7), 541–50.

Brown, G. W. and Harris, T. O. (1978). *Social Origins of Depression: A Study of Psychiatric Disorder in Women*. London: Tavistock.

Cantor-Graae, E. and Selten, J. P. (2005). Schizophrenia and migration: a meta-analysis and review. *American Journal of Psychiatry*, **162** (1), 12–24.

Carr, V., Halpin, S., Lau, N. *et al.* (2000). A risk factor screening and assessment protocol for schizophrenia and related psychosis. *Australian and New Zealand Journal of Psychiatry*, **34** (suppl.), s170–s180.

Caspi, A., McClay, J., Moffitt, T. E. *et al.* (2002). Role of genotype in the cycle of violence in maltreated children. *Science*, **297**, 851–4.

Caspi, A., Sugden, K., Moffitt, T. E. *et al.* (2003). Influence of life stress on depression: moderation by a polymorphism in the 5-HTT gene. *Science*, **301**, 386–9.

Castine, M. R., Meador-Woodruff, J. H. and Dalack, G. W. (1998). The role of life events in onset and recurrent episodes of schizophrenia and schizoaffective disorder. *Journal of Psychiatric Research*, **32** (5), 283–8.

Cotter, D. and Pariante, C. M. (2002). Stress and the progression of the developmental hypothesis of schizophrenia. *British Journal of Psychiatry*, **181**, 363–5.

Elman, I., Adler, C. M., Malhotra, A. K. *et al.* (1998). Effect of acute metabolic stress on pituitary-adrenal axis activation in patients with schizophrenia. *American Journal of Psychiatry*, **155** (7), 979–81.

Fan, J. B., Zhang, C. S., Gu, N. F. *et al.* (2005). Catechol-O-methyltransferase gene Val/Met functional polymorphism and risk of schizophrenia: a large-scale association study plus meta-analysis. *Biological Psychiatry*, **57** (2), 139–44.

Garner, B., Pariante, C. M., Wood, S. J. *et al.* (2005). Pituitary volume predicts future transition to psychosis in individuals at ultra-high risk of developing psychosis. *Biological Psychiatry*, **58** (5), 417–23.

Glaser, J. P., van Os, J., Portegijs, P. J. M. *et al.* (2006). Childhood trauma and emotional reactivity to daily life stress in adult frequent attenders of the General Practitioner. *Journal of Psychosomatic Research*, **61** (2), 229–36.

Glatt, S. J., Faraone, S. V. and Tsuang, M. T. (2003). Association between a functional catechol-O-methyltransferase gene polymorphism and schizophrenia: meta-analysis of case-control and family-based studies. *American Journal of Psychiatry*, **160** (3), 469–76.

Grace, A. A. (1991). Phasic versus tonic dopamine release and the modulation of dopamine system responsivity: a hypothesis for the etiology of schizophrenia. *Neuroscience*, **41** (1), 1–24.

Hanssen, M., Bak, M., Bijl, R. *et al.* (2005). The incidence and outcome of sub-clinical psychotic experiences in the general population. *British Journal of Clinical Psychology*, **44** (2), 181–91.

Henquet, C., Krabbendam, L., Spauwen, J. *et al.* (2005). Prospective cohort study of cannabis use, predisposition for psychosis, and psychotic symptoms in young people. *British Medical Journal*, **330**, 11.

Hirsch, S., Bowen, J., Emami, J. *et al.* (1996). A one year prospective study of the effect of life events and medication in the aetiology of schizophrenic relapse. *British Journal of Psychiatry*, **168** (1), 49–56.

Horan, W. P., Ventura, J., Nuechterlein, K. H. *et al.* (2005). Stressful life events in recent-onset schizophrenia: reduced frequencies and altered subjective appraisals. *Schizophrenia Research*, **75** (2–3), 363–74.

Jansen, L. M., Gispen de Wied, C. C., Gademan, P. J. *et al.* (1998). Blunted cortisol response to a psychosocial stressor in schizophrenia. *Schizophrenia Research*, **33** (1–2), 87–94.

Janssen, I., Hanssen, M., Bak, M. *et al.* (2003). Discrimination and delusional ideation. *British Journal of Psychiatry*, **182**, 71–6.

Johns, L. C. and van Os, J. (2001). The continuity of psychotic experiences in the general population. *Clinical Psychology Review*, **21** (8), 1125–41.

Johns, L. C., Cannon, M., Singleton, N. *et al.* (2004). Prevalence and correlates of self-reported psychotic symptoms in the British population. *British Journal of Psychiatry*, **185**, 298–305.

Kanner, A. D., Coyne, J. C., Schaefer, C. *et al.* (1981). Comparison of two modes of stress measurement: daily hassles and uplifts versus major life events. *Journal of Behavioral Medicine*, **4** (1), 1–39.

Kapur, S. (2003). Psychosis as a state of aberrant salience: a framework linking biology, phenomenology, and pharmacology in schizophrenia. *American Journal of Psychiatry*, **160** (1), 13–23.

Krabbendam, L. and van Os, J. (2005). Schizophrenia and urbanicity: a major environmental influence – conditional on genetic risk. *Schizophrenia Bulletin*, **31** (4), 795–9.

Laruelle, M. (2000). The role of endogenous sensitization in the pathophysiology of schizophrenia: implications from recent brain imaging studies. *Brain Research Review*, **31** (2–3), 371–84.

Laruelle, M. and Abi-Dargham, A. (1999). Dopamine as the wind of the psychotic fire: new evidence from brain imaging studies. *Journal of Psychopharmacology*, **13** (4), 358–71.

Lieb, R., Isensee, B., von Sydow, K. *et al.* (2000). The Early Developmental Stages of Psychopathology study (EDSP): a methodological update. *European Addiction Research*, **6** (4), 170–82.

Malla, A. K., Cortese, L., Shaw, T. S. *et al.* (1990). Life events and relapse in schizophrenia. *Social Psychiatry and Psychiatric Epidemiology*, **25**, 221–4.

Marcelis, M., Cavalier, E., Gielen, J. *et al.* (2004). Abnormal response to metabolic stress in schizophrenia: marker of vulnerability or acquired sensitisation? *Psychological Medicine*, **34**, 1103–11.

Mason, O., Startup, M., Halpin, S. *et al.* (2004). Risk factors for transition to first episode psychosis among individuals with 'at-risk mental states'. *Schizophrenia Research*, **71** (2–3), 227–37.

Mazure, C. M., Quinlan, D. M. and Bowers, M., Jr (1997). Recent life stressors and biological markers in newly admitted psychotic patients. *Biological Psychiatry*, **41** (8), 865–70.

Miller, P., Lawrie, S. M., Hodges, A. *et al.* (2001). Genetic liability, illicit drug use, life stress and psychotic symptoms: preliminary findings from the Edinburgh study of people at high risk for schizophrenia. *Social Psychiatry and Psychiatric Epidemiology*, **36** (7), 338–42.

Mitropoulou, V., Goodman, M., Sevy, S. *et al.* (2004). Effects of acute metabolic stress on the dopaminergic and pituitary-adrenal axis activity in patients with schizotypal personality disorder. *Schizophrenia Research*, **70** (1), 27–31.

Moffitt, T. E., Caspi, A. and Rutter, M. (2005). Strategy for investigating interactions between measured genes and measured environments. *Archives of General Psychiatry*, **62** (5), 473–81.

Monroe, S. M. (1983). Major and minor life events as predictors of psychological distress: further issues and findings. *Journal of Behavioral Medicine*, **6** (2), 189–205.

Munafo, M. R., Bowes, L., Clark, T. G. *et al.* (2005). Lack of association of the COMT (Val158/108Met) gene and schizophrenia: a meta-analysis of case-control studies. *Molecular Psychiatry*, **10** (8), 765–70.

Myin-Germeys, I. and van Os, J. (2007). Stress-reactivity in psychosis: evidence for an affective pathway to psychosis. *Clinical Psychology Review*, **17** (4), 409–24.

Myin-Germeys, I., van Os, J., Schwartz, J. E. *et al.* (2001). Emotional reactivity to daily life stress in psychosis. *Archives of General Psychiatry*, **58** (12), 1137–44.

Myin-Germeys, I., Krabbendam, L., Delespaul, P. A. E. G. *et al.* (2003). Do life events have their effect on psychosis by influencing the emotional reactivity to daily life stress? *Psychological Medicine*, **33** (2), 327–33.

Myin-Germeys, I., Spauwen, J., Jacobs, N. *et al.* (2004). The aetiological continuum of psychosis. In *Search for the Causes of Schizophrenia*, vol. 5, ed. W. F. Gattaz and H. Häfner. Berlin: Springer-Verlag, pp. 342–66.

Myin-Germeys, I., Delespaul, P. and van Os, J. (2005a). Behavioural sensitization to daily life stress in psychosis. *Psychological Medicine*, **35** (5), 733–41.

Myin-Germeys, I., Marcelis, M., Krabbendam, L. *et al.* (2005b). Subtle fluctuations in psychotic phenomena as functional states of abnormal dopamine reactivity in individuals at risk. *Biological Psychiatry*, **58** (2), 105–10.

Norman, R. M. G. and Malla, A. K. (1991). Subjective stress in schizophrenic patients. *Social Psychiatry and Psychiatric Epidemiology*, **26** (5), 212–16.

Norman, R. M. G. and Malla, A. K. (1993). Stressful life events and schizophrenia I: a review of the research. *British Journal of Psychiatry*, **162**, 161–6.

Nuechterlein, K. H. and Dawson, M. E. (1984). A heuristic vulnerability/stress model of schizophrenic episodes. *Schizophrenia Bulletin*, **10** (2), 300–12.

Palmatier, M. A., Kang, A. M. and Kidd, K. K. (1999). Global variation in the frequencies of functionally different catechol-O-methyltransferase alleles. *Biological Psychiatry*, **46** (4), 557–67.

Pariante, C. M., Vassilopoulou, K., Velakoulis, D. *et al.* (2004). Pituitary volume in psychosis. *British Journal of Psychiatry*, **185**, 5–10.

Pariante, C. M., Dazzan, P., Danese, A. *et al.* (2005). Increased pituitary volume in antipsychotic-free and antipsychotic-treated patients of the ÆSOP first-onset psychosis study. *Neuropsychopharmacology*, **30** (10), 1923–31.

Ryan, M. C., Sharifi, N., Condren, R. *et al.* (2004). Evidence of basal pituitary-adrenal over-activity in first episode, drug naive patients with schizophrenia. *Psychoneuroendocrinology*, **29** (8), 1065–70.

Spauwen, J., Krabbendam, L., Lieb, R. *et al.* (2006a). Impact of psychological trauma on the development of psychotic symptoms: relationship with psychosis proneness. *British Journal of Psychiatry*, **188**, 527–33.

Spauwen, J., Krabbendam, L., Lieb, R. *et al.* (2006b). Evidence that the outcome of developmental expression of psychosis is worse for adolescents growing up in an urban environment. *Psychological Medicine*, **36** (3), 407–15.

van Os, J. (2004). Does the urban environment cause psychosis? *British Journal of Psychiatry*, **184**, 287–8.

van Os, J., Bak, M., Hanssen, M. *et al.* (2002). Cannabis use and psychosis: a longitudinal population-based study. *American Journal of Epidemiology*, **156** (4), 319–27.

van Os, J., Hanssen, M., Bak, M. *et al.* (2003). Do urbanicity and familial liability coparticipate in causing psychosis? *American Journal of Psychiatry*, **160** (3), 477–82.

van Os, J., Pedersen, C. B. and Mortensen, P. B. (2004). Confirmation of synergy between urbanicity and familial liability in the causation of psychosis. *American Journal of Psychiatry*, **161** (12), 2312–14.

van Os, J., Krabbendam, L., Myin-Germeys, I. *et al.* (2005). The schizophrenia envirome. *Current Opinion in Psychiatry*, **18** (2), 141–5.

van Winkel, R. Henquet, C. Rosa, A. *et al.* (in press) Evidence that the COMT Val158Met polymorphism moderates sensitivity to stress: an experience sampling study. *American Journal of Medical Genetics B*.

Ventura, J., Nuechterlein, K. H., Subotnik, K. L. *et al.* (2000). Life events can trigger depressive exacerbation in the early course of schizophrenia. *Journal of Abnormal Psychology*, **109** (1), 139–44.

Verdoux, H. and Cougnard, A. (2006). Who is at risk? Who is a case? *International Clinical Psychopharmacology*, **21** (suppl. 2), s17–s19.

Verdoux, H. and van Os, J. (2002). Psychotic symptoms in non-clinical populations and the continuum of psychosis. *Schizophrenia Research*, **54** (1–2), 59–65.

Walker, E. F. and Diforio, D. (1997). Schizophrenia: a neural diathesis–stress model. *Psychological Review*, **104** (4), 667–85.

Wiles, N. J., Zammit, S., Bebbington, P. *et al.* (2006). Self-reported psychotic symptoms in the general population: results from the longitudinal study of the British National Psychiatric Morbidity Survey. *British Journal of Psychiatry*, **188**, 519–26.

Wittchen, H. U. and Jacobi, F. (2005). Size and burden of mental disorders in Europe – a critical review and appraisal of 27 studies. *European Neuropsychopharmacology*, **15** (4), 357–76.

Zubin, J., Magaziner, J. and Steinhauer, S. R. (1983). The metamorphosis of schizophrenia: from chronicity to vulnerability. *Psychological Medicine*, **13** (3), 551–71.

10

Migration, ethnicity and psychosis

Kwame McKenzie, Paul Fearon and Gerard Hutchinson

Introduction

In the 1930s, Ödegaard (1932) reported that first-admission rates for schizo-phrenia were high among Norwegian migrants to the United States. Since then numerous studies in a variety of countries have investigated rates of serious mental illness in migrant groups and in different cultural and ethnic groups within countries (Cantor-Graae and Selten, 2005). In this chapter, we review the literature reporting differences in the incidence of psychosis between migrant and ethnic groups, we discuss methodological issues and, using the best-researched group, people of African and Caribbean origin in the UK, we try to build a model of how migration, culture and ethnicity affect rates of incident psychosis.

History and overview

Since high rates of mental illness among Norwegian migrants to the United States were reported in the first half of the last century (Ödegaard, 1932) there have been a number of studies investigating the incidence of psychosis in migrant and ethnic minority groups. Although the vast majority of migration is between developing countries within Africa and Asia, there is surprisingly little research on the risk of psychosis in these groups. Research into the incidence of psychosis in migrant groups is best developed in northern Europe. The most comprehensive literature on the subject concerns the high incidence of schizophrenia in people of African and Caribbean origin who migrated to the UK, mainly in the 1940s and 1950s, and in their children and grandchildren, a finding which has been consistently reported for 30 years. The various studies have reported rates of schizophrenia between 2 and 14 times greater for African-Caribbeans than for whites in the UK (Fearon and Morgan, 2006). Some of the more recent findings are shown in Table 10.1. Studies have also reported elevated rates in migrant compared with host populations in other northern European countries, including

Society and Psychosis, ed. Craig Morgan, Kwame McKenzie and Paul Fearon. Published by Cambridge University Press. © Cambridge University Press 2008.

Table 10.1 Reported incidence rates for narrowly defined schizophrenia (per 10 000 per year) in African-Caribbeans in recent UK studies and in Barbados, Trinidad and Jamaica

	Incidence rate per 10 000 per year[a]	95% confidence interval
UK (Fearon *et al.*, 2006)	7.1	(5.2–9.0)
UK (Bhugra *et al.*, 1997)	5.1	Not given
UK (Harrison *et al.*, 1997)	4.7	(1.8–7.5)
UK (King *et al.*, 1994)	5.3	(1.8–8.7)
Barbados (Mahy *et al.*, 1999)	2.8	(2.0–3.7)
Trinidad (Bhugra *et al.*, 1996)	1.6	(1.1–2.1)
Jamaica (Hickling and Rodgers-Johnson, 1995)	2.1	Not given

[a] The WHO Ten Country study found rates of narrowly defined schizophrenia that ranged from 0.7 to 1.4 per 10 000 per year (Jablensky *et al.*, 1992). The meta-analysis by McGrath *et al.* (2004) found a median incidence of 1.5 per 10 000, based on 100 incidence studies.

the Netherlands (Selten and Sijben, 1994; Selten *et al.*, 1997; Selten *et al.*, 2001), Denmark (Cantor-Graae *et al.*, 2003) and Sweden (Zolkowska *et al.*, 2001) and in Australia (Krupinski and Cochrane, 1980). Cantor-Graae's and Selten's (2005) meta-analysis demonstrated a significant increased risk of schizophrenia in all migrant groups, this being greatest in those from developing countries who migrated to developed countries and in those with black skin colour migrating to countries where the population was predominantly white.

There has been much speculation about why rates of psychosis are raised in migrant and ethnic minority groups. Ödegaard (1932) suggested that the increase might be due to selection, i.e., those with a predisposition to psychotic illness being more likely to migrate, but recent studies have refuted this hypothesis (Selten *et al.*, 2002). It seems unlikely that biological factors can explain the high rates, and because of this the focus has shifted to social experiences and conditions (Sharpley *et al.*, 2001). Over time, the reasons for migration, the processes of migration and the situations of migrants in their new host countries have all come under scrutiny as researchers have sought to explain the high rates (Sharpley *et al.*,

2001). As migrants have had children, they have also become the focus of investigation (Bhugra *et al.*, 1997; Castle *et al.*, 1991; Fearon *et al.*, 2006; Harrison *et al.*,
1988; Harrison *et al.*, 1997; McGovern and Cope, 1987; Thomas *et al.*, 1993; van
Os *et al.*, 1996). This, and the possibility that a mismatch between the culture of
migrant groups and the host population is aetiologically important, has led to
a link between the study of migration and ethnicity (see definitions below). This
said, there remain a number of methodological problems with studies of the
incidence of psychosis in migrant and ethnic minority groups, and these need to
be considered in drawing conclusions. Before doing this, it is necessary to define
some relevant concepts and terms.

Definitions of relevant concepts and terms

Migration

Migration can be considered as a process of social change in which an individual
moves from one cultural setting to another. There are many reasons for, and types
of, migration, these often being enshrined in law in host countries (e.g., temporary
workers, economic migrants, asylum seekers and refugees). A further distinction
can be drawn between primary migrants and secondary migrants who follow in
their footsteps. Three stages to the migration process have been identified (Bhugra
and Jones, 2001):

- *Pre-migration*   decision to move and planning;
- *Transition*   movement from one setting to another;
- *Post-migration* coming to terms with a new life, roles and country.

The factors that increase risk for disorder in migrant groups may operate during
any of these stages.

Race, culture and ethnicity

Race, culture and ethnicity are three related but distinct concepts. The idea that
people can be separated into racial categories on the basis of physical appearance
has a long history in the West, and the popular belief that people are separable into
distinct groups on the basis of phenotypical characteristics persists and underpins
ongoing racism (Fernando, 1991). Modern genetics has undermined the scientific
validity of racial categories. For example, it has been shown that the differences
between classically described racial groups (10% of the genetic variation) are only
slightly greater than those which exist between nations (6%), and both of these are
small compared with genetic differences within local populations (84%) (Jones,
1981). The use of racial categories has now largely disappeared from scientific
research and been replaced by the use of ethnicity. However, researchers often

categorise people into 'ethnic' groups in such a way that these are indistinguishable from racial categories, e.g., the crude dichotomy between black and white (for a review see McKenzie and Crowcroft, 1994).

There are many definitions of culture, but what is common to most is the idea that culture provides a set of socially shared guidelines or rules that shape and constrain beliefs, attitudes and behaviour. In other words, culture usually refers to the behaviours and attitudes of social groups. That said, culture is not static or homogeneous. Determined by upbringing and choice, culture is constantly changing and is notoriously difficult to measure (Fernando, 1991). Such cultural flux may be particularly important in groups who have migrated, where individuals face choices about how much of the host culture to incorporate into their own.

Of all the variables, ethnicity is probably the most difficult to define and use. Such groups are characterised by a sense of belonging or group identity (Jenkins, 1986), these being dynamic and changeable and determined by social pressures and psychological needs. Aspects of race and culture may engender a sense of common identity and so, in part, determine ethnicity. For example, as Fernando (1991) suggests, a sense of belonging may emerge from the shared experiences of discrimination in a racist society – emergent ethnicity. This may be one factor that has driven the emergence of a Caribbean identity among migrants from the culturally diverse Caribbean islands to the UK. Cultural heritage may form a significant component of ethnic identity, but it does not define it, and those who perceive themselves as belonging to an ethnic group may well differ markedly in terms of the cultural reference points that inform their beliefs and actions. This warns against the conflation of culture and ethnicity.

Ethnicity is potentially fluid and changeable over time and space, as exposure to other contexts and cultures allows for its reformulation. However, the way in which ethnicity is measured and operationalised in much epidemiological research ignores these complexities. The use of fixed, predetermined 'ethnic categories' in cross-sectional research and by governments for census purposes is problematic in that key components of ethnicity – sense of belonging and changeability – are absent. For example, in one US study, in which subjects were asked to select their ethnicity at baseline and 12 months later, one third selected a different ethnicity at the second time of asking (Leech, 1989).

Methodological problems

For all the apparent consistency of studies showing high rates of psychosis in migrant groups (Cantor-Graae and Selten, 2005), there are a number of methodological issues that need to be considered in evaluating the validity of the findings. What we are ultimately trying to do is model and understand complex social processes with multiple layers and meanings. To do this effectively, methodo-logical rigour is essential, as is caution in interpreting results.

Measuring migration, ethnicity and culture

Migration is a complex variable but many studies simplify it to being a member of a migrant group or not. Incidence studies are unable to indicate whether members of the groups are economic migrants, refugees or asylum seekers, as they rely on census estimates and categories, which do not distinguish these groups, for their denominator. Perhaps the single greatest difficulty is the measurement of context. Not only do different groups have different experiences of the first two stages of migration (see above), but they also migrate into different sociopolitical contexts. These contexts are likely to be important in more fully understanding the risks for psychosis to which migrants may be exposed. A migrant group may include different cultural or ethnic groups. If information describing the process of migration and the different ethnicities and cultures within a migrant group is lacking, it becomes difficult to understand precisely what the risk-generating exposures are.

Quantifying ethnic groups

Accurate enumeration of ethnic minority populations is an important, but prob-lematic, issue. For example, national censuses, which are often used to provide the denominator for calculations of incidence rates, have varying levels of accuracy for different ethnic groups. Many national censuses give only estimations of ethnic minority populations and the size of the error can vary significantly by ethnic minority group. For example, the 1991 UK census underestimated the population by approximately 1 million people, and those not counted in this 'missing million' were disproportionately young, male and from ethnic minority groups. Further-more, in the UK census, respondents self-assign ethnicity to predetermined groups. However, in some studies, the ethnicity of incident cases is observer-assigned (e.g., Harrison *et al.*, 1997). Self-assigned and observer-assigned ethnicity may capture different people, so when studies use the latter, their numerator (number of cases of psychosis per ethnic group) is actually measuring a different group from their denominator (number of people in the defined population per ethnic group).

Ascertainment bias

Most incidence studies of psychosis measure first-admission or first-contact cases. This produces a number of challenges. For example, people from different ethnic and cultural groups with the same diagnosis follow different pathways to care, and the risk of an inpatient stay may vary (for a review see van Os and McKenzie,

2001). This may undermine the accuracy of estimates of incidence based on first admission (van Os and McKenzie, 2001). First contact studies, which include not only first-admission but also first-presentation cases to primary care and community mental health services, have been proffered as more accurate. However, there are no studies that allow estimation of any likely error rate one way or the other. In other words, incidence rates based on treated samples of cases may differ from the 'true' population incidence; if people from ethnic minority groups are more likely to come into contact with health services when they develop psychotic symptoms this could artificially increase the 'incidence' in these groups. There are no good data that allow us to estimate the consequent error.

Validity testing and the category fallacy

There is no doubt that psychosis is present across the world. However, quantifiable differences in the aetiology and course of psychosis in ethnic minority groups have been reported, and this brings into question whether, in cross-cultural incidence studies, like is being compared with like (Harrison *et al.*, 1999; McKenzie *et al.*, 2001). The cross-cultural validity of current categorical diagnoses, and the data collection tools based on them, has not been formally tested (Alarcón *et al.*, 2002). Though it is clear that well defined core symptoms of schizophrenia can be found everywhere in the world, if we argue that a particular aetiological insult, e.g., migration, could lead to an increased risk of psychosis, this may equally point to the possibility of new aetiologies or quantifiable differences in the balance of risk factors between groups. These could produce different rates of the same illness or new forms of the illness. Hence, the tools we use must not only be cross culturally valid, but must also be able to detect and differentiate new or atypical psychoses produced by new risk factors.

A critical review of the findings

The methodological problems should rightly make us cautious in interpreting cross-cultural incidence studies, but they do not negate them. Our aim has been to identify possible limitations so that we can be judicious in the way these findings are used to generate further hypotheses. So, turning to the research in more detail, what conclusions can be drawn? In addressing this question, as the best data are on schizophrenia, we will use this to illustrate the challenges posed by the current literature.

Migration and schizophrenia: a meta-analysis

Cantor-Graae and Selten (2005) recently conducted a meta-analysis of studies of schizophrenia and migration. Their criteria for inclusion were that studies:

(1) reported schizophrenia incidence rates for one or more migrant groups residing in a particular area or provided data so that such a calculation could be performed; (2) included a correction for age differences between groups or provided data that made this correction possible; and (3) were published in an English-language, peer-reviewed scientific journal. When there were two studies on the same ethnic minority groups in the same area in the same time period, only one study was chosen.

Eighteen studies were included. Of these, eight were first-contact studies (Bhugra *et al.*, 1997; Castle *et al.*, 1991; Goater *et al.*, 1999; Harrison *et al.*, 1988; Harrison *et al.*, 1997; Rwegellera, 1977; Selten *et al.*, 2001; Zolkowska *et al.*, 2001) and ten were first-admission studies (Cantor-Graae *et al.*, 2003; Cochrane and Bal, 1987; Dean *et al.*, 1981; Hitch and Clegg, 1980; Krupinski and Cochrane, 1980; McGovern and Cope, 1987; Selten and Sijben, 1994; Selten *et al.*, 1997; Thomas *et al.*, 1993; van Os *et al.*, 1996). Only five studies included more than 100 patients from migrant groups (Cantor-Graae *et al.*, 2003; Cochrane and Bal, 1987; Dean *et al.*, 1981; Krupinski and Cochrane, 1980; Selten *et al.*, 1997). Studies often combined ethnic groups (as defined above) and groups categorised by place of birth. Only one study was conducted outside Europe and this investigated European-born migrants to Australia (Krupinski and Cochrane, 1980). Two-thirds of the studies were from the UK (Bhugra *et al.*, 1997; Castle *et al.*, 1991; Cochrane and Bal, 1987; Dean *et al.*, 1981; Goater *et al.*, 1999; Harrison *et al.*, 1988; Harrison *et al.*, 1997; Hitch and Clegg, 1980; McGovern and Cope, 1987; Rwegellera, 1977; Thomas *et al.*, 1993; van Os *et al.*, 1996).

The most common group studied was people of Caribbean origin in the UK (Bhugra *et al.*, 1997; Castle *et al.*, 1991; Cochrane and Bal, 1987; Dean *et al.*, 1981; Harrison *et al.*, 1988; Harrison *et al.*, 1997; Hitch and Clegg, 1980; McGovern and Cope, 1987; Rwegellera, 1977; Thomas *et al.*, 1993; van Os *et al.*, 1996); the next most studied group was people of South Asian origin in the UK (Bhugra *et al.*, 1997; Cochrane and Bal 1987; Dean *et al.*, 1981; Goater *et al.*, 1999; Hitch and Clegg, 1980; Thomas *et al.*, 1993). These groups are a mixture of migrants, their children and their grandchildren, although the authors did distinguish between first and subsequent generations where possible. First-contact replication studies are reported for people of Caribbean origin, but only first-admission replication studies are reported for people of South Asian origin. Only four other groups were the focus of more than one incidence study, i.e., people who migrated to the Netherlands from Surinam, Dutch Antilles, Morocco and Turkey.

The meta-analysis of these studies produced a mean weighted relative risk for developing schizophrenia among first-generation migrants (40 estimates) of 2.7 (95% CI 2.3–3.2). In a separate analysis for second-generation migrants (7 estimates) the mean weighted relative risk was 4.5 (95% CI 1.5–13.1). However, this was based on 51 people from specific ethnic groups across 6 studies and 426 people of 'mixed' ethnicity (Cantor Graae and Selten, 2005). The findings of the meta-analysis, therefore, have to be treated with a degree of caution, given that the analyses conflated first-contact and first-admission samples and ethnic groups and groups categorised by place of birth. The review reports further comparisons of subgroups. These found elevated risks of first contact or admission for schizophrenia in migrants from developing versus developed countries (relative risk (RR) 3.3, 95% CI 2.8–3.9) and for migrants from areas where the majority of the population is black (RR 4.8, 95% CI 3.7–6.2) versus white and neither black nor white.

Psychosis and migration in the UK

The diversity of the migrant or ethnic minority groups and contexts that have been studied make it difficult to interpret the findings. Though there have been some studies of similar ethnic groups (e.g., African-Caribbeans in the UK) these have used different methodologies. This lack of methodological replication inspires caution.

The research is strongest for people of Caribbean and South Asian origin in the UK. However, there are still problems with this more robust body of research. First, these are complex groups, which include primary economic migrants, secondary migrants, refugees and asylum seekers. The 'South Asian' group, for example, includes people born in the UK as well as those born in Bangladesh, Sri Lanka, Pakistan and India, and includes Sikhs, Hindus, Muslims, Buddhists and Christians. People of Caribbean origin are also a diverse group, comprising those born in different Caribbean islands and their children born in the UK. This presents a considerable challenge in accurately measuring ethnic groups and in making sense of results. Second, most second-generation and all third-generation members of these groups are not migrants; they may form culturally distinct groups with different levels of exposure to their parents. Further confusion is generated by the fact that though most people today use the phrase 'second generation' to refer to the UK-born children of primary migrants, others have also included those born abroad who migrated when they were young in this category. Third, most studies are based in urban areas, which leaves out the minority of people from these groups who live in rural or semi-rural settings, who may have different risks of presenting with a psychosis. Fourth, as noted above, context is often not measured in these studies, which makes them difficult to compare. For instance, most of the ethnic minority groups investigated have only been in the UK in significant numbers for 50 years and are not, as yet, stable. Since the first incidence study, which was 30 years ago, groups are likely to have significantly changed. In general, they are likely to have become more integrated and more dispersed. The balance of first to subsequent generations has also changed. Fifth, many of the first contact studies are small, often with less than 40 patients from migrant groups (Goater *et al.*, 1999; Harrison *et al.*, 1997; Hitch and Clegg, 1980; Rwegellera, 1977; Thomas *et al.*, 1993; van Os *et al.*, 1996).

To address some of these problems, the ÆSOP study was set up (Fearon *et al.*, 2006). Specifically, ÆSOP aimed to clarify: (1) whether the rates of psychotic disorders other than schizophrenia are also increased in African-Caribbeans in the UK; (2) whether psychosis is also increased in other ethnic minority groups in the UK; and (3) whether particular age or sex groups are especially at risk. The study included all those aged 16–64 who presented to secondary mental health services with a first episode of psychosis over specified time periods in three well defined UK urban areas. Case finding took place over a two-year period in south-east London and Nottingham and over a nine-month period in Bristol, and 568 cases were identified. Standardised incidence rates for the main ethnic groups and incidence rate ratios (IRR), which compared rates for each ethnic minority group against a white British baseline group, were calculated for all major psychosis syndromes. Data from the 2001 UK census were used to estimate population denominators for each ethnic group. Remarkably high IRRs were found for both schizophrenia and mania in African-Caribbeans (schizophrenia: IRR 9.1; manic psychosis: IRR 8.0) and black Africans (schizophrenia: IRR 5.8; manic psychosis: IRR 6.2), findings that held in men and women. Incidence rates in other ethnic minority groups were more modestly increased (IRRs ranged from 1.4–3.5), as were rates for depressive psychosis and other psychoses in all minority groups (IRRs ranged from 0.8–5.6). These raised rates were evident in all age groups between 16 and 64 years. Fearon *et al.* (2006) concluded that ethnic minority groups are at increased risk of all psychotic illnesses, but that African-Caribbeans and black Africans appear to be at especially high risk of both schizophrenia and mania.

Criticisms remain, but it is difficult to dismiss these findings or those of the research to date (see Table 10.1 for a summary of recent studies). The methodological problems are mostly not quantified, but unless there are significant problems with the validity of categorisation it is difficult to see how they could account for such high increased rates. The most accurate conclusion, given our current state of knowledge, is that being of African or Caribbean origin in the UK confers an increased risk of contact with services for a psychotic illness and this is likely to reflect a true increased incidence.

Differences in incidence as a window to aetiology?

If it is accepted that there is an increased rate of psychosis in people of African and Caribbean origin in the UK, the question is why? Addressing this question also offers an opportunity to explore the causes of psychosis in general. Differences in incidence rates between groups within the same geographical areas provide a ready means of investigating possible aetiological factors.

Variations in incidence may arise for a number of reasons. For example, they may relate to differences in (1) the pattern, ascertainment or diagnosis of the disorder; (2) social contexts; (3) susceptibility to risk factors; or (4) the type of risk exposure or the action of protective factors (Rutter, 2002). When these differences are distributed on the basis of ethnicity, it may be that social and economic inequalities underpinned by racism are the fundamental cause of these observed disease variations (McKenzie, 2006). This conceivably applies to both physical and mental illness.

Genes or environment

One starting point is to consider whether the high rates of psychosis in the Caribbean population in the UK are acquired or genetically determined. Incidence studies in three Caribbean countries, from which the bulk of Caribbean migrants to the UK have come, found no evidence of markedly elevated rates compared with the UK white British population (Bhugra *et al.*, 1996; Hickling and Rodgers-Johnson, 1995; Mahy *et al.*, 1999) (see Table 10.1). Like the UK reports, these were all first-contact studies. This suggests that migrants coming to the UK do not come from places with particularly high rates of psychosis. It puts the focus on migration and the UK environment rather than on genetic risk. Furthermore, reports of a markedly increased morbid risk in the second generation (who have mostly not themselves migrated) moves the focus away from migration per se and more towards the presence of some specific risk-increasing factors, or conversely the loss of some protective factors, that operate in the UK environment (Sharpley *et al.*, 2001). However, this does not rule out the possibility of an increased genetic susceptibility that may only become apparent when there are sufficient environmental stressors.

Social factors

It is increasingly accepted that social factors are important in the genesis of psychotic disorders. Such factors include urbanicity, social isolation, disrupted familial environments in early childhood, language and cultural maladjustment, childhood abuse and persistent experiences of victimisation and discrimination (Sharpley *et al.*, 2001). The mechanisms through which these factors act are obscure. However, given the size of the rate increase in migrant groups and the relatively modest associations when risk factors are investigated singly, it is likely that they act synergistically or that their effects are magnified across the life course. Clearly, if we accept that psychosis has a physical basis then social factors must interact with genes and biological development in aetiology.

The three most often cited possible social reasons for increased rates of psychosis in migrant groups are socioeconomic factors, racism and the urban environment. Disentangling these three is difficult.

Socioeconomic factors and racism

Non-white groups in the UK, particularly those of African descent, endure significantly more social adversity than their white counterparts. Caribbean migrants with the same potential are more likely to be unemployed, live in poorer housing, do worse academically and are more likely to be excluded from school (e.g., Modood *et al.*, 1997).

The persistence of such disparities has been attributed to racial discrimination. Cross-sectional research has demonstrated an association between perceived racism and psychosis, and longitudinal research has reported an association between perceived discrimination and delusional ideation (Janssen *et al.*, 2003; Karlsen *et al.*, 2005). The association of perceived racism and discrimination with mental illness demonstrates how risk factors can interact at a number of levels. The perpetuation of socioeconomic disparities due to racism increases exposure to known risk factors for psychosis. But, at another level, the perception of racism and its experience in more than one domain could affect the victim's interaction with the world and self-perception in that world. At an individual level delusions are more common in those who have suffered discrimination, and at a community level psychotic symptoms are more common in groups such as African-Caribbeans who are subject to racism (Janssen *et al.*, 2003; Johns and van Os, 2001). Could these multilevel associations explain why the rates of schizophrenia in those who migrate from predominantly black countries to white countries is significantly greater than the risk for those who migrate from predominantly white countries to other predominantly white countries?

Urban environment

Over 90% of the African and Caribbean population in the UK live in urban environments. This may be independently important in the increased risk of psychosis in this population.

The role of the urban environment in increasing the risk for psychosis continues to be suggested as a possible explanation for variations in the incidence of schizophrenia (see Chapter 6). The inability to pinpoint a specific risk factor that defines urbanicity may indicate a confluence of factors that characterise the urban environment. For migrant groups it may be that the rate of social and population change is more acute in urban environments, causing an instability in the norms that allow people to ground themselves in a novel environment (Hutchinson and Morgan, 2004). This may be the origin of the difficulty in person–environment fit described by van Os *et al.* (2000). A different scenario might be one in which the host culture is more rigid and resistant to post-modern city life in general and does not welcome 'multi-cultural migrants' who are seen to promote the rapid social change that cities represent. Social isolation is frequently a characteristic of city life. The absence of social support that facilitates resilience in the face of the challenges of life could be an important risk factor in psychosis.

A synthesis

There are many ways that these social factors could work in concert to increase rates of psychosis in the population of African and Caribbean origin in the UK. The increased incidence could rise from the potentiation of risk by social and economic difficulties encountered in the UK, and from a disruption of family networks and perceived discrimination. The disruption would be magnified in the second generation for a number of reasons: they would not have had the early grounding that their parents had, they would be more attached to the UK and so thwarted aspirations would be felt more keenly, as would continuing social and developmental adversity experienced in education. Second and subsequent generations also have to cope with both a higher familial liability due to increased psychosis rates in the first generation and other risk factors, such as poverty, and a loss of protective factors, such as socially supportive networks (Krabbendam and van Os, 2005). Similar processes may be operating to a similar or lesser degree in all migrant and ethnic minority groups.

Interaction of risk factors

However, it is likely that a more complex model is needed. The major explanatory model is the vulnerability–stress model. Vulnerability is classically considered to be genetic, but it could equally arise from a range of developmental templates, both biological and social, while the stress can be founded on any subsequent physical, chemical or social adversity.

There is evidence that those predisposed to psychosis and who subsequently develop the disorder exhibit more socially maladaptive behaviour during childhood, including social anxiety, social withdrawal and problems socialising with peers and siblings, leading to greater social isolation (Glatt *et al.*, 2006). People who develop psychosis are also likely to experience more victimising experiences, including childhood abuse (see Chapter 7). However, it is unclear which comes first; the behaviour or the victimisation. It might be that people who develop psychosis have more social adversity across their life course, but the impact of this social adversity is likely to be informed by the state of one's social environment. Such social adversity includes life events and daily chronic hassles (see Chapter 9), which may be more common among those from ethnic minority groups and those of low socioeconomic class. Other relevant forms of social adversity may include increased social isolation and early separation from parents (Morgan *et al.*, 2007). Further, the finding that the risk of psychosis increases for African-Caribbeans when they live in environments where they comprise a smaller proportion of the population may reflect the impact of perceived social isolation (Boydell *et al.*, 2001). Indeed, it may be that the same life events have a more disruptive and damaging impact because of perceived helplessness or a lack of proximal social support. All of this suggests a need for alternative ways of measuring the impact of life experiences in groups living in diverse social contexts. The wider context has to be factored into analyses. This points to a need for multilevel studies, as the determinants of variations in risk between individuals within a population may be very different from the determinants of variations across populations (see Chapter 4).

An additional consideration is substance use, which may amplify the predisposition to psychosis in the absence of some protective social factors. Over 40% of the first admissions to a general hospital psychiatric unit in Trinidad were substance-use related (Hutchinson and Murray, 2006). However, there is little evidence of increased substance misuse among young UK African-Caribbeans.

Finally, there is the ambivalence of identity and belonging described by Naipaul (Naipaul, 1987), which may also be passed on to the children of Caribbean migrants. This might affect their perception of any negative experiences. This ambivalence has been described as a disturbance in racial identification and as a direct outcome of the historical relationship between the UK and the English speaking Caribbean (Hickling and Hutchinson, 1999). Further research needs to evaluate the healthy population to determine the presence of risk factors for psychosis and to characterise phenomenologically the tendency for Caribbean subjects to experience psychotic-like symptoms.

Sociodevelopmental model of psychosis

A sociodevelopmental model would suggest that ongoing negative social experiences, acting on a template of social deprivation and urbanicity, cause changes in social adjustment which predispose to further negative social experiences and which ultimately result in psychosis. The challenge is to identify the factors within and outside of the individual that mediate such a long-term outcome. The relevance of experience expectant programming or experience adaptive programming in brain development will also have to be considered in this context (Rutter, 2002). How psychosocial insults impact on gene function to increase vulnerability, or conversely resilience, is being investigated and there are signs that, for example, absence of maternal attachment can predispose to negative brain changes during development, leading to the expression of mental disorder in adolescence and adulthood. This has been described as the pathology of experience (Frith, 2004). The ways in which migrant communities are vulnerable to psychosis across generations offers the opportunity to clarify these gene–environment interactions in the genesis of psychosis.

Other factors that are applicable in this context are high levels of early family disruption and separation from primary caregivers (Morgan *et al.*, 2007), which inevitably lead to a lack of support in the context of a hostile environment. Perceived and real victimisation, and the problems of parents battling with decreased economic and social opportunity, mean that children often grow up with an acute sense of their own vulnerability in the presence of hostile non-accommodating environments. This is further reinforced by their own interaction with symbols of societal authority and expressed in the inability to establish income or social equity.

It is possible to speculate about the impacts of this on the individual. The impact on cognition, memory and the way in which experiences are deemed to be salient are all consistent with the hypothesis that accumulated experience can orient the thinking of individuals in ways that predispose to psychosis and, indeed, are amenable to psychological intervention. The interpretation of reality allows for a re-expression in ways that may be perceived to be socially maladaptive, which in turn may increase the risk of, and sensitivity to, persecution. It also increases vulnerability to the negative sequelae of substance abuse and the social unease that lead to more conflictual and, therefore, more negative life events.

This offers the beginnings of a model that can help shape and focus the next generation of research studies that seek to investigate the high rates of psychosis in migrant and ethnic minority populations.

Conclusions

Despite the methodological problems outlined above, it is reasonable to assume that migrant groups have an increased risk of developing psychotic disorders, especially schizophrenia. There may be no specific increased biological vulnerability, but cumulative negative social experience may be important. On an individual level, this may affect cognition and the application of salience in a way that predisposes to ongoing social unease and establishes a continuum from healthy paranoia to persecutory ideation and referential ideation that ends in psychotic behaviour and presentations to mental health services.

The implications of such a model are profound. It suggests that the prevention of psychosis in adulthood would lie with improved social and mental health services for children, an expansion of, and institutional support for, social networks, and an increased cultural sensitivity to difference. The education system would have to be sensitised to these issues so that children can teach their parents to be less alienated as well as causing the white majority to be more tolerant. This would result in less discrimination and racism and less coercion in social interactions. It would also lead to less deviant behaviour among those who currently feel disenfranchised, and would achieve a balance of holistic mental health.

REFERENCES

Alarcón, R. D., Alegria, M., Bell, C. C. *et al.* (2002). Beyond the funhouse mirrors: research agenda on culture and psychiatric diagnosis. In *A Research Agenda for DSMV*, ed. D. J. Kupfer, M. B. First and D. A. Regier. Washington, DC: APA, pp. 219–82.

Bhugra, D. and Jones, P. (2001). Migration and mental illness. *Advances in Psychiatric Treatment*, **7**, 216–23.

Bhugra, D., Hilwig, M., Hosein, B. *et al.* (1996). First contact incidence rates of schizophrenia in Trinidad and one year follow-up. *British Journal of Psychiatry*, **169**, 587–92.

Bhugra, D., Leff, J., Mallett, R. *et al.* (1997). Incidence and outcome of schizophrenia in whites, African-Caribbeans and Asians in London. *Psychological Medicine*, **27**, 791–8.

Boydell, J., van Os, J., McKenzie, K. *et al.* (2001). Incidence of schizophrenia in ethnic minorities in London: ecological study into interactions with environment. *British Medical Journal*, **323** (7325), 1336–8.

Cantor-Graae, E. and Selten, J. P. (2005). Schizophrenia and migration: a meta-analysis and review. *American Journal of Psychiatry*, **162** (1), 12–24.

Cantor-Graae, E., Pedersen, C. B., McNeil, T. F. *et al.* (2003). Migration as a risk factor for schizophrenia: a Danish population based cohort study. *British Journal of Psychiatry*, **182**, 117–22.

Castle, D., Wessely, S., Der, G. *et al.* (1991). The incidence of operationally defined schizophrenia in Camberwell, 1965–84. *British Journal of Psychiatry*, **159**, 790–4.

Cochrane, R. and Bal, S. S. (1987). Migration and schizophrenia: an examination of five hypotheses. *Social Psychiatry*, **22**, 181–91.

Dean, G., Walsh, D., Downing, H. *et al.* (1981). First admissions of native-born and immigrants to psychiatric hospitals in south-east England, 1976. *British Journal of Psychiatry*, **139**, 506–12.

Fearon, P. and Morgan, C. (2006). Environmental factors in schizophrenia: the role of migrant studies. *Schizophrenia Bulletin*, **32**, 405–8.

Fearon, P., Kirkbride, J. K., Morgan, C. *et al.* (2006). Incidence of schizophrenia and other psychoses in ethnic minority groups: results from the MRC ÆSOP study. *Psychological Medicine*, **36** (11), 1541–50.

Fernando, S. (1991). *Mental Health, Race and Culture*. London: Macmillan.

Frith, C. (2004). The pathology of experience. *Brain*, **127**, 239–42.

Glatt, S. J., Stone, W. S., Faraone, S. V. *et al.* (2006). Psychopathology, personality traits and social development of young first degree relatives of patients with schizophrenia. *British Journal of Psychiatry*, **189**, 337–45.

Goater, N., King, M., Cole, E. *et al.* (1999). Ethnicity and outcome of psychosis. *British Journal of Psychiatry*, **175**, 34–42.

Harrison, G., Owens, D., Holton, A. *et al.* (1988). A prospective study of severe mental disorder in Afro-Caribbean patients. *Psychological Medicine*, **18**, 643–57.

Harrison, G., Glazebrook, C., Brewin, J. *et al.* (1997). Increased incidence of psychotic disorders in migrants from the Caribbean to the United Kingdom. *Psychological Medicine*, **27**, 799–806.

Harrison, G., Amin, S., Singh, S. P. *et al.* (1999). Outcome of psychosis in people of African-Caribbean family origin. *British Journal of Psychiatry*, **175**, 43–9.

Hickling, F. W. and Hutchinson, G. (1999). Roast breadfruit psychosis. *Psychiatric Bulletin*, **23**, 132–4.

Hickling, F. W. and Rodgers-Johnson, P. (1995). The incidence of first contact schizophrenia in Jamaica. *British Journal of Psychiatry*, **167**, 193–6.

Hitch, P. J. and Clegg, P. (1980). Modes of referral of overseas immigrant and native born first admissions to psychiatric hospital. *Social Science and Medicine*, **14A**, 369–74.

Hutchinson, G. and Morgan, C. (2004). Social development, urban environment and psychosis. *British Journal of Psychiatry*, **186**, 76–7.

Hutchinson, G. and Murray, R. (2006). Risk factors for first-episode schizophrenia in Trinidad and Tobago. *Schizophrenia Research*, **81** (suppl.), 238.

Jablensky, A., Sartorius, N., Ernberg, G. *et al.* (1992). Schizophrenia: manifestations, incidence and course in different cultures. A World Health Organization ten-country study. *Psychological Medicine. Monograph Supplement*, **20**, 1–97.

Janssen, I., Hanssen, M., Bak, M. *et al.* (2003). Discrimination and delusional ideation. *British Journal of Psychiatry*, **182**, 71–6.

Jenkins, R. (1986). Social anthropological models of inter-ethnic relations. In *Theories of Race and Ethnic Relations*, ed. J. Rex and D. Mason. Cambridge: Cambridge University Press, pp. 170–86.

Johns, L. C. and van Os, J. (2001). The continuity of psychotic experiences in the general population. *Clinical Psychology Review*, **21** (8), 1125–41.

Jones, J. S. (1981). How different are human races? *Nature*, **293**, 188–90.

Karlsen, S., Nazroo, J., McKenzie, K. *et al.* (2005). Racism, psychosis and common mental disorder among ethnic minority groups in England. *Psychological Medicine*, **35** (12), 1795–803.

King, M., Coker, E., Leavey, G. *et al.* (1994). Incidence of psychotic illness in London: comparison of ethnic minority groups. *British Medical Journal*, **309**, 1115–19.

Krabbendam, L. and van Os, J. (2005). Schizophrenia and urbanicity: a major environmental influence – conditional on genetic risk. *Schizophrenia Bulletin*, **31** (4), 795–9.

Krupinski, J. and Cochrane, R. (1980). Migration and mental health – a comparative study. *Journal of Intercultural Studies*, **1**, 49–57.

Leech, K. (1989). *A Question in Dispute: The Debate About an 'Ethnic' Question in the Census.* Runnymede research report. London: Runnymede Trust.

Mahy, G. E., Mallett, R., Leff, J. *et al.* (1999). First contact incidence rate of schizophrenia in Barbados. *British Journal of Psychiatry*, **175**, 28–33.

McGovern, D. and Cope, R. (1987). First psychiatric admission rates of first and second generation Afro-Caribbeans. *Social Psychiatry*, **22**, 139–49.

McGrath, J., Saha, S., Wellham, J. *et al.* (2004). A systematic review of the incidence of schizophrenia: the distribution of rates and the influence of sex, urbanicity, migrant status, and methodology. *BMC Medicine*, **2**, 13.

McKenzie, K. (2006). Racial discrimination and mental health. *Psychiatry*, **5** (11), 383–7.

McKenzie, K. and Crowcroft, N. S. (1994). Race, ethnicity, culture and science. *British Medical Journal*, **309**, 286–7.

McKenzie, K., Samele, C., van Horn, E. *et al.* (2001). A comparison of the course and treatment of psychosis in patients of Caribbean origin and British whites. *British Journal of Psychiatry*, **178**, 160–5.

Modood, T., Berthoud, R., Lakey, J. *et al.* (1997). *Ethnic Minorities in Britain: Diversity and Disadvantage*. London: Policy Studies Institute.

Morgan, C., Kirkbride, J., Leff, J. *et al.* (2007). Parental separation, loss and psychosis in different ethnic groups: a case-control study. *Psychological Medicine*, **37** (4), 495–505.

Naipaul, V. S. (1987). *The Enigma of Arrival*. London: Alfred A. Knopf.

Ödegaard, Ö. (1932). Emigration and insanity. *Acta Psychiatrica et Neurologica Scandinavica*, **7** (suppl. 4), 1–206.

Rutter, M. (2002). The interplay of nature, nurture and developmental influences. *Archives of General Psychiatry*, **59**, 996–1000.

Rwegellera, G. G. (1977). Psychiatric morbidity among West Africans and West Indians living in London. *Psychological Medicine*, **7**, 317–29.

Selten, J. P. and Sijben, N. (1994). First admission rates for schizophrenia in immigrants to the Netherlands. *Social Psychiatry and Psychiatric Epidemiology*, **29**, 71–7.

Selten, J. P., Slaets, J. P. J. and Kahn, R. S. (1997). Schizophrenia in Surinamese and Dutch Antillean immigrants to the Netherlands: evidence of an increased incidence. *Psychological Medicine*, **27**, 807–11.

Selten, J. P., Veen, N., Feller, W. *et al.* (2001). Incidence of psychotic disorders in immigrant groups to the Netherlands. *British Journal of Psychiatry*, **178**, 367–72.

Selten, J. P., Cantor-Graae, E., Slaets, J. *et al.* (2002). Ödegaard's selection hypothesis revisited: schizophrenia in Surinamese immigrants to the Netherlands. *American Journal of Psychiatry*, **159**, 669–71.

Sharpley, M., Hutchinson, G., McKenzie, K. J. *et al.* (2001). Understanding the excess of psychosis among the African Caribbean population in England. Review of the current hypotheses. *British Journal of Psychiatry*, **178** (suppl. 40), s60–s68.

Thomas, C. S., Stone, K., Osborn, M. *et al.* (1993). Psychiatric morbidity and compulsory admission among UK-born Europeans, Afro-Caribbeans and Asians in central Manchester. *British Journal of Psychiatry*, **163**, 91–9.

van Os, J. and McKenzie, K. (2001). Cultural differences in pathways to care and service use. In *New Oxford Textbook of Psychiatry*, ed. M. Gelder, J. Lopez-Ibor and N. Andreasen. London: Oxford University Press, pp. 1899–904.

van Os, J., Castle, D. J., Takei, N. *et al.* (1996). Psychotic illness in ethnic minorities: clarification from the 1991 census. *Psychological Medicine*, **26**, 203–8.

van Os, J., Driessen, G., Gunther, N. *et al.* (2000). Neighbourhood variation in incidence of schizophrenia – evidence for person-environment interaction. *British Journal of Psychiatry*, **176**, 243–8.

Zolkowska, K., Cantor-Graae, E. and McNeil, T. F. (2001). Increased risk of psychosis among immigrants to Sweden: is migration a risk factor for psychosis? *Psychological Medicine*, **21**, 669–778.

Part III

Social factors and the outcome of psychosis

11

Social factors as a basis for treatment

Richard Warner

Introduction

Service delivery programmes in psychiatry are usually developed as a solution to a specific problem. Assertive community treatment, for example, was devised by Stein and Test (1980) as an answer to the hospital revolving-door problem that resulted from the radical deinstitutionalisation that took place in the USA in the 1960s. The psychosocial clubhouse was developed as a solution to the boredom and social exclusion that many people with mental illness experience when they achieve a stable existence in the community (Beard *et al.*, 1982). The specificity of the programme models as solutions to contextual problems explains why different psychosocial treatment models have been successful in different systems of care at different times.

For this reason, it is useful to explore how social difficulties have led to different treatment and rehabilitation solutions, and how they might lead to new treatment approaches in the future. Let me list some of the social problems that people with mental illness confront:

- *Unemployment*   Only 10–20% of people with serious mental illness in most Western countries are employed (Marwaha and Johnson, 2004).
- *Poverty*   Most people with mental illness must survive on disability benefits, below the poverty level.
- *Homelessness*   The proportion of people with psychosis among the homeless in Britain and the USA varies depending on the population selected, but ranges around 10–30% (Warner, 2004).
- *Incarceration*   The proportion of those in jail who suffer from a psychosis in Britain and the USA is around 10%, and, in Britain, is increasing (Warner, 2004).
- *Isolation*   Many people with mental illness have few social contacts or supports.
- *Powerlessness*   The lack of control over many aspects of their lives worsens the course of illness for people with mental illness.

Society and Psychosis, ed. Craig Morgan, Kwame McKenzie and Paul Fearon. Published by Cambridge University Press. © Cambridge University Press 2008.

• *Stigma*   People with mental illness are subject to stigma and discrimination in hiring, accommodation and participation in the larger community (see Chapter 12).

Many programmes have been developed or proposed to solve these problems. To illustrate these, this chapter will focus on unemployment, poverty, homelessness, incarceration and isolation (see Chapter 12 for a discussion on stigma).

Unemployment

For many people with mental illness, and their friends and family members, work is a fundamental measure of recovery. A job can bring increased income, expanded social contacts and a sense of meaning in life, while unemployment carries risks of alienation, apathy, substance abuse, physical ill-health and isolation (Bond, 2004; Warr, 1987). In recent decades, however, rates of employment for people with psychosis enrolled in treatment in the USA and most European countries have rarely exceeded 10–20% (Marwaha and Johnson, 2004). Over the years, there have been several obstacles to employment for people with mental illness – periods of high general unemployment; ineffective vocational rehabilitation programmes; disincentives to employment fostered by disability pension systems; and the stigma of mental illness, leading to hiring discrimination. People with mental illness themselves may hold back from working, or family members or therapists may discourage it. The stereotype of schizophrenia breeds the assumption, accepted even by those afflicted with the illness, that work is not feasible. In a sample of Colorado residents with schizophrenia interviewed by me in 2005, 84% reported that they had held back from applying for work because of their diagnosis, 50% to a great extent.

Disincentives to employment

Fifty to sixty percent of people with psychosis are capable of work in the competitive workforce, as evidenced by various observations. In northern Italian cities in the mid-1990s, 50% or more of people with schizophrenia were working, 20–25% of them full-time (Warner *et al.*, 1998). This is due, in part, to the fact that Italian disability benefits impose fewer work disincentives. In studies of supported employment programmes for people with serious mental illness in the USA, moreover, 50–60% of participants routinely achieve competitive employment. In a recent study in Chennai, India, 67% of people with chronic schizophrenia were employed, mostly in mainstream jobs (Srinivasan and Tirupati, 2005), and in another 20-year follow-up of men with schizophrenia in Madras (now Chennai), 76% were employed (Thara, 2004). Clearly, it is not psychosis per se which imposes high rates of idleness, but the economic system. People with mental illness in the developed world face significant financial disincentives to work if they are receiving disability benefits (Rosenheck *et al.*, 2006; Warner, 2000). These disincentives are more severe in Britain and the USA than in Italy, with the result that a much smaller proportion of people with mental illness are employed in these English-speaking countries.

Disability pension systems can be designed to minimise disincentives. In the USA there are two major governmental disability support programmes – Supplemental Security Income (SSI) and Social Security Disability Income (SSDI). Under both programmes, support payments decline when people accept employment. Recipients of SSI lose 50 cents of benefits for each dollar earned when earnings exceed a small amount. Recipients of SSDI lose nothing until they earn a much greater amount, but then lose it all. In practice, SSDI creates fewer disincentives to work, as recipients continue to collect the full benefit as long as they don't earn too much.

In Britain, disincentives are worse, as disabled people run the risk of losing all their incapacity benefit if they earn more than a small weekly amount, and an earnings disregard is permitted for only a few months. Since a full benefits package is worth significantly more than a full-time minimum-wage job, there is little financial incentive for the psychiatrically disabled in Britain to work part-time or full-time (Grove *et al.*, 2004). Attempts have been made to alleviate disincentives in the UK. One measure allows a person to retain benefits if the job ends within a year, and another tops up incomes for those who earn only a little. Nevertheless, fewer than 5% of those receiving incapacity benefit for two years return to the labour market (Grove *et al.*, 2004).

In Italy, work disincentives are less severe than in the USA or Britain because (1) fewer people with mental illness qualify for benefits and (2) Italian disabled people often manage to retain benefits while working. The Italian disability pension is substantially lower than in Britain, but this is not the critical issue – to receive the benefit the person must be 80% disabled (Fioritti, 2004). A system like this is only possible because 80–90% of Italians with psychosis are living with, and being supported by, their families (Warner, 2000). The lack of formal income support for many people with mental illness increases the incentive to make use of the work opportunities, which are often quite comprehensive, for people with mental illness in Italy, especially in the north. Beyond these formal system features, however, many Italians who receive disability benefits continue to work in the 'black market' labour force – along the beaches in summer and on family farms (Fioritti, 2004).

Econometric labour-supply models (Moffit, 1990) can forecast the effects of changes in benefits policy. Averett *et al.* (1999) gathered economic information from over 200 people with psychosis in Colorado and examined the result of modifying SSI regulations. The model revealed that increasing the earnings disregard or offering a wage subsidy led to increased hours of work.

A simpler answer is to advise clients about the remedies that are already in place to ease disincentives. Grove *et al.* (2004) report success in Britain with the use of personal advisors who provide clients with information about return-to-work benefits. Tremblay and colleagues (2006), in the USA, demonstrated that people with psychiatric disabilities who were provided with benefits counselling improved their income by $1250 a year more than control subjects. Where benefits counsellors are not available, case managers can be trained to understand benefits regulations well enough to help clients make good decisions about work and income.

Supported employment

Vocational programmes were unsuccessful in improving long-term employment outcomes for people with psychosis until the 1970s (Bond, 1992; Lehman, 1995). Traditional 'train and place' vocational services designed for people with physical disabilities have proven ineffective for people with serious mental illness (Noble *et al.*, 1997; US General Accounting Office, 1993), but, in the 1970–80s, vocational programmes designed for people with psychiatric disorders were successful in placing clients in sheltered jobs or transitional employment positions, and in helping them hold down those jobs. With the introduction of supported employment in the 1990s, competitive, mainstream employment became a viable option for people with mental illness.

Transitional employment programmes (TEPs), developed in the 1970s, were the precursors of supported employment. In a TEP, a job coach locates a job in a local business, learns how to do it, trains a client with mental illness and places him or her in the position for a limited period, usually six months. The worker is supported on the job by the coach and can attend weekly support meetings. If the disabled person cannot work for any reason the job coach will find someone else to work that day. The principle behind TEP is that the disabled person learns basic job skills in a transitional position that will help him or her get a permanent, unsupported job in the competitive marketplace. In fact, research does not support the belief that TEP workers are more likely to secure competitive employment (Lehman, 1995). For the person with a mental illness, a supported employment model – similar to the TEP approach except that the job is permanent – is more suitable.

A refinement of the supported employment model has been named individual placement and support (IPS). Bond has outlined several evidence-based principles of this approach (Bond, 1998; Bond, 2004):

- Eligibility is based on consumer choice. No clients are excluded because of a poor prior work record, or lack of 'work readiness'. People with mental illness have better outcomes in supported employment regardless of diagnosis, substance abuse or prior frequency of hospitalisation (McGurk and Mueser, 2003; Sengupta *et al.*, 1998).

- Integration of vocational rehabilitation and mental health services. Supported employment programmes are more likely to be successful if vocational and clinical staff coordinate their activities (Drake *et al.*, 2003; Gowdy *et al.*, 2003).
- Rapid job search and placement. Eight of nine randomised controlled studies demonstrate better work outcomes for clients who embark on rapid job search and placement instead of being offered vocational assessment, training and counselling (Bond, 2004).
- Attention to the mentally ill person's preferences. Matching the person to the job on such preferences as type of work and hours results in higher rates of job placement and longer job tenure (Becker *et al.*, 1998).
- Continuous assessment and support. Sustained employment is more likely for clients who receive ongoing support (McHugo *et al.*, 1998).

Eleven US randomised controlled studies have all shown substantial advantages for supported employment, with competitive employment rates in the supported employment cohorts averaging 60% and in the control groups 21% (Bond, 2004). Studies of the effectiveness of converting six New England day programmes to supported employment found similar results (Becker *et al.*, 2001; Drake *et al.*, 1996; Gold and Marrone, 1998). A recent British study of supported employment for people recovering from their first episode of psychosis demonstrated an increase in employment from 10% to 41% (Rinaldi *et al.*, 2004).

Social firms

An alternative vocational model is gaining ground in Europe. Social firms, or affirmative businesses, as they are known in North America, are businesses created with a dual mission – to employ people with disabilities and to provide a needed product or service. The model was developed for people with psychiatric disabilities in Italy in the 1970s and, by diffusion, has gained prominence in Europe. Principles of the model include: (1) over a third of employees are people with a disability or labour-market disadvantage, (2) every worker is paid a fair-market wage, and (3) the business operates subsidy-free. Independent of European influence, social firms have also developed in Canada, the USA, Japan and elsewhere.

The first European social firm was developed as a worker-cooperative for ex-hospital-patients in 1973 in Trieste in north-eastern Italy. The business provided employment in cleaning public buildings (Dell'Acqua and Dezza, 1985). By 2004, the annual income of the Trieste cooperatives had reached $14 million and several additional social cooperatives had been established by non-governmental agencies. The Hotel Tritone, one of the original social firms, has proven particularly successful and a franchising venture is planned. All office-cleaning and street-cleaning contracts for the municipality of Trieste are currently awarded to social firms. Other enterprises include shopping for the homebound, landscaping and bookbinding. The businesses employ a workforce of disabled or disadvantaged and non-disadvantaged workers in a 50:50 proportion (Warner, 2004). About 300 disabled or disadvantaged people, half with mental illness, are employed in the Trieste cooperatives earning a full market wage, and another 180 people with mental illness hold training positions reimbursed by governmental stipend. The model has diffused widely in Italy (Warner, 2004; www.cefec.org).

In the last decade, there has been an increase in interest in social firms in Europe, partly due to the transfer of technology fostered by support organisations in Italy and elsewhere. By 2005 there were over 8000 social firms in Europe with about 80 000 workers, 30 000 of whom had psychiatric or other disabilities (Seyfried and Ziomas, 2005). The largest number of social firms outside Italy is in Germany. In 2005 there were over 500 such companies with a combined workforce of 16 500, producing foods, technical products or services such as moving and house painting. Typically, 30% of German social firm income is derived from government wage supplements for disabled workers (Seyfried and Ziomas, 2005; Stastny, P., Gelman, R. and Mayo, H. *The European Experience with Social Firms in the Rehabilitation of Persons with Psychiatric Disabilities*. Unpublished report, Albert Einstein College of Medicine, 1992). Prior to 1997 there were just six social firms in Britain. Since then, with the assistance of the support group, Social Firms UK, the number has grown to 49, plus 70 'emerging' social firms. In 2005, British social firms were employing over 1500 people, two-thirds being disabled, mostly with mental disabilities. Catering and horticulture, the largest business sectors, accounted for 13% of operations (www.socialfirms.co.uk; Grove, R., personal communication). Several social firms have been developed in Sweden (Seyfried and Ziomas, 2005), the Netherlands, Spain and Greece (Schwartz and Higgins, 1999).

The success of individual social firms is enhanced by locating the right market niche, selecting labour-intensive products, building up the public orientation of the business and forming links with treatment services. The growth of the social-firm movement is aided by an advantageous legal framework for the businesses, policies favouring employment of the disabled and support entities that facilitate technology transfer. Advantages of the social-firm model include opportunities for empowerment, the development of a sense of community in the workplace and worker commitment resulting from the organisation's social mission.

Poverty

In most developed countries a large proportion of people with serious mental illness live in poverty. In the 1990s in Canada, for example, 27% of adults with mental illness were living in poverty, more than double the rate for non-disabled people, and the proportion of people with serious mental illness was undoubtedly much greater (Wilton, 2004). Income from disability benefits in the USA and Canada is routinely below poverty levels. Norwegians with mental illness report that poverty, unemployment and substandard living conditions are among their greatest obstacles to recovery (Borg *et al.*, 2005). In Ontario, interviews with people with mental illness reveal that chronic poverty leads to disturbances of social and family relations, leisure and self-esteem (Wilton, 2004). Poverty limits the disabled person's ability to find decent housing in a safe neighbourhood (Carling and Curtis, 1997) and restricts opportunities to develop social networks (Nelson *et al.*, 2001). Living in poverty also appears to worsen outcome from illness. It is associated, for example, with increased demand for inpatient psychiatric care (Abas *et al.*, 2003), and, while poverty and substance abuse are not necessarily related, poverty often increases the degree of harm that occurs at any given level of substance use (Room, 2005).

Poverty traps people with mental illness into inadequate housing or homelessness, low quality health care, poor educational attainment, increased risks of committing a crime or becoming a victim of crime and restricted employment prospects (Draine *et al.*, 2002). These factors worsen the quality of life and outcome from illness for people with psychiatric problems. Treating the mental illness adequately will not necessarily protect them from negative consequences; it is necessary also to respond to the problem of poverty. Commentators have suggested a number of social policy changes: better income support, more employment accommodations and enhanced supports to reduce the risk of criminal behaviour (Draine *et al.*, 2002). Another option is the economic development approach outlined here.

An economic development approach

People with serious mental illness are an economically disadvantaged group with reservoirs of untapped productive capacity and consumer power, but their economic power can be turned to their advantage, creating employment opportunities and improving their social and financial welfare. An evaluation of the economic life of a group of people with serious mental illness in Colorado in 1992 found that their total consumption – the combination of their cash expenses and the non-cash income of goods and services with which they were provided – was considerable, at over $2000 a month (£1300 in 1992). The top four areas of consumption were: psychiatric treatment ($1116 a month), rent ($295), food and prepared meals ($179), and medication ($90). Reviewing these data, economists might suggest a number of consumer-employing enterprises that could be developed that would serve people with mental illness and exploit their consumption power, for example, (1) employing people with mental illness within the treatment system, (2) housing cooperatives, (3) food cooperatives or (4) a consumer-oriented pharmacy (Warner and Polak, 1995). Some of these options have, in fact, proven feasible; two will be presented here.

Employing consumers in the psychiatric service system

A Denver-based group, the Regional Assessment and Training Center, developed a programme to train people with serious mental illness to become case-manager aides, residential facility staff and job coaches in the mental health centres across Colorado. The programme closed recently after 20 years of operation, during which time it enrolled trainees – people who had made good recoveries from mental illness – in six weeks of classroom education and then placed them in on-the-job internships for three months, working in community mental health teams. Graduates were hired throughout the mental health system at standard rates of pay. As case manager aides they helped their clients with a variety of tasks, such as applying for welfare entitlements and finding housing, and coun-selling them around issues of day-to-day living (Sherman and Porter, 1991). Well over a hundred consumer mental health workers have been placed in employment throughout the service system, providing models of successful recovery from mental illness for patients and staff alike. Two-thirds of the trainees continue to be successfully employed in the mental health system two years after graduation. The programme has been replicated in several cities and states across the USA.

In many mental health services, increasing numbers of consumers are being employed in a variety of roles. Around 10% of the workforce of the Pathfinder Trust in London are people with mental illness. At the Mental Health Center of Boulder County, in Colorado, consumers are employed as therapists, case man-ager aides, residential counsellors, job coaches, psychosocial clubhouse staff, office workers, consumer organisers and research interviewers. A mental health agency can also shift services that are currently contracted to outside enterprises (such as courier services or medical record transcription) to a consumer enterprise. In 1993, the mental health agency in Boulder started a property repair business to maintain the agency's buildings and residences, employing a non-disabled fore-man and a number of part-time consumer workers.

A consumer-oriented pharmacy

In 2002, a consumer-oriented pharmacy was opened at the Mental Health Center of Boulder County with the intent of providing employment and other benefits to the agency's clients. Four consumers are employed as pharmacy technicians alongside three pharmacists. Pharmacy profits, amounting to nearly $200 000 (£105 000) a year, are used to support other rehabilitation programmes. Customers and staff receive more education from the pharmacist on the effects of medication than they would from a high-street pharmacy, pharmacy services are much better coordinated with treatment services and prices are low. The model is now being franchised.

Homelessness

In the early 1980s, around half of inner-city homeless men in New York City, Los Angeles, Philadelphia, Boston and St. Louis were found to be suffering from psychosis, their numbers swollen by former state hospital patients who were receiving inadequate community services. Since then, the average proportion of homeless men suffering from psychosis has dropped to about a quarter (Warner, 2004). Advocates point to economic factors, such as low disability benefits, which inflate the proportion of disabled among the homeless (National Coalition for the Homeless, 1999). In 14 US states and 69 cities, the total disability pension is less than the fair-market rent for a one-bedroom apartment (Kaufman, 1997).

The number of homeless in Britain doubled during the 1980s, but the proportion of the homeless with psychosis remained high at around 20–40%. Observers complained that the expansion of community mental health services had failed to keep pace with hospital closures. A 1990 study of homeless mentally ill people in Britain revealed that a large majority had been discharged from hospital without any discussion of their housing needs (Medical Campaign Project, 1990). Some reduction in the proportion of mentally ill among homeless British men, to 10–15%, was noted in the 1990s, though the proportion among homeless women remained very high (Warner, 2004).

Apartments and supervision

Cooperative apartments, or group homes, work well for people with long-term mental illness leaving mental hospital after several years and for younger mentally ill clients. Group living offers a substitute family to those who have difficulty setting up a stable family or living with relatives. For those who are volatile, disruptive or subject to relapse, supervision is often required. By providing increasing amounts of staff support on the premises, it is possible to develop a range of community living arrangements for clients with progressively lower levels of functioning.

Some residential settings provide security and support for residents by developing a sense of community and employing consumers in staff positions. A cooperative housing project of this type, the clustered apartment project of Santa Clara County Mental Health Department, designed to build community among clients living independently in apartments in the same neighbourhood, encouraged staff to abandon traditional roles and to become community organisers. As the project took shape, each community developed different strengths. In one program, staff were drawn from the consumer group. In another, the programme developed a sense of community around its Latino identity. In a third, community members provided respite care in a crisis apartment to members who were acutely disturbed. The programmes were all successful in building a sense of empowerment among the residents (Mandiberg, 1995).

Cooperatively-owned housing

Housing cooperatives could become a viable response to the homelessness of people with mental illness and, simultaneously, improve their economic situation and quality of life. Cooperatives can provide long-term affordable housing, help residents develop a feeling of community and build leadership skills among members (Davis and Thompson, 1992). For various reasons, however, there are relatively few successful examples of cooperative homeownership by people with mental illness. Lenders and potential residents may be put off by the cooperative governance. Being somewhat mobile, undercapitalised and at risk of prolonged hospitalisation, people with mental illness may be unable to make the required payment. Despite difficulties, however, housing cooperatives for the mentally ill can be viable. Chapters of the National Alliance for the Mentally Ill (a US advocacy organisation) have established non-profit housing trusts, the residents usually being relatives of the investors.

Incarceration

From the 1980s until recently, an average of 8% of inmates of local jails in the USA have been diagnosed with schizophrenia (Warner, 2004). The 1991 Epidemiologic Catchment Area Study determined the prevalence of schizophrenia in US prisons to be 5% (Keith et al., 1991). Many Americans suffering from psychosis remain in jail because hospital or community care is not available. In Britain, the number of incarcerated mentally ill prisoners has been increasing dramatically in recent years – from 2–3% of male inmates in the decades leading up to 1980, to 6% of male inmates in 1990, to 7–10% of male inmates and 14–20% of women prisoners in 1997 (Singleton et al., 1998; Warner, 2004).

Under the ever-present threat of litigation, services for the mentally ill in US jails have improved in recent years. Intake screening to detect mental illness and case management services for mentally ill inmates are now provided in four-fifths of the jails in the country (Goldstrom et al., 1998). Various diversion programmes, including the establishment of special mental health courts, have been proposed. Here, I will present a successful programme, which is being replicated in other areas of the United States.

A jail diversion programme

People suffering from both substance abuse disorder and serious mental illness form a significant component of the jail population. The usual office-based treatment is often not successful for such people because substance abuse interferes with treatment of the psychiatric illness and vice versa. A modification of the assertive community treatment model, however, can prevent such people cycling repeatedly through jail. The approach requires collaboration between the mental health, criminal justice and correctional systems. A programme of this type, the PACE programme, established in Boulder, Colorado, in 2000, coordinates treatment planning between judges, attorneys and mental health professionals, with psychiatric and probation services provided on the same site. The programme also offers daily administration of medications, sobriety testing, case management to help clients obtain housing, financial benefits and medical care, and job placement and support. In the first year of operation, the PACE programme reduced clients' jail time from an average of nine days a month before enrolment to two days a month afterwards. There were associated improvements in sobriety and employment and big cost savings for the criminal justice system (www.mhcbc.org).

Social isolation

People with mental illness have restricted social networks – 20–30% of the average of others in the community; a third have no friends at all. They have relationships that are more one-sided, dependent and lacking in complexity of content and diversity of interconnections. Although family relationships deteriorate less than contact with friends, a significant disintegration does occur (Warner, 2004). Family members also experience social isolation, which is associated with decreased social support and increased burden for the family (Magliano et al., 2006).

Social isolation is associated with poor outcome for people with schizophrenia, including an increased risk of suicide (Montross et al., 2005) and heart disease (Gegenava and Kavtaradze, 2006). Regardless of the severity of their symptoms, people with schizophrenia in New York City boarding homes were less likely to be readmitted to hospital if they had broader and more complex social networks (Cohen and Sokolovsky, 1978). The psychosocial clubhouse seeks to address both the problems of social isolation and powerlessness of people with mental illness.

The psychosocial clubhouse

Organisations such as Fountain House, in New York City, and Thresholds, in Chicago, have gained international prominence by establishing a model in which people with mental illness are involved in running a programme that meets many of their social and vocational needs. In these programmes, clients are referred to as 'members' and work with staff in running the operations of the clubhouse – putting together the daily newsletter, working in the food service or staffing the reception desk. The clubhouse is open evenings, weekends and holidays, providing refuge for people who may live in cramped housing and sometimes cannot fit in well in other social settings. Psychiatric treatment is not part of the programme; instead the emphasis is on developing work skills and job opportunities for members. The clubhouse is not for everyone. Some lower-functioning clients may be scared off by the emphasis on work and many higher-functioning clients are not keen to mingle with other mentally ill people. Improvement in quality of life and reductions in service utilisation have been demonstrated for those who do participate (Warner *et al.*, 1998).

The first clubhouse, Fountain House, was founded in 1947 by ex-patients of Rockland State Hospital and for 30 years was the only one of its kind, enjoying an international reputation and entertaining hundreds of visitors each year. In 1976, Fountain House launched a national training programme and in 1988, a national expansion effort. The International Center for Clubhouse Development was established in 1994, launching a programme to certify clubhouses that met operational standards (Macias *et al.*, 2001). By 2003, there were over 300 certified clubhouses worldwide, 191 in the USA, 29 in Scandinavia, 23 in Canada, 22 in the British Isles and others in Australia, New Zealand, Japan, Korea and some European countries (ICCD, 2004).

The basic components of the clubhouse model include the 'work-ordered day' – a structured eight-hour day, in which members and staff work side-by-side on clubhouse work units. New members are only required to volunteer for work when they feel ready but, since they are assigned to a work group upon enrolment, gentle pressure to become involved is always present. Another element is the democratic mode of decision-making: members and staff meet in open session to discuss policy and planning; and no staff-only or member-only meetings are permitted. Other basic components include employment programmes, and community support and reach-out to members (ICCD, 2004; Macias *et al.*, 2001).

The attractions of the model for people with mental illness, most of whom are not well off, include good, cheap food; a comfortable social environment; mutual support; empowerment, which flows from the democratic philosophy; and access to employment. Observers point out weaknesses, however. The clubhouse movement has conducted almost no controlled trials and has a weak evidence base. It is unclear, therefore, which clubhouse elements are effective and which standards are necessary for success.

Conclusion

Social factors can affect the course and outcome of mental illness. Programmes that attempt to ameliorate the effect of such social problems as unemployment, poverty, homelessness, incarceration and isolation have proven effective in improving outcome, quality of life and social inclusion for people with serious mental illness.

REFERENCES

Abas, M., Vanderpyl, J., Robinson, E. *et al.* (2003). More deprived areas need greater resources for mental health. *Australia and New Zealand Journal of Psychiatry*, **37**, 437–44.

Averett, S., Warner, R., Little, J. *et al.* (1999). Labor supply, disability benefits and mental illness. *Eastern Economic Journal*, **25**, 279–88.

Beard, J. H., Probst, R. and Malamud, T. J. (1982). The Fountain House model of psychiatric rehabilitation. *Psychosocial Rehabilitation Journal*, **5**, 47–53.

Becker, D. R., Bebout, R. R. and Drake, R. E. (1998). Job preferences of people with severe mental illness: a replication. *Psychiatric Rehabilitation Journal*, **22**, 46–50.

Becker, D. R., Bond, G. R., McCarthy, D. *et al.* (2001). Converting day treatment centers to supported employment programs in Rhode Island. *Psychiatric Services*, **52**, 351–7.

Bond, G. R. (1992). Vocational rehabilitation. In *Handbook of Psychiatric Rehabilitation*, ed. R. P. Liberman. New York: Macmillan Press, pp. 244–63.

Bond, G. R. (1998). Principles of individual placement and support. *Psychiatric Rehabilitation Journal*, **22**, 11–23.

Bond, G. R. (2004). Supported employment: evidence for an evidence-based practice. *Psychiatric Rehabilitation Journal*, **27**, 345–59.

Borg, M., Sells, D., Topor, A. *et al.* (2005). What makes a house a home: the role of material resources in recovery from severe mental illness. *American Journal of Psychiatric Rehabilitation*, **8**, 243–56.

Carling, P. and Curtis, L. (1997). Implementing supported housing: current trends and future directions. *New Directions in Mental Health Services*, **74**, 79–94.

Cohen, C. I. and Sokolovsky, J. (1978). Schizophrenia and social networks: ex-patients in the inner city. *Schizophrenia Bulletin*, **4**, 546–60.

Davis, M. and Thompson, B. (1992). *Cooperative Housing: A Development Primer*. Washington, DC: National Cooperative Business Association.

Dell'Acqua, G. and Dezza, M. G. C. (1985). The end of the mental hospital: a review of the psychiatric experience in Trieste. *Acta Psychiatrica Scandinavica*, **316** (suppl.), 45–69.

Draine, J., Salzer, M. S., Culhane, D. P. *et al.* (2002). Role of social disadvantage in crime, joblessness, and homelessness among persons with serious mental illness. *Psychiatric Services*, **53**, 565–73.

Drake, R. E., Becker, D. R., Beisanz, B. A. *et al.* (1996). Day treatment versus supported employment for persons with severe mental illness: a replication study. *Psychiatric Services*, **47**, 1125–7.

Drake, R. E., Becker, D. R., Bond, G. R. *et al.* (2003). A process analysis of integrated and non-integrated approaches to supported employment. *Journal of Vocational Rehabilitation*, **18**, 51–8.

Fioritti, A. (2004). Disincentives to work within the Italian disability pension system. *World Psychiatry*, **3** (suppl. 1), 57. (Paper presented at the WPA International Congress on Treatments in Psychiatry: An Update, Florence, Italy.)

Gegenava, M. and Kavtaradze, G. (2006). Risk factors for coronary heart disease in patients with schizophrenia. *Georgian Medical News*, **134**, 55–8.

Gold, M. and Marrone, J. (1998). *Mass Bay Employment Services (A Service of Bay Cove Human Services, Inc.): A Story of Leadership, Vision, and Action Resulting in Employment for People with Mental Illness*. Vol. 1 of *Roses and Thorns from the Grassroots* (spring vol.). Boston, MA: Institute for Community Inclusion.

Goldstrom, I., Henderson, M., Male, A. *et al.* (1998). Jail mental health services: a national survey. In *Mental Health: United States, 1998*, ed. R. W. Manderscheid and M. A. Sonnenschein. Washington, DC: Department of Health and Human Services, pp. 176–87.

Gowdy, E. A., Carlson, L. S. and Rapp, C. A. (2003). Practices differentiating high-performing from low-performing supported employment programs. *Psychiatric Rehabilitation Journal*, **26**, 232–9.

Grove, R., Secker, J. and Seebohm, P. (ed.) (2004). *New Thinking about Mental Health and Employment*. Oxford: Radcliffe Publishing.

ICCD (2004). *International Clubhouse Directory 2003*. New York: International Center for Clubhouse Development.

Kaufman, T. L. (1997). *Out of Reach: Rental Housing at What Cost?* Washington, DC: National Low Income Housing Coalition.

Keith, S. J., Regier, D. A. and Rae, D. S. (1991). Schizophrenic disorders. In *Psychiatric Disorders in America: The Epidemiologic Catchment Area Study*, ed. L. N. Robins and D. A. Regier. New York: Maxwell Macmillan International, pp. 33–52.

Lehman, A. F. (1995). Vocational rehabilitation in schizophrenia. *Schizophrenia Bulletin*, **21**, 645–56.

Macias, C., Barriera, P., Alden, M. *et al.* (2001). The ICCD benchmarks for clubhouses: a practical approach to quality improvement in psychiatric rehabilitation. *Psychiatric Services*, **52**, 207–13.

Magliano, L., Fiorillo, A., Malangone, C. *et al.* (2006). Social network in long-term diseases: a comparative study in relatives of persons with schizophrenia and physical illnesses versus a sample from the general population. *Social Science and Medicine*, **62**, 1392–402.

Mandiberg, J. (1995). Can interdependent mutual support function as an alternative to hospitalization? The Santa Clara County Clustered Apartment Project. In *Alternatives to the Hospital for Acute Psychiatric Treatment*, ed. R. Warner. Washington, DC: American Psychiatric Press, pp. 193–210.

Marwaha, S. and Johnson, S. (2004). Schizophrenia and employment: a review. *Social Psychiatry and Epidemiology*, **39**, 337–49.

McGurk, S. R. and Mueser, K. T. (2003). Cognitive functioning and employment in severe mental illness. *Journal of Nervous and Mental Disease*, **191**, 789–98.

McHugo, G. J., Drake, R. E. and Becker, D. R. (1998). The durability of supported employment effects. *Psychiatric Rehabilitation Journal*, **22**, 55–61.

Medical Campaign Project (1990). *A Paper Outlining Good Practice on Discharge of Single Homeless People with Particular Reference to Mental Health Units*. London: Policy Studies Institute.

Moffit, R. (1990). The econometrics of kinked budget constraints. *Journal of Economic Perspectives*, **4**, 119–39.

Montross, L. P., Zisook, S. and Kasckow, J. (2005). Suicide among patients with schizophrenia: a consideration of risk and protective factors. *Annals of Clinical Psychiatry*, **17**, 173–82.

National Coalition for the Homeless (1999). *Fact Sheet Number 5*. Washington, DC: National Coalition for the Homeless.

Nelson, G., Lord, J. and Ochocka, J. (2001). *Shifting the Paradigm in Community Mental Health: Towards Empowerment and Community*. Toronto: University of Toronto Press.

Noble, J. H., Honberg, R. S., Hall, L. L. *et al.* (1997). *A Legacy of Failure: The Inability of the Federal-State Vocational Rehabilitation System to Serve People with Severe Mental Illnesses*. Arlington, VA: National Alliance for the Mentally Ill.

Rinaldi, M., McNeil, K., Firn, M. *et al.* (2004). What are the benefits of evidence-based supported employment for patients with first-episode psychosis? *Psychiatric Bulletin*, **28**, 281–4.

Room, R. (2005). Stigma, social inequality and alcohol and drug use. *Drug and Alcohol Review*, **24**, 143–55.

Rosenheck, R., Leslie, D., Keefe, R. *et al.* (2006). Barriers to employment for people with schizophrenia. *Psychiatric Services*, **163**, 411–17.

Schwartz, G. and Higgins, G. (1999). *Marienthal: The Social Firms Network*. Redhill, Surrey: Netherne Printing Services and Social Firms UK.

Sengupta, A., Drake, R. E. and McHugo, G. J. (1998). The relationship between substance use disorder and vocational functioning among persons with severe mental illness. *Psychiatric Rehabilitation Journal*, **22**, 41–5.

Seyfried, E. and Ziomas, D. (2005). Pathways to social integration for people with mental health problems: the establishment of social co-operatives in Greece. *Peer Review in the Field of Social Inclusion Policies*. Available at www.peer-review-social-inclusion.net/peer-reviews/2005/review-25/05_EL_disc_en_050924.pdf.

Sherman, P. S. and Porter, R. (1991). Mental health consumers as case management aides. *Hospital and Community Psychiatry*, **42**, 494–8.

Singleton, N., Meltzer, H., Gatward, R. *et al.* (1998). *Psychiatric Morbidity Among Prisoners in England and Wales*. London: Office of National Statistics.

Srinivasan, L. and Tirupati, S. (2005). Relationship between cognition and work functioning among patients with schizophrenia in an urban area of India. *Psychiatric Services*, **56**, 1423–8.

Stein, L. I. and Test, M. A. (1980). Alternative to mental hospital treatment: I. Conceptual model, treatment program, and clinical evaluation. *Archives of General Psychiatry*, **37**, 392–7.

Thara, R. (2004). Twenty-year course of schizophrenia: The Madras Longitudinal Study. *Canadian Journal of Psychiatry*, **49**, 564–9.

Tremblay, T., Smith, J., Xie, H. *et al.* (2006). Effect of benefits counseling services on employment outcomes for people with psychiatric disabilities. *Psychiatric Services*, **57**, 816–21.

US General Accounting Office (1993). *Evidence for Federal Program's Effectiveness is Mixed. GAO/PEMD-93-19.* Washington, DC: US Government Printing Office, August.

Warner R. (2000). *The Environment of Schizophrenia: Innovations in Practice, Policy and Communications.* London: Brunner-Routledge.

Warner, R. (2004). *Recovery from Schizophrenia: Psychiatry and Political Economy*, 3rd edn. Hove: Brunner-Routledge.

Warner, R. and Polak, P. (1995). The economic advancement of the mentally ill in the community: economic opportunities. *Community Mental Health Journal*, **31**, 381–96.

Warner, R., de Girolamo, G., Belelli, G. *et al.* (1998). The quality of life of people with schizophrenia in Boulder, Colorado, and Bologna, Italy. *Schizophrenia Bulletin*, **24**, 559–68.

Warr, P. (1987). *Work, Unemployment and Mental Health.* Oxford: Oxford University Press.

Wilton, R. (2004). Putting policy into practice? Poverty and people with serious mental illness. *Social Science and Medicine*, **58**, 25–39.

12

Public attitudes, stigma and discrimination against people with mental illness

Graham Thornicroft and Aliya Kassam

Introduction

Many people with mental illness are subjected to systematic disadvantages in most areas of their lives. Why should this be so? What can we learn from other conditions whose image may have changed over time? Should we fatalistically accept that these processes of exclusion are somehow tribal, deeply rooted and resistant to change? Or is it realistic to see stigma and discrimination as cultural constructions, which we can collectively change if we understand them clearly and commit ourselves to tackle them? These issues are at the core of this chapter.

The starting point: stigma

The unavoidable starting point for this discussion is the idea of stigma. This term (plural, stigmata) was originally used to refer to an indelible dot left on the skin after stinging with a sharp instrument, sometimes used to identify vagabonds or slaves (Cannan, 1895; Hobbes of Malmesbury, 1657). The resulting mark led to the metaphorical use of 'stigma' to refer to stained or soiled individuals who were in some way morally diminished (Gilman, 1985). In modern times stigma has come to mean 'any attribute, trait or disorder that marks an individual as being unacceptably different from the 'normal' people with whom he or she routinely interacts, and that elicits some form of community sanction' (Goffman, 1963; Scambler, 1998).

Stigma and physical conditions

While this chapter is concerned specifically with people who have diagnoses of mental illnesses, the stigma concept has also been used extensively for some particular physical conditions (Mason, 2001). What can we learn from this work?

Society and Psychosis, ed. Craig Morgan, Kwame McKenzie and Paul Fearon. Published by Cambridge University Press. © Cambridge University Press 2008.

Box 12.1 Service user accounts (1)

'Perhaps the reason that science struggles in the face of mental illness is that the illness is somehow bound up with their personality. This I think is dead central to the stigma issue. If the illness is in some way related to your personality, then haven't you in some way brought it on yourself? If your personality has grown to become bound up with illness, then why would anyone want to be around such an influence? Based on this, it's no wonder that people try to steer clear of the mentally ill.' Robert

'Often I have heard comments, either said to me or about people with depression, as 'lazy'. I was constantly tired and at low periods I would take to my bed and isolate myself from the outside world.' Tania

People with HIV or AIDS have perhaps been most often described in recent years as suffering from the effects of stigmatisation (Klitzman and Bayer, 2003). The prominent themes in these discussions have been how far the individuals concerned are responsible (and, therefore, to blame) for their status (e.g., Kelly *et al.*, 1987), and the balance between the need to protect the public health and to respect the confidentiality and human rights of people with this diagnosis (Goldin, 1994; Herek *et al.*, 2003). It is particularly important to note that during the 1990s inaccurate beliefs about the risks posed by casual social contact with people with HIV and AIDS increased, as did the belief that people with AIDS deserve their illness, but overt expression of stigma declined through this decade (Herek *et al.*, 2002). In other words, it was not necessary for factual knowledge or moral attitudes to improve for behaviour to change in a positive way (see Box 12.1).

Degrees of rejection

What do we know about how far stigma applies to people with mental illnesses compared with other conditions? In brief, very little. Most of the literature on stigma and discrimination focuses on: theories of psychological processes, attitude scales, opinion surveys, links with violence and portrayals in the media. Comparative stigma is one of the many areas about which very little has been written (Weiss, 2001).

There have been several studies of social distance (e.g., Corrigan *et al.*, 2001). These typically present a vignette or a hypothetical scenario of a person with a particular condition, and ask whether you would want to live next door to that person, whether you would let that person act as a childminder to your children or whether you would allow your son or daughter to marry such a person (e.g., Angermeyer *et al.*, 2003). A series of such surveys in Germany found high levels of social distance expressed towards people with schizophrenia, and even higher levels to those with alcohol dependence (Angermeyer and Matschinger, 1997). A revealing US study asked employers about job-offer intentions, and found that ex-convicts were seen to be more acceptable than people with mental illness, and the only group less favoured by employers were those with tuberculosis (Brand, Jr and Clairborn, 1976). Such high levels of concern were also found in a sample of over 1500 members of the general UK population who were asked about their attitudes to people with five different conditions. Their concern levels were: stress or depression, 34%; epilepsy, 19%; heart attack, 17%; facial disfigurement, 9%; or use of a wheelchair, 4% (Jacoby *et al.*, 2004).

In a very detailed comparison in Kansas, over 100 undergraduate psychology students were asked to compare 66 different medical conditions in 13 dimensions, including social distance. Overall, five of these dimensions predicted rejection: severity of the condition, contagiousness, behavioural causality, availability and sexual transmission, where the last four were all closely linked to personal control. In other words, how far is the individual directly or indirectly at fault in developing the condition? In an important conclusion, the authors stated, 'Severity and behavioural causality account for a significant amount of the socially shared representation of what makes an illness stigmatisable.' (Crandall and Moriarty, 1995, p. 74.) Care is needed here. It may not necessarily follow, for example, that emphasising the biological basis of mental illnesses will reduce stigma by reducing blame for a condition over which the person affected is assumed to have little responsibility. Indeed a German survey found the opposite (Dietrich *et al.*, 2004). Stigma can also be assessed indirectly. One particularly intriguing approach is to see whether people with a particular physical condition are treated differently if they do or do not also have a diagnosis of mental illness (Murray and Lopez, 1996). For people with diabetes, for example (which is more common in people treated with some types of antipsychotic medication), the quality of care was assessed by five key indicators: annual foot inspection, foot-pulse examination, foot sensory examination, retina examination and a specific blood test (glycated haemoglobin). The study found that people with mental illness (particularly substance misuse) were less likely to receive these recommended health checks (Desai *et al.*, 2002a).

In terms of treatment for heart conditions, most (but not all (Desai *et al.*, 2002b)) studies also show that people with mental illness receive inferior physical healthcare. For example, careful examination of the treatment records of over 110 000 people who had acute in-patient care in the USA found that, compared with those without a mental illness, people with such conditions were prescribed appropriate medications less often (Druss *et al.*, 2001) and also received fewer surgical procedures (Druss *et al.*, 2000). These care deficits were associated with higher mortality rates after heart attacks (Druss *et al.*, 2001). This strongly suggests that some form of direct or indirect discrimination is in operation.

Understanding stigma

There is now a voluminous literature on stigma (e.g., Corrigan, 2005; Goffman, 1963; Heatherton *et al.*, 2003; Link *et al.*, 1989; Mason, 2001; Pickenhagen and Sartorius, 2002; Sartorius and Schulze, 2005; Wahl, 1999). The stigma of mental illness is the subject of many hundreds of scientific papers (Pickenhagen and Sartorius, 2002). The most complete model of the component processes of stigmatisation has four key components (Link and Phelan, 2001): (1) labelling, in which personal characteristics are signalled or noticed as conveying an important difference; (2) stereotyping, which is the linkage of these differences to undesirable characteristics; (3) separating, the categorical distinction between the mainstream or normal group and the labelled group as being in some respects fundamentally different; and (4) status loss and discrimination, i.e., devaluing, rejecting and excluding the labelled group. Interestingly, more recently, the authors of this model have added a revision to include the emotional reactions which may accompany each of these stages (Link *et al.*, 2004).

Another way to look at stigma is to think of six dimensions along which it can vary: (1) concealability or visibility, (2) its course over time, (3) the strain on interpersonal relationships, (4) related aesthetic qualities, (5) the cause of the disorders and (6) the peril or danger to others associated with the condition (Jones *et al.*, 1984).

Shortcomings of stigma models

A number of features have limited the usefulness of these theories. First, while these processes are undoubtedly complex, the approach taken by academics has been dominated by those within social psychology or sociology (Corrigan, 2005; Goffman, 1963; Heatherton *et al.*, 2003; Mason, 2001) and, in particular, there have been relatively few connections with the fields of disability policy (Penn and Wykes, 2003; Sayce, 2000) or clinical practice. For example, legislation such as the Americans with Disabilities Act in the USA and the Disability Discrimination Act in the UK, have been applied relatively infrequently to cases involving mental illness (Appelbaum, 1998; Glozier, 2004).

The focus on the core concept of stigma, rather than on prejudice and discrimination, has also separated the field of mental illness from the mainstream of disability-related policy and, in particular, the stigma idea has offered policy-makers and politicians few recommendations for action. Further, few lessons have been drawn from other areas of unequal treatment such as for HIV and AIDS (Aggleton, 2002) or sexually transmitted diseases (Breitkopf, 2004).

Overwhelmingly, most work on mental illness and stigma has been descriptive, commonly describing the results of attitude surveys or relating to the portrayal of mental illness by the media. Very little is known about effective interventions to reduce stigma (Pinfold *et al.*, 2005). There have been notably few contributions to this literature from service users themselves. Little has been written about the actual experiences of rejection or exclusion by people with mental illness (Crossley and Crossley, 2001; Dinos *et al.*, 2004). There has been an underlying pessimism that stigma is deeply historically rooted and difficult to change (Porter, 1998).

In stigma theories, the relationship between 'perceiver' and 'target' has focused research attention on the level of one-to-one or small-group interactions (Heatherton *et al.*, 2003). Sometimes, such theories come close to seeing those who are disadvantaged as victims (Heatherton *et al.*, 2003). This tends to de-emphasise any analysis of cultural or social factors. In particular, such theories rarely pay attention to questions of power in relation to people with mental illness (Morone, 1997). Further stigma theories have paid little attention to the structural factors that manifest the low value given to disadvantaged groups, such as relatively low levels of investment in mental health services (Corrigan *et al.*, 2004b).

A further limitation of stigma-related research is that it has rarely connected to the domains of civil liberties and human rights (Amnesty International, 2000; Bindman *et al.*, 2003). For this reason there has been little use of international declarations and conventions to improve psychiatric treatment and care, especially for those undergoing compulsory treatment (Kingdon *et al.*, 2004). Further, stigma research has tended to focus on single conditions (predominantly schizophrenia) and has shown scant regard for people who have two or more diagnoses. In particular, one whole area of research that is largely absent refers to people with two forms of disadvantage, for example in relation to mental illness and ethnicity, or among mentally ill offenders. Finally, an emphasis on individual psychological factors has meant that less attention has been given to environmental factors, for example to how reasonable adjustments at work can prevent impairments from becoming disabilities (Ustun *et al.*, 1995).

Recently, there have been early signs in the research literature of a developing focus on discrimination. This can be seen as the behavioural consequences of stigma that act to the disadvantage of service users (Corrigan *et al.*, 2004a; Sayce, 2000; 2003). The importance of discriminatory behaviour has been clear for many years in terms of the personal experiences of service users, in terms of devastating effects upon personal relationships, parenting and childcare, education, training, work and housing (e.g., Becker and Drake, 2003; Dear and Wolch, 1992; Thornicroft *et al.*, 2004). These voices have said that the rejecting behaviour of others may bring greater disadvantage than the primary condition itself (Corrigan *et al.*, 2001; Sartorius and Schulze, 2005).

We shall consider later what needs to be done to give people with mental illnesses a full opportunity for social participation. First of all, we need to have a clear map to know where we are and where we want to go.

The three core problems

Stigma theories have not been enough to understand the feelings and experiences of people with mental illness, nor to know what practical steps are needed to reverse social exclusion (Social Exclusion Unit, 2004). Rather, 'stigma' can be seen as an overarching term that contains three important elements: problems of knowledge (ignorance); problems of attitudes (prejudice); and problems of behaviour (discrimination). In terms of social psychology, these are referred to as the cognitive, affective and behavioural domains (Dovidio et al., 1996; Dovidio et al., 2000), and each will now be discussed.

But first a word is necessary here about attitudes, as much of the literature on stigma consists of attitude theories and surveys (Crocker et al., 1998; Fiske, 1998). While, on the face of it, the idea of attitudes towards mental illness is clear, on closer examination it becomes less straightforward. 'Attitude' can be defined as consisting of four aspects: cognitive (consciously held beliefs or opinions), affective (emotional tone or feeling), evaluative (positive or negative) and cognitive (tendency towards action) (Reber and Reber, 2001). The concept of attitude, therefore, mixes, often in a rather unclear and general way (as does the stigma concept), the separate elements that are discussed in this chapter.

Ignorance: the problem of knowledge

As we have seen above, while some information is available on knowledge about mental illnesses in non-Western nations, the vast majority of stigma and discrimination information stems from the more economically developed countries. A surprisingly consistent picture emerges: wherever it has been studied, it is found that general levels of knowledge about mental illness are remarkably low. One common misunderstanding, for example, is that schizophrenia means 'split-mind', usually misinterpreted to mean a 'split-personality' (as in the 'Dr Jekyll and Mr Hyde' story by Robert Louis Stevenson). Surveys of over 12 000 individuals in several European countries have discovered that such views are common, and are supported by many or most people in: Austria (29%), Germany (80%), Greece (81%), Poland (50%), Slovakia 61%) and Turkey (39%) (Gaebel et al., 2002; Sartorius and Schulze, 2005). Commonly, older people are less knowledgeable than younger people (Stuart and Arboleda-Florez, 2001).

At a time when there is an unprecedented volume of information in the public domain about health problems in general, the level of general knowledge about mental illnesses is universally meagre. In one population survey in England, for example, most people (55%) believed that the statement 'someone who cannot be held responsible for his or her own actions' describes a person who is mentally ill

(Department of Health, 2003). Most (63%) thought that fewer than 10% of the population would experience a mental illness at some time in their lives. In Northern Italy, it was found that people who had more information about mental illnesses were less fearful and more willing to favour working with people with a history of mental illness (Vezzoli *et al.*, 2001), and exactly the same finding came from a Canadian study (Stuart and Arboleda-Florez, 2001). Most such studies agree with the findings of a Swiss survey that age matters: older people are both less well informed about mental illness and less favourable towards people with mental illnesses, although these are relatively small effects (Lauber *et al.*, 2000). Women also tend to offer more favourable views about people with mental illness in most Western surveys (Madianos *et al.*, 1999), such as one large study throughout Australia (Jorm *et al.*, 1999).

There are also striking knowledge gaps about how to find help. In Scotland most children did not know what to do if they had a mental health problem or what to recommend to a friend with mental health difficulties: only 1% mentioned school counselling, 1% nominated helplines, 4% recommended talking with friends, 10% said that they would turn to a doctor, but over a third (35%) were unsure where to find help (See Me Scotland, 2004).

The public level of knowledge about mental illnesses and their treatments has sometimes been called 'mental health literacy' (Jorm *et al.*, 1997). In Australia, over 2000 adults were asked about the features of two mental illnesses and their treatment. Most (72%) could identify the key characteristics of depression, but relatively few (27%) could accurately recognise schizophrenia. Many standard psychiatric treatments (such as antidepressant and antipsychotic medication, or admission to a psychiatric ward) were more often rated as harmful than as helpful, and most people more readily recommended the use of vitamins (Jorm *et al.*, 1997). Similarly, although most people in a nationwide survey in the USA agreed that psychiatric medications are effective, the majority were not willing to take such drugs themselves (Croghan *et al.*, 2003). Also, among people with depression, many had strong and often ambivalent feelings about taking antidepressant drugs, although, interestingly, the rate of acceptance was higher among people who had taken them for a previous episode of depression (Sirey *et al.*, 1999; Sirey *et al.*, 2001).

Such findings have led many, especially in Australia where much of this work has been pioneered, to conclude that it is necessary to provide far more public information on the nature of conditions, such as depression, and on the treatment options that are available, so that both the general population and those people who are depressed can make decisions about getting help on a fully informed basis (Jorm, 2000; Jorm *et al.*, 2003; Parslow and Jorm, 2002). In other words, the best remedy for ignorance is information.

Is stigma getting better or worse? As we have seen elsewhere in this chapter, sometimes the literature is voluble (for example on risk and violence) and sometimes it whispers or even remains silent. Trends in stigma are a quiet zone. There has been active research about stigma for over half a century (Allport, 1954; Crocker *et al.*, 1998; Fiske, 1998; Nunnally, 1961) and over most of this time public attitude surveys have been carried out (Cumming and Cumming, 1965; Star, *What the Public Thinks About Mental Health and Mental Illness*, Paper presented at the annual meeting of the National Association of Mental Health, Indianapolis, Indiana, 1952). Indeed most of the published work on mental health and stigma consists of attitude surveys, but very few have been repeated over time to see if attitudes are becoming more or less favourable.

What evidence we do have about trends is contradictory. In Greece, a comparison was made between public views about mental illness in 1980 and 1994 (Madianos *et al.*, 1999). Significant improvements were identified for social discrimination, restrictiveness and social integration. For example, more people said that they would accept a mentally ill person as a neighbour or work colleague at the second time point. In contrast, a long-term comparison of popular views about mental illness in Germany has found a hardening of opinion against people with schizophrenia (Angermeyer and Matschinger, 2005b), but no change towards people with depression (Angermeyer and Matschinger, 2004). There are also some indirect indications that popular views of mental illness have changed, for example the fact that increasing numbers of people in many countries do now seek help for mental illnesses (Phelan *et al.*, 2000), although the majority still do not (Kessler *et al.*, 2005).

An important study in the USA compared popular views of mental illness in 1950 and 1996 (Phelan *et al.*, 2000). Over this period, it found evidence that there was a broadening of what was seen as mental illness, to include non-psychotic disorders and socially deviant behaviour. The second focus of the study was on 'frightening characteristics', and the results here were less heartening. There was a significant increase (almost twofold) over the 46 year period in public expectations linking mental illness to violence in terms of extreme, unstable, excessive, unpredictable, uncontrolled or irrational behaviour. This link was especially marked for public views of psychotic disorders, whereas dangerousness was mentioned less often as typical of non-psychotic conditions in 1996. In other words, depression and anxiety-related disorders had become 'less alien and less extreme', while schizophrenia and similar conditions had grown in their perceived threat (Phelan *et al.*, 2000). The authors examined the hypothesis that closing large psychiatric hospitals had led to this greater disapproval and rejection. In fact, they found the opposite: those who reported frequently seeing people in public who seemed to be mentally ill were significantly less likely to perceive them as dangerous (Link *et al.*, 1994). The authors concluded that 'something has occurred in our culture that has increased the connection between psychosis and violence in the public mind' (Phelan *et al.*, 2000, p. 203).

There have also been changes in public views about mental illness in Germany. A series of surveys between 1990 and 2001 found that the German public became more ready to recommend seeking help from psychiatrists or psychotherapists for people with schizophrenia or depression. In particular, there was a greater willingness to accept drug treatment and psychotherapy, especially for schizophrenia. Intriguingly, respondents just as often recommended that mediation or yoga should be used (Angermeyer and Matschinger, 2005b). The results suggested that the gap between professional and popular views on treatment was closing (Angermeyer and Matschinger, 2005a).

There is evidence that deliberate interventions to improve public knowledge about depression can be successful. In a campaign in Australia to increase knowledge about depression and its treatment, some states and territories received this coordinated programme, while others did not (Hickie, 2004). In areas that had received the programme, people recognised the features of depression more often, and were more likely to support seeking help for depression or to accept treatment with counselling and medication (Jorm *et al.*, 2005).

In Great Britain, there have been conflicting findings on trends in attitudes to mental illness. A series of government surveys has been carried out from 1993 to 2003 and give a mixed picture (Department of Health, 2000). On one hand, there are some clear improvements, for example, the proportion thinking that people with mental illness can be easily distinguished from 'normal people' fell from 30% to 20% (Department of Health, 2003). On the other hand, views became significantly less favourable over this decade for the following items:

- It is frightening to think of people with mental problems living in residential neighbourhoods (increased from 33% to 42%);
- Residents have nothing to fear from people coming into their neighbourhood to obtain mental health services (decreased from 70% to 55%);
- Mental illnesses are far less of a danger than most people suppose (decreased from 65% to 58%);
- Less emphasis should be placed on protecting the public from people with mental illness (decreased from 38% to 31%).

How is it possible that different studies show that public attitudes seem to be becoming both more favourable and more rejecting at the same time? One key seems to be diagnosis. Before and after its campaign, *Changing Minds*, the UK Royal College of Psychiatrists commissioned national opinion polls of nearly 2000 adults, asking about mental illness (Crisp *et al.*, 2004). Unusually, they asked each of the key questions separately for a series of different diagnoses. Significant changes were reported in the percentage of people who agreed with the following items between 1998 and 2003:

- 'Danger posed to others': depression (fell from 23% to 19%), schizophrenia (fell from 71% to 66%), but no change for alcoholism or drug addiction;
- 'Hard to talk to': depression (fell from 62% to 56%), schizophrenia (fell from 58% to 52%), alcoholism (fell from 59% to 55%);
- 'Never fully recover': schizophrenia (decrease from 51% to 42%), eating disorders (increase from 11% to 15%), alcoholism (increase 24% to 29%) and drug addiction (increase from 23% to 26%);
- 'Feel different from us': depression (decrease 43% to 30%), schizophrenia (decrease 57% to 37%), dementia (decrease 61% to 42%).

It is clear from these trends that a complicated picture emerges of both favourable and unfavourable change across a wide spectrum of conditions (Crisp *et al.*, 2005). These variations suggest that public opinion surveys, which ask about 'the mentally ill' in general terms, are likely to produce a composite and possibly uninformative response, which summarises these conflicting trends. Overall, it seems that popular views about depression appear to be improving in some Western countries, in terms of less social rejection, but the evidence about views about people with psychotic disorders is too confused to give a clear picture.

Common myths about disability and mental illness

It is clear that lay opinions about what mental illnesses are, and how people with these conditions should be helped, are often very different from professional views. A series of common beliefs about mental illnesses have developed, which are firmly held but not based firmly on evidence. These are often described by experts as 'myths'. Some such myths are held to apply to all disabled people (Fine and Asch, 1988), including those listed in Table 12.1. Other myths apply in particular to people with mental illness (Hegner, 2000; Social Exclusion Unit, 2004), such as those listed in Table 12.2.

Table 12.1 Some myths about people with a disability

Disability is solely the result of biological causes.
When a disabled person faces problems, it is assumed that the impairment causes them.
It is assumed that the disabled person is a 'victim'.
It is assumed that disability is central to the disabled person's self-concept.
It is assumed that having a disability is synonymous with needing help and social support.

Table 12.2 Some myths about people with a mental illness

Schizophrenia means a split personality.

All 'schizophrenics' are violent and dangerous.

People with serious mental illness are completely disabled.

Having schizophrenia means that you can never do anything with your life.

Schizophrenia represents a form of creative imagination or 'inner journey'.

They're lazy and not trying.

It's all the fault of the genes.

They can't work.

They are incapable of making their own decisions.

There's no hope for people with mental illnesses.

Mental illnesses cannot affect me.

Mental illness is the same as mental retardation.

Once people develop mental illnesses, they will never recover.

Mental illnesses are brought on by a weakness of character.

Psychiatric disorders are not true medical illnesses like diabetes.

Mental illness is the result of bad parenting.

Depression results from a personality weakness or character flaw.

They could just snap out of it if they tried hard enough.

Depression is a normal part of the aging process.

If you have a mental illness, you can will it away, and being treated for a psychiatric disorder means you have in some way 'failed' or are weak.

That many of these ideas still have a common currency shows that the factual understanding of mental illnesses among most members of the general population is still very weak. In the presence of ignorance, myths abound (see Box 12.2).

Prejudice: the problem of negative attitudes

If ignorance is the first great hurdle faced by people with mental illness, prejudice is the second. Although the term prejudice is used to refer to many social groups that experience disadvantage, for example, minority ethnic groups, it is rarely employed in relation to people with mental illness (Corrigan *et al.*, 2001; Veltro *et al.*, 2005). Social psychologists have focused upon thoughts (cognition) rather than feelings (affect). In particular they have long been interested in stereotypes (widely held and fixed images about a particular type of person) and degrees of social distance to such stereotypes (Allport, 1954; Fiske, 1998). However, the reactions of a host majority acting with prejudice in rejecting a minority group usually involve not just negative thoughts but also emotionally laden attitudes involving anxiety, anger, resentment, hostility, distaste or disgust (Link *et al.*,

Box 12.2 Service user accounts (2)

'I think that the reason for the stigma is, first, that the mentally ill can cause serious social problems including violence, threats of violence. They can be continually morose, talk endless streams of nonsense. They can be manipulative, attention-seeking, obsessive, arrogant. They can seem extremely lazy. These are all traits of people that nobody could like to be around, whether or not this is due to an illness. What is happening to them has no properly understood step-by-step solution, so when we see somebody in a state that is clearly abnormal, we are scared because we are aware that nobody really knows how they got that way, how to get them out of this state, or whether it will even be possible for them to be returned to a more normal state. I think it is much more scary to see a man with an amputated leg than a man with a leg in plaster, because we know that the leg in plaster is getting better, whereas we know that the amputated leg will not return as far as science allows. I think if science did allow the amputated leg to 'grow back' then there would be no fear of looking at an amputee. Similarly I don't think that the stigma and conflicting views of the mentally ill would exist if science allowed all the sufferers to rapidly return to health by a fairly unstoppable means.' Robert

2004). In fact, prejudice may more strongly predict discrimination than do stereotypes (Dovidio *et al.*, 1996).

So-called 'gut-level' prejudices (Fiske, 1998) stem from anticipated threats, in other words, how far a member of an 'out-group' is seen to threaten the goals or the interests of the person concerned. Anticipating harm may provoke anger (if the person seen to threaten harm does so unjustifiably), fear (if the harm is in the certain future), anxiety (if the harm is in the uncertain future) or sadness (if the harm is in the past) (Fiske, 1998). Some writers have made a distinction between 'hot' prejudice, in which strong emotions are more prominent than negative thoughts, and 'cold' forms of rejection, for example, in failing to promote a member of staff, when stereotypes are activated in the absence of negative feelings (Fiske, 1993).

Prejudiced emotional reactions may also be a consequence of direct contact with the 'other' group. This can be experienced as discomfort, anxiety, ambivalence or a rejection of intimacy (Crocker *et al.*, 1998). Such feelings have been shown to be stronger in individuals who have a relatively authoritarian personality, and among people who believe that the world is basically just (and so people get what they deserve) (Crandall and Eshleman, 2003; Crandall *et al.*, 2002). Such emotional aspects of rejection have been studied extensively in the fields of HIV and AIDS (Herek *et al.*, 2002), and in those conditions that produce visible marks which contravene aesthetic conventions (Hahn, 1988), such as the use of catheters or colostomies (MacDonald and Anderson, 1984; Wilde, 2003).

Interestingly, probably because research on exclusion and mental health has been almost entirely carried out using the concept of stigma rather than prejudice, there is almost nothing published about emotional reactions to people with mental illness apart from that which describes a fear of violence (Corrigan *et al.*, 2001; Lauber *et al.*, 2000). One fascinating exception to this is work carried out in the south-eastern region of the USA, in which students were asked to imagine meeting people who either did or did not have a diagnosis of schizophrenia. All three physiological measures of stress (brow muscle tension, palm skin conductance and heart rate) were raised during imagery with 'labelled' compared with 'non-labelled' individuals. Such tension was also associated with self-reported negative attitudes of stigma towards people with schizophrenia. The authors concluded that one reason why individuals avoid those with mental illness is physiological arousal, which is experienced as unpleasant feelings (Graves *et al.*, 2005).

Conclusion: discrimination – the problem of rejecting and avoidant behaviour

We have seen earlier in this chapter that most research on stigma and mental illness consists of attitude surveys. Much of this is concerned with asking people, usually either students or members of the general public, about what they would do in imaginary situations or what they think 'most people' would do, for example, when faced with a neighbour or work colleague with mental illness. Important lessons have flowed from these findings, as discussed earlier in this chapter. At the same time, this work has emphasised what 'normal' people say rather than the actual experiences of people with mental illness themselves. It also assumes that such statements (usually on knowledge, attitudes or behavioural intentions) are linked with actual behaviour, rather than assessing such behaviour directly. In short, with some clear exceptions, it has focused on hypothetical rather than real situations (Sayce, 2000), shorn of emotions and feelings (Crocker *et al.*, 1998; Fiske, 1998), divorced from context (Corrigan *et al.*, 2004a), indirectly rather than directly experienced (Repper and Perkins, 2003), and without clear implications for how to intervene to reduce social rejection (Corrigan, 2004). In short, most work on stigma has been beside the point.

If we deliberately shift the focus from stigma to discrimination, there are a number of distinct advantages. First, attention moves from attitudes to actual behaviour; not if an employer would hire a person with mental illness, but if he or she does. Second, interventions can be tried and tested to see if they change behaviour towards people with mental illness, without necessarily changing knowledge or feelings. Third, people who have a diagnosis of mental illness can expect to benefit from all the relevant anti-discrimination policies and laws in their country or jurisdiction, on a basis of parity with people with physical disabilities. Fourth, a discrimination perspective requires us to focus not upon the 'stigma-tised' but upon the 'stigmatiser'. In summary, this means sharpening our sights on

> **Box 12.3 Service user accounts (3)**
> 'I remember the first time a psychiatrist told me that if I had broken my leg, it would take a long time to heal and that your mind can take a long time to heal too. The day that the stigma against mental illness is the same as the stigma against a broken leg will be the time to stop talking about it, and until then I think that although the mentally ill can be a pest during the peaks of their suffering, but that if people are treated with respect just like you might help someone with a broken leg to walk up some stairs, that people may be able to recover quicker, and feel less isolated after.' Robert

human rights, on injustice and on discrimination as actually experienced by people with mental illness (Chamberlin, 2005; Kingdon *et al.*, 2004; see Box 12.3).

Acknowledgement

This chapter is an edited version of an extract from Thornicroft, G. (2006) *Shunned: Discrimination Against People with Mental Illness.* Oxford: Oxford University Press.

REFERENCES

Aggleton, P. (2002). Barcelona 2002: law, ethics, and human rights. HIV/AIDS-related stigma and discrimination: a conceptual framework. *Canadian HIV/AIDS Policy and Law Review*, **7** (2–3), 115–16.

Allport, G. (1954). *The Nature of Prejudice.* New York: Doubleday Anchor Books.

Amnesty International (2000). *Ethical Codes and Declarations Relevant to the Health Professions.* London: Amnesty International.

Angermeyer, M. C. and Matschinger, H. (1997). Social distance towards the mentally ill: results of representative surveys in the Federal Republic of Germany. *Psychological Medicine*, **27** (1), 131–41.

Angermeyer, M. C. and Matschinger, H. (2004). Public attitudes to people with depression: have there been any changes over the last decade? *Journal of Affective Disorders*, **83** (2–3), 177–82.

Angermeyer, M. and Matschinger, H. (2005a). The stigma of mental illness in Germany: a trend analysis. *International Journal of Social Psychiatry*, **51** (3), 276–84.

Angermeyer, M. C. and Matschinger, H. (2005b). Have there been any changes in the public's attitudes towards psychiatric treatment? Results from representative population surveys in Germany in the years 1990 and 2001. *Acta Psychiatrica Scandinavica*, **111** (1), 68–73.

Angermeyer, M. C., Beck, M. and Matschinger, H. (2003). Determinants of the public's preference for social distance from people with schizophrenia. *Canadian Journal of Psychiatry*, **48** (10), 663–8.

Appelbaum, P. S. (1998). Discrimination in psychiatric disability coverage and the Americans with Disabilities Act. *Psychiatric Services*, **49** (7), 875–6.

Becker, D. R. and Drake, R. E. (2003). *A Working Life for People with Severe Mental Illness*. Oxford: Oxford University Press.

Bindman, J., Maingay, S. and Szmukler, G. (2003). The Human Rights Act and mental health legislation. *British Journal of Psychiatry*, **182**, 91–4.

Brand, R. C., Jr and Clairborn, W. L. (1976). Two studies of comparative stigma: employer attitudes and practices toward rehabilitated convicts, mental and tuberculosis patients. *Community Mental Health Journal*, **12** (2), 168–75.

Breitkopf, C. R. (2004). The theoretical basis of stigma as applied to genital herpes. *Herpes*, **11** (1), 4–7.

Cannan, E. (1895). The stigma of pauperism. *Economic Review*, 380–91.

Chamberlin, J. (2005). User/consumer involvement in mental health service delivery. *Epidemiologia e Psichiatria Sociale*, **14**, 10–14.

Corrigan, P. W. (2004). Target-specific stigma change: a strategy for impacting mental illness stigma. *Psychiatric Rehabilitation Journal*, **28** (2), 113–21.

Corrigan, P. (2005). *On the Stigma of Mental Illness*. Washington, DC: American Psychological Association.

Corrigan, P. W., Edwards, A. B., Green, A. *et al.* (2001). Prejudice, social distance, and familiarity with mental illness. *Schizophrenia Bulletin*, **27** (2), 219–25.

Corrigan, P. W., Markowitz, F. E. and Watson, A. C. (2004a). Structural levels of mental illness stigma and discrimination. *Schizophrenia Bulletin*, **30** (3), 481–91.

Corrigan, P. W., Watson, A. C., Warpinski, A. C. *et al.* (2004b). Stigmatizing attitudes about mental illness and allocation of resources to mental health services. *Community Mental Health Journal*, **40** (4), 297–307.

Crandall, C. S. and Eshleman, A. (2003). A justification-suppression model of the expression and experience of prejudice. *Psychology Bulletin*. **129** (3), 414–46.

Crandall, C. S. and Moriarty, D. (1995). Physical illness, stigma and social rejection. *British Journal of Social Psychology*, **34** (1), 67–83.

Crandall, C. S., Eshleman, A. and O'Brien, L. (2002). Social norms and the expression and suppression of prejudice: the struggle for internalization. *Journal of Personality and Social Psychology*, **82** (3), 359–78.

Crisp, A. H., Cowan, L. and Hart, D. (2004). The College's anti-stigma campaign 1998–2003. *Psychiatric Bulletin*, **28**, 133–6.

Crisp, A. H., Gelder, M. G., Goddard, E. *et al.* (2005). Stigmatization of people with mental illnesses: a follow-up study within the Changing Minds campaign of the Royal College of Psychiatrists. *World Psychiatry*, **4**, 106–13.

Crocker, J., Major, B. and Steele, C. (1998). Social stigma. In *The Handbook of Social Psychology*, 4th edn, ed. D. Gilbert, S. T. Fiske and G. Lindzey, Boston, MA: McGraw-Hill, pp. 504–33.

Croghan, T. W., Tomlin, M., Pescosolido, B. A. *et al.* (2003). American attitudes toward and willingness to use psychiatric medications. *Journal of Nervous and Mental Disease*, **191** (3), 166–74.

Crossley, M. L. and Crossley, N. (2001). 'Patient' voices, social movements and the habitus; how psychiatric survivors 'speak out'. *Social Science and Medicine*, **52** (10), 1477–89.

Cumming, J. and Cumming, E. (1965). On the stigma of mental illness. *Community Mental Health Journal*, **1**, 135–43.

Dear, M. and Wolch, J. (1992). *Landscapes of Despair*. Princeton: Princeton University Press.

Department of Health (2000). *Attitudes to Mental Illness Summary Report 2000*. London: Department of Health.

Department of Health (2003). *Attitudes to Mental Illness 2003 Report*. London: Department of Health.

Desai, M. M., Rosenheck, R. A., Druss, B. G. *et al.* (2002a). Mental disorders and quality of diabetes care in the veterans health administration. *American Journal of Psychiatry*, **159** (9), 1584–90.

Desai, M. M., Rosenheck, R. A., Druss, B. G. *et al.* (2002b). Mental disorders and quality of care among post-acute myocardial infarction outpatients. *Journal of Nervous and Mental Disease*, **190** (1), 51–3.

Dietrich, S., Beck, M., Bujantugs, B. *et al.* (2004). The relationship between public causal beliefs and social distance toward mentally ill people. *Australian and New Zealand Journal of Psychiatry*, **38** (5), 348–54.

Dinos, S., Stevens, S., Serfaty, M. *et al.* (2004). Stigma: the feelings and experiences of 46 people with mental illness. Qualitative study. *British Journal of Psychiatry*, **184**, 176–81.

Dovidio, J., Brigham, J. C., Johnson, B. T. *et al.* (1996). Stereotyping, prejudice and discrimination: another look. In *Stereotypes and Stereotyping*, ed. N. McCrae, C. Stangor and M. Hewstone. New York: Guilford Press, pp. 276–319.

Dovidio, J., Major, B. and Crocker, J. (2000). Stigma: introduction and overview. In *The Social Psychology of Stigma*, ed. T. F. Heatherton, R. E. Kleck, M. R. Hebl and J. G. Hull. New York: Guilford Press, pp. 1–28.

Druss, B. G., Bradford, D. W., Rosenheck, R. A. *et al.* (2000). Mental disorders and use of cardiovascular procedures after myocardial infarction. *Journal of the American Medical Association*, **283** (4), 506–11.

Druss, B. G., Bradford, W. D., Rosenheck, R. A. *et al.* (2001). Quality of medical care and excess mortality in older patients with mental disorders. *Archives of General Psychiatry*, **58** (6), 565–72.

Fine, F. and Asch, A. (1988). Disability beyond stigma: social interaction, discrimination, and activism. *Journal of Social Issues*, **44** (1), 3–23.

Fiske, S. T. (1993). Social cognition and social perception. *Annual Review of Psychology*, **44**, 155–94.

Fiske S. T. (1998). Stereotyping, prejudice and discrimination. In *The Handbook of Social Psychology*, 4th edn, ed. D. Gilbert, S. T. Fiske. and G. Lindzey, Boston, MA: McGraw-Hill, pp. 357–411.

Gaebel, W., Baumann, A., Witte, A. M. *et al.* (2002). Public attitudes towards people with mental illness in six German cities: results of a public survey under special consideration of schizophrenia. *European Archives of Psychiatry and Clinical Neuroscience*, **252** (6), 278–87.

Gilman, S. L. (1985). *Difference and Pathology: Stereotypes of Sexuality, Race and Madness*. Ithaca: Cornell University Press.

Glozier, N. (2004). The Disability Discrimination Act 1995 and psychiatry: lessons from the first seven years. *Psychiatric Bulletin*, **28**, 126–9.

Goffman, I. (1963). *Stigma: Notes on the Management of Spoiled Identity*. Harmondsworth, Middlesex: Penguin Books.

Goldin, C. S. (1994). Stigmatization and AIDS: critical issues in public health. *Social Science and Medicine*, **39** (9), 1359–66.

Graves, R. E., Cassisi, J. E. and Penn, D. L. (2005). Psychophysiological evaluation of stigma towards schizophrenia. *Schizophrenia Research*, **76** (2–3), 317–27.

Hahn, H. (1988). The politics of physical differences: disability and discrimination. *Journal of Social Issues*, **44**, 39–47.

Heatherton, T. F., Kleck, R. E., Hebl, M. R. *et al.* (2003). *The Social Psychology of Stigma*. New York: Guilford Press.

Hegner, R. E. (2000). Dispelling the myths and stigma of mental illness: the Surgeon General's report on mental health. *Issue Brief National Health Policy Forum*, **754**, 1–7.

Herek, G. M., Capitanio, J. P. and Widaman, K. F. (2002). HIV-related stigma and knowledge in the United States: prevalence and trends, 1991–1999. *American Journal of Public Health*, **92** (3), 371–7.

Herek, G. M., Capitanio, J. P. and Widaman, K. F. (2003). Stigma, social risk, and health policy: public attitudes toward HIV surveillance policies and the social construction of illness. *Health Psychology*, **22** (5), 533–40.

Hickie, I. (2004). Can we reduce the burden of depression? The Australian experience with beyondblue: the national depression initiative. *Australasian Psychiatry*, **12** (suppl.), s38–s46.

Hobbes of Malmesbury, T. (1657). ΣΤΙΓΜΑΙ Αγεομετρίας, Αγροικίας, Αντιπολιείας, Αμαθείας; *or Markes of the Absurd Geometry, Rural Language, Scottish Church Politicks, and Barbarismes of John Wallis Professor of Geometry and Doctor of Divinity*. London: Andrew Crooke.

Jacoby, A., Gorry, J., Gamble, C. *et al.* (2004). Public knowledge, private grief: a study of public attitudes to epilepsy in the United Kingdom and implications for stigma. *Epilepsia*, **45** (11), 1405–15.

Jones, E., Farina, A., Hastorf, A. *et al.* (1984). *Social Stigma: The Psychology of Marked Relationships*. New York: W. H. Freeman and Co.

Jorm, A. F. (2000). Mental health literacy. Public knowledge and beliefs about mental disorders. *British Journal of Psychiatry*, **177**, 396–401.

Jorm, A. F., Korten, A. E., Jacomb, P. A. *et al.* (1997). 'Mental health literacy': a survey of the public's ability to recognise mental disorders and their beliefs about the effectiveness of treatment. *Medical Journal of Australia*, **166** (4), 182–6.

Jorm, A. F., Korten, A. E., Jacomb, P. A. *et al.* (1999). Attitudes towards people with a mental disorder: a survey of the Australian public and health professionals. *Australian and New Zealand Journal of Psychiatry*, **33** (1), 77–83.

Jorm, A. F., Griffiths, K. M., Christensen, H. *et al.* (2003). Providing information about the effectiveness of treatment options to depressed people in the community: a randomized controlled trial of effects on mental health literacy, help-seeking and symptoms. *Psychological Medicine*, **33** (6), 1071–9.

Jorm, A. F., Christensen, H. and Griffiths, K. M. (2005). The impact of beyondblue: the national depression initiative on the Australian public's recognition of depression and beliefs about treatments. *Australian and New Zealand Journal of Psychiatry*, **39** (4), 248–54.

Kelly, J. A., St Lawrence, J. S., Smith, S. Jr *et al.* (1987). Stigmatization of AIDS patients by physicians. *American Journal of Public Health*, **77** (7), 789–91.

Kessler, R. C., Demler, O., Frank, R. G. *et al.* (2005). Prevalence and treatment of mental disorders, 1990 to 2003. *New England Journal of Medicine*, **352** (24), 2515–23.

Kingdon, D., Jones, R. and Lonnqvist, J. (2004). Protecting the human rights of people with mental disorder: new recommendations emerging from the Council of Europe. *British Journal of Psychiatry*, **185**, 277–9.

Klitzman, R. and Bayer, R. (2003). *Mortal Secrets: Truth and Lies in the Age of AIDS*. Baltimore: The Johns Hopkins University Press.

Lauber, C., Nordt, C., Sartorius, N. *et al.* (2000). Public acceptance of restrictions on mentally ill people. *Acta Psychiatrica Scandinavica*, **102** (407) (suppl.), 26–32.

Link, B. G. and Phelan, J. C. (2001). Conceptualizing stigma. *Annual Review of Sociology*, **27**, 363–85.

Link, B. G., Cullen, F. T., Struening, E. L. *et al.* (1989). A modified labeling theory approach in the area of mental disorders: an empirical assessment. *American Sociological Review*, **54**, 100–23.

Link, B. G., Susser, E., Stueve, A. *et al.* (1994). Lifetime and five-year prevalence of homelessness in the United States. *American Journal of Public Health*, **84** (12), 1907–12.

Link, B. G., Yang, L. H., Phelan, J. C. *et al.* (2004). Measuring mental illness stigma. *Schizophrenia Bulletin*, **30** (3), 511–41.

MacDonald, L. D. and Anderson, H. R. (1984). Stigma in patients with rectal cancer: a community study. *Journal of Epidemiology and Community Health*, **38** (4), 284–90.

Madianos, M. G., Economou, M., Hatjiandreou, M. *et al.* (1999). Changes in public attitudes towards mental illness in the Athens area (1979/1980–1994). *Acta Psychiatrica Scandinavica*, **99** (1), 73–8.

Mason, T. (2001). *Stigma and Social Exclusion in Healthcare*. London: Routledge.

Morone, J. A. (1997). Enemies of the people: the moral dimension to public health. *Journal of Health Politics, Policy and Law*, **22** (4), 993–1020.

Murray, C. and Lopez, A. (1996). *The Global Burden of Disease*. Vol. 1 of *A Comprehensive Assessment of Mortality and Disability from Diseases, Injuries and Risk Factors in 1990, and Projected to 2020*. Cambridge, MA: Harvard University Press.

Nunnally, J. C. (1961). *Popular Conceptions of Mental Health*. New York: Holt, Rinehart and Winston.

Parslow, R. A. and Jorm, A. F. (2002). Improving Australians' depression literacy. *Medical Journal of Australia*, **177** (suppl.), s117–s121.

Penn, D. and Wykes, T. (2003). Stigma, discrimination and mental illness. *Journal of Mental Health*, **12**, 203–8.

Phelan, J. C., Link, B. G., Stueve, A. *et al.* (2000). Public conceptions of mental illness in 1950 and 1996: what is mental illness and is it to be feared? *Journal of Health and Social Behavior*, **41**, 188–207.

Pickenhagen, A. and Sartorius, N. (2002). *The WPA Global Programme to Reduce Stigma and Discrimination Because of Schizophrenia*. Geneva: World Psychiatric Association.

Pinfold, V., Thornicroft, G., Huxley, P. *et al.* (2005). Active ingredients in anti-stigma pro-grammes in mental health. *International Review of Psychiatry*, **17** (2), 123–31.

Porter, R. (1998). Can the stigma of mental illness be changed? *Lancet*, **352**, 1049–50.

Reber, A. S. and Reber, E. S. (2001). *Dictionary of Psychology*, 3rd edn. London: Penguin.

Repper, J. and Perkins, R. (2003). *Social Inclusion and Recovery*. Edinburgh: Billière Tindall.

Sartorius, N. and Schulze, H. (2005). *Reducing the Stigma of Mental Illness. A Report from the Global Programme Against Stigma of the World Psychiatric Association*. Cambridge: Cambridge University Press.

Sayce, L. (2000). *From Psychiatric Patient to Citizen. Overcoming Discrimination and Social Exclusion*. Basingstoke: Palgrave.

Sayce, L. (2003). Beyond good intentions. Making anti-discrimination strategies work. *Disability and Society*, **18**, 625–42.

Scambler, G. (1998). Stigma and disease: changing paradigms. *Lancet*, **352**, 1054–5.

See Me Scotland (2004). *The Second National Public Attitudes Survey, 'Well? What do you think?'* Edinburgh: Scottish Executive.

Sirey, J. A., Meyers, B. S., Bruce, M. L. *et al.* (1999). Predictors of antidepressant prescription and early use among depressed outpatients. *American Journal of Psychiatry*, **156** (5), 690–6.

Sirey, J. A., Bruce, M. L., Alexopoulos, G. S. *et al.* (2001). Perceived stigma as a predictor of treatment discontinuation in young and older outpatients with depression. *American Journal of Psychiatry*, **158** (3), 479–81.

Social Exclusion Unit (2004). *Mental Health and Social Exclusion*. London: Office of the Deputy Prime Minister.

Stuart, H. and Arboleda-Florez, J. (2001). Community attitudes toward people with schizo-phrenia. *Canadian Journal of Psychiatry*, **46**, 245–52.

Thornicroft, G., Tansella, M., Becker, T. *et al.* (2004). The personal impact of schizophrenia in Europe. *Schizophrenia Research*, **69** (2–3), 125–32.

Ustun, T. B., Cooper, J. E., Duuren-Kristen, S. *et al.* (1995). Revision of the ICIDH: mental health aspects. WHO/MNH Disability Working Group. *Disability and Rehabilitation*, **17** (3–4), 202–9.

Veltro, F., Raimondo, A., Porzio, C. *et al.* (2005). [A survey on the prejudice and the stereotypes of mental illness in two communities with or without psychiatric residential facilities]. *Epidemiologia e Psichiatria Sociale*, **14** (3), 170–6. (In Italian, with English abstract.)

Vezzoli, R., Archiati, L., Buizza, C. *et al.* (2001). Attitude towards psychiatric patients: a pilot study in a northern Italian town. *European Psychiatry*, **16** (8), 451–8.

Wahl, O. F. (1999). *Telling is a Risky Business: Mental Health Consumers Confront Stigma*. New Jersey: Rutgers University Press.

Weiss, M. G. (2001). Cultural epidemiology. *Anthropology and Medicine*, **8**, 5–29.

Wilde, M. H. (2003). Life with an indwelling urinary catheter: the dialectic of stigma and acceptance. *Qualitative Health Research*, **13**, 1189–204.

13

Outcomes elsewhere: course of psychosis in 'other cultures'

Kim Hopper

Introduction

In the mid-1970s, a fledgling anthropologist and her family landed in Dublin, ready to tackle the runes and riddles of 'Gaelic sexuality'. Fortune had other plans. Within days of her arrival, a chance meeting with a psychiatrist convinced Nancy Scheper-Hughes to try her hand at a more consequential topic, runaway rates of schizophrenia in rural Ireland. Settling down in a seafaring village on the Dingle peninsula, she set out (as she would later put it) to 'study madness among bachelor farmers as a projection of cultural themes' (Kreisler, 1999). Drawing on Bateson's notion of pathogenic paradoxical communication snares (Bateson *et al.*, 1956), she made good on the dare. Hospitalised Patrick was one of many last-born sons 'crippled by his parents' double-binding attempts' to keep him in reserve (single, at home, on call for their old age). Commonplace in this 'demoralised, dying, western village' (Scheper-Hughes, 1979, p. 190), these desperate parental gambits were late expressions of 'the breakdown of traditional patterns of Irish familialism'. Patrick's plaintive 'I am their dead son' was less psychotic delusion than dreary, de facto truth.

When *Saints, Scholars and Schizophrenics* was published in 1979, it caused a sensation, one that has yet to fade entirely. Alternately hailed and denounced as breakthrough ethnography and heart-breaking exposé, its place in medical anthropology's canon was quickly secured. Complaints about its inaccuracies and betrayals aside, the book was plagued by a more fundamental methodological difficulty. At the heart of the argument lay a self-subverting couplet that had long harried cross-cultural studies of mental disorder. Scheper-Hughes aimed to unriddle an epidemiological puzzle – elevated rates of schizophrenia among marginalised rural bachelors – using the interpretive tools of an anthropology premised upon distinctive 'sociocultural' constructions of psychiatric disorder. But the original puzzle exists only if we assume that rates of disorder, based on standardised

Society and Psychosis, ed. Craig Morgan, Kwame McKenzie and Paul Fearon. Published by Cambridge University Press. © Cambridge University Press 2008.

assessments of pathology, can legitimately be subjected to cross-cultural inquiry. In effect, the logic that makes for the arresting anomaly was itself called into question by the tools used to unravel it.

In this instance, prosaic artefactual realities would ultimately do in elegant ethnographic theorising, as the author herself (to her credit) later acknowledged. In the 20th anniversary edition of *Saints, Scholars and Schizophrenics*, Scheper-Hughes reviews critical responses to the book that convincingly demolish its starting premise. What looked like elevated rates of schizophrenic disorder were in fact the false flags of unreliable hospital records and the catch-all nature of psychiatric facilities as 'indiscriminate repositories of social problems' (Finnerty *et al.*, 2007). More rigorous examinations of the data did show that these celibate denizens of blighted rural areas were prone to higher rates of depression and suicide, and Scheper-Hughes revises her account accordingly. But the original puzzle is still cultural in nature. Like the asylum in nineteenth century America (or, for that matter, in colonial Nigeria (Sadowsky, 1999, p. 53)), the Irish hospital was a multipurpose facility prone to misuse, 'a convenient way of getting rid of inconvenient people' (Scull, 1977, p. 33). The whole assemblage of double count-ing, slipshod records, extended lengths of stay and elastic diagnoses had to be taken sceptically and read sociologically. The ethnographic question had less to do with psychopathology than with what made this institutional option acceptably con-venient, a question with which anthropologists continue to grapple (Biehl, 2005; Saris, 1996). Scheper-Hughes' stranded bachelors, like their counterparts in south-western France (Bourdieu and Wacquant, 1992, p. 165), may have been 'caught between old and new social systems and moral economies' (Scheper-Hughes, 2000, p. 49), but they were not, by that token alone, on the road to madness. At the same time, she insisted that the damaged men of An Clochán – not just those hospitalised, but those whose profound strangeness and heartbreaking isolation were locally tolerated – are specific casualties, of a hard time and unbending place, with signifying value.

But precisely *how* should they signify? Psychiatry has generally favoured the epidemiological road in answering that question, plying an ever more refined technology of comparative analysis to assess local incidence and outcome of well defined disorders. In that sweeping cross-cultural enterprise, one anomaly has held firm since it first appeared in the 1960s: the claim that persons with schizophrenia in 'developing' countries consistently enjoyed better outcomes than their counter-parts in more 'developed' settings. How well has that evidence stood the test of time? And how, in any event, should we read it? But a second, less prominent (even self-effacing) interpretive tradition takes another route. Like Scheper-Hughes – unrepentant for all her travails, revising on the spot to pry signifying value out of reworked epidemiological data – these anthropological analysts are more concerned with meaning and practice than with rates and measures. Forlorn, dishevelled, lost not least of all to themselves, local madmen (though not all of them and not all of the time) may be figures of prophetic import. Wittingly or not, mute or frenzied, heeded or ignored, such people offer critical commentary shaped by their own trying times and tuned to the fault-lines of their fractious cultures. The analyst's job is to hear and decipher it. If cultures are arguments over what kind of collective life a people will commit to (Douglas, 2004, p. 94), then some of the mad, some of the time, constitute a defecting Greek chorus of one, declaiming what may be painfully obvious from without if invisible (or forbidden) from within. Discredit and dismissal are the usual price they pay for the dubious privilege. What might we learn from this alternative, sectarian tradition of reading outcome differently?

The epidemiological record

Upbeat descant to the descending bass-line of progressive deterioration in the West, the course of schizophrenia in 'other cultures' has long claimed pride of place among the curiosities of cross-cultural psychiatry, a stature neither wholly earned (rates of recovery in the West are by no means uniformly bad) nor unanimously subscribed to (indeed, it is one of the favoured targets of sceptical commentators). Before reviewing the untidy particulars of that story, however, it is worth noting how durable the caricatures in this call-and-response have proven. On the one hand, molecular myopia can lead some researchers to make (what seem) wilfully uninformed pronouncements such as this one: 'Once the symptoms of schizophrenia occur (usually in young adulthood) they persist for the entire lifetime of the patient and are almost totally disabling' (Sawa and Snyder, 2002, p. 692). On the other hand, the WHO international outcome studies are some-times misread as damning witness to Western psychiatry's single-handed reliance on medication, which is then taken to explain the poor showing of 'developed' centres in that research (Whitaker, 2001). Neurobiological determinism faces off against psychopharmacological imperialism. Neither troubles itself with the bulk of evidence inconveniently lying elsewhere.

The rumour of recovery from schizophrenia in other cultures made innocent rounds in early ethnographic circles only to be roundly discredited in clinical corridors. It took two forms. The first, ignorant (or dismissive) of Kraepelin's (1919) own south-east Asian reconnaissance in the early twentieth century, alleged low (or no) incidence of severe psychopathology in traditional societies, even while recognising idiopathic (culture-specific) disorders (Faris, 1934). For these investigators, in Demerath's (1942, p. 703) mocking formula, 'The functional pathologies are the peculiar curse of civilised man.' Course of illness was immaterial when incidence was near zero. Such bold speculation, built on an admittedly thin evidentiary base, was countered strongly by reports suggesting that the notion of idyllic pathology-free regions was wistful fiction (Laubscher, 1937; Winston, 1934). But tantalising inconsistency was the rule (Gillin, 1939). For every dogmatic assertion, a sceptical demurral could also be found. Lopez (1932) reported that schizophrenia was indeed found among displaced Brazilian Indians living on the coast, but not in the then-undisturbed interior. Seligman (1929) found no insanity in untouched Papua New Guinean villages, but definite instances in those where 'white influence' was felt. Benedict (1934) described whole cultures built on routine trafficking between dream and everyday realities. And Mead reported that the imported wives of Manus men in the Admiralty Islands are 'noticeably schizoid'; such women were 'taken from their own villages to live among the people of their husbands and in that group they are *always outsiders*' (recounted by Faris, 1934, p. 31, emphasis added).

Overreaching aside, the field validity of specific reports was hard to contest. Aggregated and more attentive to methods, they took on more persuasive power. By mid-century, variation in the 'true' community prevalence of severe disorders was apparent even in European studies (Hammer and Leacock, 1961). The argument had undeniable relativist appeal: that *what we don't see*, even on close sustained examination, may be telling us *both* that it doesn't occur *and* to look elsewhere to detect trace effects. What derails reason on the home front may be otherwise accommodated elsewhere. How else to account for the argument, made by an NIMH researcher (the same year WHO launched the International Pilot Study of Schizophrenia), that the occupational availability of shamanism in some cultures may channel disruptive identity crises that might otherwise find expression as reactive schizophrenia (Silverman, 1967)? In such settings, resolution of these nominally 'psychotic' episodes is 'effectively channelled by the prevailing institutional structures or may perform a given function in relation to the total culture' (Silverman, 1967, p. 23). Like the 'mazeway resynthesis' earlier proposed as the breakthrough ordeal of the protagonist of a cultural revitalisation movement among the Seneca Indians, the success of extreme states of reintegration depends on 'both the resources of the individual and the support his effort is given by the community' (Wallace, 1961, p. 192).

The second version frankly admitted that phenotypically close approximations of garden-variety (Western) psychoses can be found almost everywhere, and went on to make the case for qualitatively better outcomes in more traditional societies. Murphy and Raman's (1971) 12-year follow-up study in Mauritius set the stage for what the suite of WHO studies would shortly (and problematically) establish: that in pre-industrial cultures, 'acute, short-lasting psychosis'– indistinguishable from textbook schizophrenia *but for* its brief course and good prognosis – may be the rule. What further distinguished this study was its attention to comparative rigour. Per capita hospital bed rates were roughly on a par with European ones (but treatment was a decade behind and aftercare non-existent), only first admissions were included, and follow-up assessments were intensive and standardised. The upshot: nearly two-thirds (60%) of the Mauritian cohort 'were functioning normally ... and had no history of relapses in the period since leaving hospital' (Murphy and Raman, 1971, p. 495). The comparable rate in the closest British equivalent (Brown, 1966), a 5-year follow-up study, was at best 40%. Intriguingly, somewhat less than a third of both samples showed continuous, crippling illness. Murphy and Raman hypothesised that, facilitating factors in Mauritius aside, the less severe (and better prognosis) European patients may be 'trapped' in chronicity by an incapacitating sick role. The lingering effects of 'institutionalism' among discharged patients of that era offer indirect corroboration (Wing and Brown, 1970).

For their part, the WHO studies (Harrison et al., 2001; Hopper et al., 2007a; Jablensky et al., 1992; WHO, 1973, 1979) have consistently shown (with a few exceptions) that both short-term and long-term courses favoured subject cohorts in 'developing' centres. The finding is remarkably robust. It extends across three generations of WHO collaborative studies. It holds for brief and long-term follow-up, for distinctive diagnostic groupings (ICD-9, converted to ICD-10 and all psychoses), and for different groupings of 'developed' and 'developing' countries. And, by one reckoning, the differential is relatively constant – an odds of recovery ratio of roughly 1.5 favouring the non-industrial group.

During this period, too, independent reports from other 'developing' regions continued to appear, employing a host of methods and making for a decidedly mixed picture (e.g., Kebede et al., 2005; Kurihara et al., 2000; Ran et al., 2001). If a salient impression were to be hazarded from this assortment, it would be something like this: be wary of glib optimism in relation to outcomes elsewhere. Clinical status (especially among untreated cohorts) is likely to be poor, even when coupled with high, necessity-driven rates of social functioning. But these are neither long-term nor fully reported, in the main. Cohort studies are expensive, logistically demanding, and require extensive training and coordination over time; not surprisingly, few get done.

How to take stock of so varied and contentious a legacy? For our purposes, a recent authoritative review captures the difficulty neatly. As Bresnahan and colleagues (2003) assess the evidence, 'It appears that some aspect of the economic or cultural circumstance in developing countries may provide a more therapeutic context for recovery' (p. 29). They go on to round up the 'usual suspects' commonly assembled to operationalise (if only plausibly) that nondescript phrase 'some aspect' – involved families present for the long haul, informal economies and flexible work demands, desegregated treatment and community cohesion. Conspicuously absent is treatment, and that (as we will see) may be an unwarranted omission.

At the same time, it would be unwise to ignore persistent criticisms of the WHO studies. Nagging questions have been raised about selection bias ('leakage' in case identification), diagnostic elasticity (over-inclusion of reactive psychoses, with better prognosis, in developing centres), unacceptable rates of drop-out in developing centres, anecdotal accounts of gross mistreatment and searing stigma, crude classification of participating cohorts as 'developed' and 'developing', and blackboxing of culture. Some of these objections, those pertaining to potential confounds owing to composition of cohorts or follow-up irregularities, have been addressed by strong-inference analyses of the long-term results of the International Study of Schizophrenia (ISoS) (Hopper and Wanderling, 2000). Others go yet unanswered.

Consider 'culture'. For all the potential explanatory power packed into the concept, it becomes clear that 'culture' is both a constant presence in the WHO corpus and a ghostly one, nimbly stepping in to claim (if not account for) otherwise 'unexplained variance' (Edgerton and Cohen, 1994; Hopper, 2003). The WHO investigators have wisely skirted the long-running civil wars in anthropology over its meaning and use, but a working notion of culture is discernible in the write-ups themselves and their contending interpreters. Off-stage but everhovering, an insistent prompt and script-doctor, culture provides both institutional armature and internalised programme for collective living. It puts in place a local moral world and its array of supporting practices within which an illness episode and its aftermath are embedded. This capacious understanding has long made for profligate, if not always well specified or documented, hypotheses for why outcomes elsewhere are better: exculpatory beliefs, less-complex cognitive demands, extended family support, accommodating work regimens, absent stigma (Cohen, 1993; Cooper and Sartorius, 1977; Hopper, 1991; Warner, 2003). But, as Bresnahan and colleagues (2003) are careful to note (even as they rehearse the list), evidence for these is uneven at best. Even were a factor to be shown to be relevant, the messy, inevitably improvised particulars of *how local culture works to shape recovery*, the detailed close-ups and extended exposures that the documentary record would require to show how disability is averted and resumption of valued social roles accomplished, remain missing – if for no better reasons than (1) the epidemiological design of the studies was not up to the task and (2) relevant secondary accounts are scarce.

But other factors are surely relevant, though they too have proven refractory to focused, single-take documentation. If culture is both shaping and shifting, so too, it turns out, is treatment. Of the two Indian sites that account for the 'developing' country side of the ISoS divide, one is remarkable for the tenacity of its clinical follow-up and both had conducted interim follow-up studies on their own initiative. In one, as a side benefit of this research interest, subjects 'were in close contact with the centre and were very closely monitored', their clinical status and life circumstances were commonly known, and they 'remained on active follow-up and treatment' (Varma and Malhotra, 2007, p. 125). At the other, the Schizophrenia Research Foundation (SCARF, the Chennai research centre) is renowned for its insistent attention to work and informed family involvement, while its psychiatrists are unflinching in their adherence to a Western 'biomedical model' of mental illness. Medications are provided free to poor patients (Miller, 2006; Thara *et al.*, 2007). Aside from such well established clinical operations as these, and much harder to include in the usual array of instruments and debriefings that go into follow-up studies, are parallel or 'complementary' ethnomedical and religious healing modalities. Plural treatment options and multiple therapeutic use – sequentially or concurrently, if rarely with cross-consultation – are the rule throughout South India (Campion and Bhugra, 1998; Kapur, 1979). In rural areas, religious temples provide respite and asylum to people suffering from disabling disorders; many people show marked improvement after (Pakaslahti, 1998; Raguram, 2002). Elsewhere, an ad hoc syncretism holds sway, driven pragmatically by family treatment management teams. In Kerala, Halliburton's (2004) informants were families with afflicted members whose expressive and behavioural features were strongly suggestive of psychosis: 'nonsensical speech, flat affect, delusions, repeated acts of violence and morbid self-neglect' (p. 86). Interviewed at various stages in their illness careers, they had sought treatment – and reported differential relief – from Western (allopathic), ayurvedic and religious healers. Obviously, this makes compiling an accurate record of interventions over time difficult, to say nothing of apportioning beneficial effect.

Still, the most profound challenge to the robust ISoS irregularity of better outcomes elsewhere may be the protest lodged by researchers, themselves experienced students of and practitioners in their own 'developing' settings, who insist that an approach that more accurately limned the full span of illness course and consequence would yield a more faithful – and unsettling – picture of local realities (Patel *et al.*, 2006). This position challenges not only the hidebound orthodoxy of neurobiological fundamentalism, but also the insurgent corrective that could be read as finding therapeutic virtue in collective hardship. Empirically, the case is compelling if still incomplete. Mortality among those diagnosed with schizophrenia with poor early course of illness can be highly elevated – by 47% in the rural Chandigarh ISoS cohort (Mojtabai *et al.*, 2001); by 17% over 20 years, less steep but still high, in the Chennai cohort (Thara, 2004). Evidence of human rights abuses, less systematically documented than wrenchingly recounted, is steadily mounting. Globalisation's rippling impact and accelerating social change introduce fresh uncertainty into already precarious livelihoods; spikes in suicide rates are one index (Phillips *et al.*, 1999; Sundar, 1999). Increased risk of mental disorders more generally must surely be counted among the casualties and further complications of poverty (Patel and Kleinman, 2003).

In other cultural registers, too, the evidence points to ethnographic extremes that are washed out in statistical averages. Take the case of marriage in India. A recent interpretive analysis of the ISoS material (Hopper *et al.*, 2007b) rehearses the extraordinary rates of marital success in the Indian ISoS cohorts, especially when compared with their European, American and Japanese counterparts. That picture holds for both newly contracted unions (arranged post-psychosis) and durable ones (those who were married at the time of first break and remain so at follow-up). The relevant ethnographic literature strongly suggests that, despite the intense stigma attached to mental illness – indeed, in part *motivated* by that stigma – families redouble their efforts to negotiate marriages for afflicted members, and then contrive to secure and support them to preserve the lineage. *Dharma* overrides stigma but at the cost of great effort and long commitment. The net effect is substantially to boost this social strut of self-respect for the post-psychotic partner, to provide an offsetting anchor of moral worth to counter the discrediting pull of madness (as history or prospect). Yet even here, the dark complement to this uplifting picture is the wretched plight of women whose marriages fail – doubly disgraced and abandoned, for all intents and purposes, to a social death (Thara *et al.*, 2003a, 2003b).

At the very least, then, cross-cultural psychiatric epidemiologists will need to provide more complete pictures of course and outcome, and the consequences that accompany them, if informative comparisons are to be made both elsewhere and on the well trodden, more familiar terrain of Euro-American aftercare as well. The self-same complaint, if for different reasons, comes from the anthropological front.

The discursive school: outcome read differently

The WHO studies draw implicitly on the well aged convention of culture as a local model for living, circulating as 'institutionalised canonicity' and embodied as native bent and propensity. Convention's completing counterpart, and that which captures the vital meaning-making that is part-and-parcel of the everyday interpretive work of its members, is culture as 'imagined possibility' (Amsterdam and Bruner, 2000, pp. 217–45). Less obviously in play in the epidemiological record, it is everywhere apparent in that literature's shadow self, what I will call the discursive tradition of cross-cultural psychiatry. (This is a useful fiction,

I should stress, neither known nor subscribed to by the authors discussed here.) In closely attending to the 'idioms of madness' (Vaughan, 1983), these analysts have charted a distinctively different, avowedly interpretive, route into the signifying value of psychosis, often using the somewhat arcane toolkits of sociolinguistics and hermeneutic analysis. Nor, unlike most of the former, have they shied away from drawing explicit lessons for application on the home front. Following Karp's early lead, this notional school may be said to read psychosis as unauthorised (and often transgressive) cultural *commentary* (Karp, 1985). Deeply contextualised intrigue and code-shifting, disguised and bitter resentment, and the embedded pragmatics of communication (Watzlawick *et al.*, 1967) – not clinical outcome – are its governing concerns. Its practitioners are less interested in recovery than in legibility; not how it turns out when all is said and done, but how what is said and done along the way can be read meaningfully as vernacular critique or resistance. This is long-term translational work: seeking first to discern, and then finding ways to learn from, the elusive 'coherence in psychotic discourse' (Ribeiro, 1994).

The discursive school is still a cottage industry, bearing little of the institutional support or clinical imprimatur that underwrites cross-cultural epidemiology. Exemplars in this literature have, often enough, an explicitly derivative provenance. Shorter, pressured postscripts to longer sober tracts, most of the dozen or so examples I have drawn upon are products of engagements that could not be refused, even if their telling had to be postponed. They range widely: Wilson's (1974) wryly affectionate recounting of homeless Oscar's antics on Providencia, Spence's (1988) quixotic account of the star-crossed eighteenth century Chinese catechist John Hu, Swartz's and Swartz's (1987) linguistic analysis of conversation failure on a locked South African ward, Littlewood's (1993) account of the 'imitation of madness' in the founding community of a Trinidadian priestess, Desjarlais' (1997) and Lovell's (1997) forays into the elusive speech-worlds of homeless-trafficked urban streets and shelters, Corin's unpacking of 'the play of signifiers' in psychosis in Toronto and Chennai (Corin, 1990; Corin *et al.*, 2004), Lester's visionary Mexican nun (Lester, R. Where time and space are broken: dissociation and metaphysical critique in the experience of a Mexican nun. Paper presented at *Annual Meeting of the American Anthropological Association*, Washington, DC, 2 December, 2005), Biehl's (2005) lovingly rendered account of Catarina, adrift in one of the new 'zones of abandonment' cropping up haphazardly in the Southern Cone, Wilce's (2000, 2003) meticulous analysis of the 'poetics of madness' in a Bangladeshi village, Lucas' (2003) walkabout account of the uses of culture in identity work by persons diagnosed with schizophrenia in an Australian city, Estroff's (2003) exegesis of first-person 'c/s/x' (consumer/survivor/ex-patient) poetry, protest and pamphleteering. These are all close-hauled dispatches from the troubled fronts of unreason, shorn of familiar clinical dressings and format

Working for interpretation and against diagnosis, these (undeclared) reclamation projects amount to painstaking attempts to restore intention to discredited moral agents, to retrieve meaning otherwise disavowed and dismissed. The aim, simply said, is to reinstate claims for intelligibility – if only the right register, depth of field and willing audience can be found – for performances that seem scripted to repudiate it.

If the analysis is arduous, the founding premise is simplicity itself: read properly, psychotic screed can be rich coded commentary on the knotted ground-rules of social intercourse and personal identity. The 'privileged obscenity', destruction of property, neologisms and flamboyantly transgressive performances are best viewed, Karp (1985) taught us, as 'socially constituted vehicles . . . for communicating that self-society relations' had become 'problematic' (p. 222). Damaged and fearful, madness' preferred dialect is badinage; indirection and caricature its favoured terms of exchange. Taking on 'social facts that are too encompassing, or too much a part of the taken-for-granted fabric of normal social existence, for the average person even to notice' (Sass, 1992, p. 7), the mad perversely court scorn and rejection. Unaccredited anthropologists in their home cultures, psychotics are unwelcome as meddlesome scribes or scolds, feared as unsummoned replacements for familiar others, spurned as marginal and dangerous. Diagnosis domesticates even as it certifies (wittingly or not) the seal of unintelligibility. (But not always: Jaspers acknowledged the clairvoyance of Old Testament Ezekiel, and still considered him schizophrenic.)

Schizophrenia remains 'psychiatry's quintessential other' (Sass, 1992, p. 19), but then *others* are anthropology's stock-in-trade, 'learn[ing] to grasp what we cannot embrace' (Geertz, 1985) its watchword and creed. Making sense of their words and actions – of the lightning-fast code shifting, the referential obscurity, table-turning conversational antics, off-stage family entanglements, self-effacements and many layered meanings – requires the commitment and time that, thankfully, the protocols of ethnography demand. (Again, these accounts are often by-products of long-term field projects.) All too commonly, patience is rewarded not by mutual breakthroughs of understanding but by deeper insight on the outsider's part into the wellsprings of suffering, and how clinical and social responses can compound or redirect it. Both Wilson (1974) and Littlewood (1993) explore how cultural dissonance, born of unaccommodating history (and, in the latter, organic ailment), is refracted in maddening efforts to marry the dictates of 'respectability' to the local means of repute. But where Oscar finds marginality and a grudging recognition of the hard truths he speaks, Mother Earth's trial by madness gives birth to new community.

What impresses the reader of such accounts is the *labour* invested, both in enduring the ordeal of madness and, where it (too rarely) applies, in taking on the 'work of recovery' (Davidson and Strauss, 1992). That labour, it turns out, may provide one key to intervention. In refusing to accept her confinement as just, Catarina provokes and enlists Biehl's own disbelief (Biehl, 2005). In reconstructing this obscure miscarriage of care, he lays bare the slow death of kinship's claim, the veiled negotiations between family and state surrogate to arrive at a mutually acceptable disposition of a troubled or troubling member (what he calls 'social psychosis'). When Desjarlais (1997) describes how a local 'ethic of listening' can trump the staff's 'ethic of understanding' when sitting alongside shelter residents 'talking ragtime' (p. 195), he stumbles upon a crucial tool in the street-worker's outreach kit. Swartz's and Swartz's (1987) determination to seek clues to 'conversation failure' in 'talk about talk' on a locked ward proved fruitful, showing how such failures are often the fault of the clinical interlocutor. And if the effort chastens (it is hugely labour-intensive), it also beckons: locating the patient's verbal cubism in the unsecured slippage between context and discourse opens fresh possibilities for listening and understanding. Similarly, when Estroff (2003) channels the rage and pain of 'c/s/x' communiqués, she means not merely to indict but to challenge: the point is not to read and weep (though that is difficult not to do), but to take the necessary action that would turn these durable refrains of neglect to preventive account. This means finding the time and devoting the labour needed to engage with respect and attentiveness. Inescapably, too, such counsel amounts to a plea, no less daunting for being unstated, to transform present-day systems of care (which one US state mental commissioner has characterised as 'a shambles') into arrangements more conducive to such engagements.

Conclusion: border crossings

'If social restitution constitutes our criterion, we have to consider some factors which lie beyond the patient's control.' (Bleuler, 1950 [1911], p. 255)

'If I become psychotic, I'd rather be in India than in Switzerland.' (Shekhar Saxena, Director of Mental Health Research, World Health Organization, 27/01/06)

For too long, attempts to explain the anomalous WHO findings have reverted, for want of anything better, to one of two alternatives. One option was adamant agnosticism, in which 'culture' (as our critics have rightly remarked) does double duty for 'unexplained variance' (Edgerton and Cohen, 1994); the other, the hopeful notion of 'developing' regions as *thérapeutiques tropiques*, inventing flexible means of inclusion within the confines of hard necessity. If not quite 'virtuous peasants, as yet uncorrupted by Western culture' (Evans, 2002, p. 3), it could come perilously close at times. Neither will suffice today. Accelerating global flows of all sorts are converting cultural edges into liquid interfaces churning with appropriations and blends (Appadurai, 1996, pp. 27–47). Ever at heart a 'noun of process' (Williams, 1976, p. 77), *culture* is increasingly less place-and-people than matrix-and-mix. In such a 'creolising' world, problems of cultural pluralism, of 'fragmented referential models' in the construction of viable selves, are unavoidable (Bibeau, 1997). To address them, the hand-me-down geographic premises of cross-cultural epidemiology need to be rethought. One puzzle in particular is forcing the issue.

Dislocations and fusions have redrawn global coordinates to such an extent that *migrancy* is fast becoming a modal form of membership. In being elsewhere uprooted and relocated here, the migrant is the prototypical 'amalgamated other' (Sassen, 1993): market commodity, social suspect, vexed citizen. In the last two decades, with progressively refined research attempts to take clinical measure of migrant mental health, a 'renaissance' in social psychiatry has occurred (e.g., Cooper, 2005; Harrison, 2004; McGrath, 2007; van Os, 2003). In the event, the ground has been re-seeded for the type of collaborative, interdisciplinary work that Murphy and Raman called for so long ago. But it was epidemiology, not anthropology, which got there first.

Early reports that African-Caribbean migrants to the UK had elevated incidence rates of schizophrenia (Harrison *et al.*, 1988) have since been borne out in a series of studies in England, the Netherlands and Sweden (Boydell *et al.*, 2001; Selten *et al.*, 1997; Sharpley *et al.*, 2001; Zolkowska *et al.*, 2001). Not only elevated incidence but also compromised course and outcome are at stake (Harrison *et al.*, 1999). The gathering consensus (Bhugra, 2006; Fearon and Morgan, 2006; Selten and Cantor-Graae, 2005) is that these results (and especially the even higher rates seen among second-generation immigrants) cannot be explained away by diagnostic bias, shoddy study methodology, selective migration, prenatal exposures or home country rates of psychosis. Social and cultural factors in the receiving country must be implicated. Given the risk gradient for discrepant skin colour among migrants (Cantor-Graae and Selten, 2005), persistent interpersonal and structural discrimination is a strong candidate. 'Social defeat' is another. Borrowed from ethology and defined (less resonantly than the phrase itself) as 'a subordinate position or as 'outsider status'' (Selten and Cantor-Graae, 2005), social defeat may be taken to refer to the repeated experience of failure in socially consequential settings, where something of value is at stake with respect to social standing, routine problem-solving, developmental milestones, the usual adult challenges or public repute. Social defeat is the enacted reminder – subtle, gross or structural – that one does not really belong or measure up.

If prolonged and unyielding, social defeat undermines the slow march of mastery, hobbles the formation of durable life plans, pre-empts the regard of others, and sabotages self-respect. Rawls (1971) considered 'the social bases of self-respect' the most important 'primary good' that a just society should guarantee. Denied the conditions necessary for its development, we flounder – bereft of self-confidence in our ability to carry through on intentions, 'plagued by failure and self-doubt, [unable] to continue our endeavours, finding [neither] our person [nor] our deeds confirmed by others' (Rawls, 1971, p. 440). Building 'the secure conviction that [one's] conception of the good, [one's] plan of life, is worth carrying out' (Rawls, 1971, p. 440) begins early and recruits the developing brain on its behalf. Because its delay or derailment can be so consequential, Eaton and Harrison (2000) see it as critical to ethnic disadvantage as it relates to schizophrenia. Staged life transitions may compound the danger. Convention-governed preparations, established counsellors on hand to guide, and the settled expectation that transitions will be successfully negotiated: such are the usual protocols of rites of passage. All may be missing where a migrant group's foothold is tenuous. In the event, capacity to aspire (Appadurai, 2004) and ability to plan are both jeopardised. Cultural limbo takes up residence where orchestrated liminality was once the rule.

That much granted, the conceptual work, documentary evidence and comparative ethnography needed to flesh out this notional process are still fragmentary. Substantial headway was made some time ago (Estroff, 1981) and fresh inquiry is now under way (Luhrmann, 2006). (And even as the epidemiology is being sorted out and plausible biological pathways proposed, a suggestion from the speculative wilds of evolutionary psychology has reintroduced the *soixante-huitard* figure of the 'prophet' into the mix (see Price, 2006; Stevens and Price, 2000).) But the quest for a hybrid framework, an ethnopsychiatry sufficient to the task of specifying the deprivations (absent resources and withheld opportunities), limning their neurological repercussions, and charting this entrained dialectic over time, continues.

None of this – neither implications for research (collaborating with professional and epistemic others, finding one's feet in a world where cultural bounds are readily permeable membranes, mixing methods and melding sensibilities), nor those for practice (setting aside the time and securing the terms of work that the c/s/x plaintive appeals call for) – will be easy. The ranks of researchers are already responding with mounting insistence for interdisciplinary inquiry. But the challenge to practice may be steeper. As Kleinman (1988) recognised some time ago, to urge this sort of attentiveness to the content of illness discourse, to take narrative repair as seriously as pharmacological redress, is tantamount to recommending that clinicians sign on to become minor-order ethnographers. However presumptuous and impractical, the invitation is real, if only because the understanding sought runs so counter to clinical training and treatment programme. In this task, anthropology may have been there first, but it's still trying to get it right:

'Comprehending that which is . . . alien to us and likely to remain so, without either smoothing it over with vacant murmurs of common humanity [or peremptorily diagnosing it] is a skill we have arduously to learn, and having learnt it, always very imperfectly, to work continuously to keep alive . . .' (Geertz, 1985, p. 274)

REFERENCES

Amsterdam, A. and Bruner, J. (2000). *Minding the Law.* Cambridge: Harvard University Press.

Appadurai, A. (1996). *Modernity at Large: Cultural Dimensions of Globalization.* Minneapolis: University of Minnesota Press.

Appadurai, A. (2004). The capacity to aspire. In *Culture and Public Action*, ed. V. Rao and M. Walton. Stanford: Stanford University, pp. 59–84.

Bateson, G., Jackson, D. D., Haley, J. *et al.* (1956). Toward a theory of schizophrenia. *Behavioral Science*, **1**, 251–64.

Benedict, R. (1934). *Patterns of Culture.* Boston: Houghton Mifflin.

Bhugra, D. (2006). Severe mental illness across cultures. *Acta Psychiatrica Scandinavica*, **113** (suppl. 429), 17–23.

Bibeau, G. (1997). Cultural psychiatry in a creolizing world. *Transcultural Psychiatry*, **34**, 9–41.

Biehl, J. (2005). *Vita.* Berkeley: University of California.

Bleuler, E. (1950). *Dementia Praecox or the Group of Schizophrenias* (translated by J. Zincs from the original German edn. *Dementia Praecox oder die Gruppe der Schizophrenien*, 1911). London: Heinemann.

Bourdieu, P. and Wacquant, L. (1992). *An Invitation to Reflexive Sociology.* Chicago: University of Chicago Press.

Boydell, J., van Os, J., McKenzie, K. *et al.* (2001). Incidence of schizophrenia in ethnic minorities in London: ecological study into interactions with environment. *British Medical Journal*, **323** (7325), 1336–8.

Bresnahan, M., Menezes, P., Varma, V. *et al.* (2003). Geographical variation in incidence, course and outcome of schizophrenia: a comparison of developing and developed countries. In *The Epidemiology of Schizophrenia*, ed. R. M. Murray, P. B. Jones, E. Susser, J. van Os and M. Cannon. Cambridge: Cambridge University Press, pp. 18–33.

Brown, G. W. (1966). *Schizophrenia and Social Care.* London: Oxford.

Campion, J. and Bhugra, D. (1998). Religious and indigenous treatment of mental illness in South India – a descriptive study. *Mental Health, Culture and Religion*, **1**, 21–9.

Cantor-Graae, E. and Selten, J. P. (2005). Schizophrenia and migration: a meta-analysis and review. *American Journal of Psychiatry*, **162**, 12–24.

Cohen, C. I. (1993). Poverty and the course of schizophrenia: implications for research and policy. *Hospital and Community Psychiatry*, **44**, 951–8.

Cooper, B. (2005). Immigration and schizophrenia: the social causation hypothesis revisited. *British Journal of Psychiatry*, **186**, 361–3.

Cooper, J. and Sartorius, N. (1977). Cultural and temporal variations in schizophrenia: a speculation on the importance of industrialization. *British Journal of Psychiatry*, **130**, 50–5.

Corin, E. E. (1990). Facts and meaning in psychiatry: an anthropological approach to the life-world of schizophrenics. *Culture, Medicine and Psychiatry*, **14** (2), 153–88.

Corin, E. E., Thara, R. and Padmavati, R. (2004) Living through a staggering world: the play of signifiers in early psychosis in South India. In *Schizophrenia, Culture and Subjectivity*, ed. J. H. Jenkins and R. J. Barrett. New York: Cambridge University Press, pp. 110–45.

Davidson, L. and Strauss, J. S. (1992). Sense of self in recovery from severe mental illness. *British Journal of Medical Psychology*, **65**, 131–45.

Demerath, N. J. (1942). Schizophrenia among primitives: the present status of sociological research. *American Journal of Psychiatry*, **98**, 703–7.

Desjarlais, R. (1997). *Shelter Blues: Sanity and Selfhood among the Homeless*. Philadelphia, PA: University of Pennsylvania Press.

Douglas, M. (2004). Traditional culture: let's hear no more about it. In *Culture and Public Action*, ed. V. Rao and M. Walton. Stanford: Stanford University, pp. 84–109.

Eaton, W. and Harrison, G. (2000). Ethnic disadvantage and schizophrenia. *Acta Psychiatrica Scandinavica*, **102** (suppl. 407), 38–43.

Edgerton, R. B. and Cohen, A. (1994). Culture and schizophrenia: the DOSMD challenge. *British Journal of Psychiatry*, **164**, 222–31.

Estroff, S. E. (1981). *Making it Crazy*. Berkeley: University of California.

Estroff, S. E. (2003). Subject/subjectivities in dispute: the poetics, politics and performance of first-person narratives of people with schizophrenia. In *Schizophrenia, Culture and Subjectivity*, ed. J. H. Jenkins and R. J. Barrett. New York: Cambridge University Press, pp. 282–302.

Evans, P. (2002). *Liveable Cities*. Berkeley: University of California Press.

Faris, R. E. L. (1934). Cultural isolation and the schizophrenic personality. *American Journal of Sociology*, **39**, 155–69.

Fearon, P. and Morgan, C. (2006). Environmental factors in schizophrenia: the role of migrant studies. *Schizophrenia Bulletin*, **32**, 405–8.

Finnerty, A., Keogh, F., O'Grady Walshe, A. *et al.* (2007). Dublin, Ireland. In *Recovery from Schizophrenia – An International Perspective*, ed. K. Hopper, G. Harrison, A. Janca and N. Sartorius. New York: Oxford, pp. 129–40.

Geertz, C. (1985). *The Uses of Diversity*. The Tanner Lectures on Human Values. University of Michigan. www.tannerlectures.utah.edu/lectures/geertz86.pdf.

Gillin, J. (1939). Personality in preliterate societies. *American Sociological Review*, **4**, 681–702.

Gureje, O. and Bamidele, R. (1999). Thirteen-year social outcome among Nigerian outpatients with schizophrenia. *Social Psychiatry and Psychiatric Epidemiology*, **34** (3), 147–51.

Halliburton, M. (2004). Finding a fit: psychiatric pluralism in South India and its implications for WHO studies of mental disorder. *Transcultural Psychiatry*, **41**, 80–98.

Hammer, M. and Leacock, E. (1961). Source material on the epidemiology of illness. In *Field Studies in the Mental Disorders*, ed. J. Zubin. New York: Grune and Stratton, pp. 418–86.

Harrison, G. (2004). Course and outcome in schizophrenia: towards a new social biology of psychotic disorders. In *Search for the Causes of Schizophrenia*, vol. 5, ed. W. F. Gattaz and H. Häfner. Darmstadt: Steinkopff Verlag, pp. 32–53.

Harrison, G., Owens, D., Holton, A. *et al.* (1988). A prospective study of severe mental disorder in Afro-Caribbean patients. *Psychological Medicine*, **18**, 643–57.

Harrison, G., Amin, S., Singh, S. P. *et al.* (1999). Outcome of psychosis in people of African-Caribbean family origin. *British Journal of Psychiatry*, **175**, 43–9.

Harrison, G., Hopper, K., Craig, T. *et al.* (2001). Recovery from psychotic illness: a 15 and 25 year international follow-up study. *British Journal of Psychiatry*, **178**, 506–17.

Hopper, K. (1991). Some old questions for the new cross-cultural psychiatry. *Medical Anthropology Quarterly* (new series), **5**, 299–330.

Hopper, K. (2003). Interrogating the meaning of 'culture' in the WHO international studies of schizophrenia. In *Schizophrenia, Culture and Subjectivity*, ed. J. H. Jenkins and R. J. Barrett. New York: Cambridge University Press, pp. 62–86.

Hopper, K. and Wanderling, J. (2000). Revisiting the developed vs developing country distinction in course and outcome in schizophrenia: results from ISoS, the WHO-Collaborative Follow-up Project. *Schizophrenia Bulletin*, **26** (4), 835–46.

Hopper, K., Harrison, G., Janca, A. *et al.* (eds) (2007a). *Recovery from Schizophrenia – An International Perspective*. New York: Oxford University Press.

Hopper, K., Wanderling, J. and Narayanan, P. (2007b). To have and to hold: a cross-cultural inquiry into marital prospects after psychosis. *Global Public Health*, **2**(3), 257–80.

Jablensky, A., Sartorius, N., Ernberg, G. *et al.* (1992). Schizophrenia: manifestations, incidence and course in different cultures. A World Health Organization ten-country study. *Psychological Medicine. Monograph Supplement*, **20**, 1–97.

Kapur, R. I. (1979). The role of traditional healers in mental health care in rural India. *Social Science and Medicine*, **13**, 27–31.

Kebede, D., Alem, A., Shibre, T. *et al.* (2005). Short-term symptomatic and functional outcomes of schizophrenia in Butajira, Ethiopia. *Schizophrenia Research*, **78**, 171–85.

Karp, I. (1985). Deconstructing culture-bound syndromes. *Social Science and Medicine*, **21**, 221–8.

Kleinman, A. (1988). *The Illness Narratives*. New York: Basic Books.

Kraepelin, E. (1919). *Dementia Praecox and Paraphrenia* (ed. G. M. Robertson); translated by R. M. Barclay. Edinburgh: E. and S. Livingstone (reprinted 1976 in Huntingdon, NY, by Robert E. Kreiger).

Kreisler, H. (1999). Habits of a militant anthropologist: conversation with Nancy Scheper-Hughes. http://globetrotter.berkeley.edu/people/Scheper-Hughes.

Kurihara, T., Kato, M., Reverger, R. *et al.* (2000). Outcome of schizophrenia in a non-industrialized society: comparative study between Bali and Tokyo. *Acta Psychiatrica Scandinavica*, **101**, 148–52.

Laubscher, B. J. F. (1937). *Sex, Custom and Psychopathology*. London: Routledge.

Littlewood, R. (1993). *Pathology and Identity: The Work of Mother Earth in Trinidad*. New York: Cambridge University Press.

Lopez, C. (1932). Ethnographische Betrachtungen über Schizophrenie. *Zeitschrift für die gesamte Neurologie und Psychiatrie*, **142**, 706–11.

Lovell, A. M. (1997). The city is my mother: narratives of schizophrenia and homelessness. *American Anthropologist* (new series), **99** (2), 355–68.

Lucas, R. (2003). In and out of culture: ethnographic means to interpreting culture. In *Schizophrenia, Culture and Subjectivity*, ed. J. H. Jenkins and R. J. Barrett. New York: Cambridge University Press, pp. 146–66.

Luhrmann, T. M. (2006). Subjectivity. *Anthropological Theory*, **6**(3), 345–61.

McGrath, J. J. (2007). The surprisingly rich contours of schizophrenia epidemiology. *Archives of General Psychiatry*, **64**, 14–16.

Miller, G. (2006). A spoonful of medicine – and a steady diet of normality. *Science*, **311**, 464–5.

Mojtabai, R., Varma, V. K., Malhotra, S. *et al.* (2001). Mortality and long-term course in schizophrenia with a poor 2-year course – a study in a developing country. *British Journal of Psychiatry*, **178**, 71–5.

Murphy, H. B. M. and Raman, A. C. (1971). The chronicity of schizophrenia in indigenous tropical peoples. *British Journal of Psychiatry*, **118**, 489–97.

Pakaslahti, A. (1998). Family centered treatment of mental health problems at the Bajaji Temple in Rajasthan. In *Changing Patterns of Family and Kinship in South Asia*, ed. A. Parpola and S. Tenhunen. Helsinki: Finnish Oriental Society, pp. 129–66.

Patel, V. and Kleinman, A. (2003). Poverty and common mental disorders in developing countries. *Bulletin of the World Health Organization*, **81**(8), 609–15.

Patel, V., Cohen, A., Thara, R. *et al.* (2006). Is the outcome of schizophrenia really better in developing countries? *Revista Brasileira Psiquiatria*, **28** (2), 129–52.

Phillips, M. R., Liu, H. Q. and Zhang, Y. P. (1999). Suicide and social change in China. *Culture Medicine and Psychiatry*, **23** (1), 25–50.

Price, P. S. (2006). Letter: social defeat and schizophrenia. *British Journal of Psychiatry*, **186**, 393.

Raguram, R. (2002). Temple healing: spiritual care is important – response. *British Medical Journal*, **325** (7370), 969.

Ran, M., Xiang, M., Huang, M. *et al.* (2001). Natural course of schizophrenia: 2-year follow-up study in a rural Chinese community. *British Journal of Psychiatry*, **178**, 154–8.

Rawls, J. (1971). *A Theory of Justice*. Cambridge, MA: Belknap Press.

Ribeiro, B. T. (1994). *Coherence in Psychotic Discourse*. Oxford: Oxford University Press.

Sadowsky, J. (1999). *Colonial Bedlam: Institutions of Madness in Colonial Southwest Nigeria*. Berkeley: University of California Press.

Saris, J. (1996). Mad kings, proper houses, and an asylum in Ireland. *American Anthropologist*, **98**, 539–54.

Sass, L. A. (1992). *Madness and Modernism*. New York: Basic Books.

Sassen, S. (1993). *Cities in a World Economy*. New York: Pine Forge/Sage.

Sawa, A. and Snyder, S. H. (2002). Schizophrenia: diverse approaches to a complex disease. *Science*, **296**, 692–5.

Scheper-Hughes, N. (1979; 2000) *Saints, Scholars and Schizophrenics*. Original and expanded edns. Berkeley: University of California.

Scull, A. (1977). *Decarceration*. Englewood Cliffs, NJ: Prentice Hall.

Seligman, C. G. (1929). Temperament, conflict and psychosis in a stone-age population. *British Journal of Medical Psychology*, **4**, 195.

Selten, J. P. and Cantor-Graae, E. (2005). Social defeat: risk factor for schizophrenia? *British Journal of Psychiatry*, **187**, 101–2.

Selten, J. P., Slaets, J. P. and Kahn, R. S. (1997). Schizophrenia in Surinamese and Dutch Antillean immigrants to the Netherlands: evidence of an increased incidence. *Psychological Medicine*, **27**, 807–11.

Sharpley, M. S., Hutchinson, G., McKenzie, K. *et al.* (2001). Understanding the excess of psychosis among the African-Caribbean population in England. *British Journal of Psychiatry*, **178** (suppl. 40), s60–s68.

Silverman, J. (1967). Shamans and acute schizophrenia. *American Anthropologist*, **69**, 21–31.

Spence, J. (1988). *The Question of Hu*. New York: Vintage.

Stevens, A. and Price, J. (2000). *Prophets, Cults and Madness*. London: Duckworth.

Sundar, M. (1999). Suicide in farmers in India. *British Journal of Psychiatry*, **175**, 585–6.

Swartz, S. and Swartz, L. (1987). Talk about talk: metacommentary and context in the analysis of psychotic discourse. *Culture, Medicine and Psychiatry*, **11**, 305–416.

Thara, R. (2004). Twenty-year course of schizophrenia: the Madras Longitudinal Study. *Canadian Journal of Psychiatry*, **49**, 564–9.

Thara, R., Kamath, S. and Kumar, S. (2003a). Women with schizophrenia and broken marriages – doubly disadvantaged. Part I: patient perspective. *International Journal of Social Psychiatry*, **49**, 225–32.

Thara, R., Kamath, S. and Kumar, S. (2003b). Women with schizophrenia and broken marriages – doubly disadvantaged. Part II: family perspective. *International Journal of Social Psychiatry*, **49**, 233–40.

Thara, R., Rajkumar, S. and Joseph, A. (2007). Chennai (Madras) India. In *Recovery from Schizophrenia: An International Perspective*, ed. K. Hopper, G. Harrison, A. Janca and N. Sartorius. New York: Oxford University Press, pp. 266–76.

van Os, J. (2003). Can the social environment cause schizophrenia? *British Journal of Psychiatry*, **182**, 291–2.

Varma, V. K. and Malhotra, S. (2007). Chandigarh, India. In *Recovery from Schizophrenia – An International Perspective*, ed. K. Hopper, G. Harrison, A. Janca and N. Sartorius. New York: Oxford University Press, pp. 115–128.

Vaughan, M. (1983). Idioms of madness: Zomba Lunatic Asylum, Nyasaland, in the colonial period. *Journal of Southern African Studies*, **9**, 218–38.

Wallace, A. F. C. (1961). *Culture and Personality*. New York: Random House.

Warner, R. (2003). *Recovery from Schizophrenia: Psychiatry and the Political Economy*, 3rd edn. London: Routledge.

Watzlawick, P., Bavelas, J. B. and Jackson, D. D. (1967). *Pragmatics of Human Communication*. New York: W. W. Norton.

Whitaker, R. (2001). *Mad in America*. New York: Perseus Publishing.

WHO (1973). *Report of the International Pilot Study of Schizophrenia*, vol. 1. Geneva: World Health Organization.

WHO (1979). *Schizophrenia. An International Follow-Up Study*. Chichester: Wiley and Sons.

Wilce, J. (2000). The poetics of 'madness': shifting codes and styles in the linguistic construction of identity in Matlab, Bangladesh. *Cultural Anthropology*, **15** (1), 3–34.

Wilce, J. (2003). To 'speak beautifully' in Bangladesh: subjectivity as Pagalami. In *Schizophrenia, Culture, and Subjectivity*, eds J. H. Jenkins and R. J. Barrett. New York: Cambridge University Press, pp. 196–218.

Williams, R. (1976). *Keywords: A Vocabulary of Culture and Society*. London: Fontana Press.

Wilson, P. (1974). *Oscar: An Inquiry into the Nature of Sanity*. New York: Random House.

Wing, J. and Brown, G. (1970). *Institutionalism and Schizophrenia*. London: Cambridge University Press.

Winston, E. (1934). The alleged lack of mental diseases among primitive groups. *American Anthropologist*, **36**, 234–8.

Zolkowska, K., Cantor-Graae, E. and McNeil, T. F. (2001). Increased risk of psychosis among immigrants to Sweden: is migration a risk factor for psychosis? *Psychological Medicine*, **21**, 669–778.

Part IV

Models and conclusions

14

Theories of cognition, emotion and the social world: missing links in psychosis

Paul Bebbington, David Fowler, Philippa Garety, Daniel Freeman and Elizabeth Kuipers

Introduction

Throughout the twentieth century, clinicians and researchers struggled to establish a convincing account of psychosis and the processes and mechanisms underlying its manifestations. This effort depended on refinements of classification and case definition over the whole course of the century. However, despite the huge investment of intellectual energy and monetary resources, results have been slow in coming and disappointingly piecemeal. It has become clear that psychosis is a phenomenon of great complexity. Recent social and cognitive models of psychosis are attempts to deal with some aspects of this complexity. We will argue for the appositeness of such models, and place them within the broader research effort in psychosis. Before doing this, we need to revisit some of the consequences of the formulation of the concept of schizophrenia, the disorder that represents the core of psychotic phenomena.

A failed category?

The idea that schizophrenia is a failed category emerges regularly in the psychiatric and psychological literature, the most prominent current advocate being Bentall (2003). This is essentially a criticism of approaching schizophrenia as a medical entity. The medical strategy of investigation involves the identification of syndromes, which, in turn, form the basis of theories. These include those relating to aetiology, pathology, outcome and treatment (Wing, 1978). Syndromes are essentially theoretical constructs: while they can be regarded as disease entities, they are never really more than tentative. Nevertheless, there is a tendency in psychiatry to

Society and Psychosis, ed. Craig Morgan, Kwame McKenzie and Paul Fearon. Published by Cambridge University Press. © Cambridge University Press 2008.

regard psychiatric syndromes as having more virtue than they actually possess. They do, however, form a useful basis for research. If theories about syndromes are refuted, consideration may be given to abandoning them. In medicine we generally reject theories, of aetiology and so on, before rejecting the theoretical construct represented by the syndrome. We may nevertheless eventually decide that the syndrome has failed, in the sense that the knowledge built up in relation to it is confused and imprecise, and there may be better ways of organising the clinical information for the purposes of research. There is current debate about whether we have reached this stage with schizophrenia.

One of the difficulties for a biomedical approach in psychiatry is the sheer cussedness of the subject matter. It is, for example, extremely difficult to construct a classification, as categories in psychiatry are notorious for overlapping one another. This is not merely a problem of imprecise definition: the subject matter is actually hierarchical rather than planar, and any attempt to construct a flat classification is thus probably doomed to failure.

The nature of psychiatric phenomena creates three crucial problems for the definition of categories like schizophrenia. The first is the *threshold problem*, that is, the point at which the syndrome becomes recognisable and distinguishable from normal experience. The second is the *boundary problem*, the difficulty of drawing valid lines between, for example, schizophrenia and bipolar disorder. Added to this is a third problem, which is both empirical and conceptual. This is that the disorder seems to be inherently difficult to explain.

One of the early authorities to grasp the problem of the threshold was Jaspers (1913). He saw schizophrenia as the battleground between opposing traditions of explanation in science. The methods of the physical sciences were concerned with *causal explanation*, whereas social sciences involved appreciation through a process of *understanding*, through meaningful connections. His view was that where understanding failed (as it seems to in people's attempts to share the experiences of those deemed to be mad), we are left only with resort to physical explanation. The implication is that in such circumstances we are facing a physical illness with physical causes. The conclusion is that there ceases to be room for explanations of the schizophrenic experience in terms of social contexts, and that cognitive accounts represent understanding at a different level from biological explanations. The resulting biological hegemony held sway in psychiatry until the last decades of the twentieth century, and is only now being replaced by a more flexible and comprehensive approach to the problems besetting scientific research in schizophrenia.

Jaspers himself never regarded schizophrenia as a no-go area for social and psychological research. He was quite happy with the idea that psychosis could be meaningfully connected to circumstances, although reluctant to see the process as *wholly* understandable. He did acknowledge that it was difficult to identify the point at which paranoia became delusional, and there is now considerable evidence confirming his view.

Psychosis as a continuum with normal experience

Modern cognitive models of psychosis actually start by postulating continuities between psychosis and normal experience. The emergence of psychotic phenomena thus reflects an abnormal concatenation of largely normal mechanisms. What is weakness in the medical category, in this theoretical formulation becomes strength. In the past, the urge to make a categorical distinction between psychosis and normality almost certainly led to a Procrustean tendency to discount unusual beliefs and experiences in people we would be reluctant to see as undergoing a psychosis. However, it became apparent by the late 1980s that paranoid ideation and anomalous experiences, such as hearing voices, were not confined to clinical groups. It is clear that the frequency of auditory hallucinosis greatly exceeds the accepted prevalence of psychosis (e.g., Wiles *et al.*, 2006). The distinguishing feature of those in contact with services is the *level of distress* occasioned by their unusual experiences (Hanssen *et al.*, 2003; van Os *et al.*, 1999).

The distribution of unusual beliefs in the populace is also extensive. Many people are convinced of the truth of ideas that are not supported by available and accessible evidence. These include beliefs in astrology, alien beings, telepathy or ghosts. Political beliefs are held with strong conviction even though they may be untried, or indeed tried and found wanting. People who hold these cherished ideas typically have a *confirmatory bias*, being unlikely to consider alternatives impartially. These beliefs shade into what would be regarded as delusional, since the thinking that underpins them is similar in style to that in people with acknowledged psychosis.

Attempts have been made to define delusions in terms that would enable them to be distinguished clearly and reliably from normal thinking. The form of words varies, but generally implies the following: they are held with a basic and compelling subjective conviction; they are not susceptible to contrary experience or to counter-argument; they are impossible, incredible or false; they lie outside the belief systems characteristic of the individual's cultural group. However, because of the overlap with 'normal' thinking, it has been impossible to construct criteria that are, individually or jointly, both necessary and sufficient for an operationalised definition (Bebbington and Broome, 2004).

The continua of beliefs in the community have been demonstrated empirically. One example concerns 'paranoid' beliefs, in other words, those relating to self-reference and threat. Freeman *et al.* (2005b) found that 30% of an internet sample

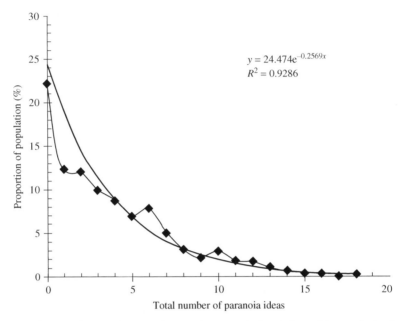

$$y = 24.474e^{-0.2569x}$$
$$R^2 = 0.9286$$

Figure 14.1 Distribution of paranoia scores in a student population (taken with permission from Freeman *et al.*, 2005b)

of students had such ideas. Moreover, the frequency distribution of individual paranoid ideas followed an exponential curve (Figure 14.1), with the relationship between them being non-hierarchical, such that more extreme ideas were predictive of those that were less extreme but not vice versa. This finding has now been corroborated using general population data (Bebbington, P. E. *et al.* The paranoia dimension in the general population (submitted to the *British Journal of Psychiatry*)). The pattern is much like that shown by affective symptoms (Melzer *et al.*, 2002; Sturt, 1981). At a single point in time the continuum is defined by differences between individuals, who are thus located at individual positions on the curve. However, people are themselves likely to vary in a way that would place them at different positions on the curve at different times, dependent on changing circumstances. In a sense, they would move along the curve.

These findings have considerable relevance to the aetiology of psychosis. They imply that in some people movement along a continuum (indeed probably more than one continuum) results in the emergence of psychosis. Thus the role of aetiology is to explain exactly why particular people make this journey at particular times in their lives. In the genetic arena, this suggests a focus on quantitative analyses (Linney *et al.*, 2003), along with the identification of quantitative trait loci (Plomin *et al.*, 1994). In the psychological domain, it implies the concatenation of different psychological attributes, some cognitive, some emotional (Hanssen *et al.*,

2005; Krabbendam and van Os, 2005; Krabbendam *et al.*, 2005). There are also implications for treatment, in particular psychological treatments, such as cognitive behaviour therapy (Kuipers *et al.*, 2006).

The boundary problem

The boundary problem, whereby schizophrenia is imprecisely separated from other psychiatric conditions, has also been a source of discomfiture. The relationship between bipolar disorder and schizophrenia, for instance, is certainly ambiguous. Clearly some individuals have mood dysregulation, and some have psychotic experiences. However, many have both, and in varying proportions. While attempts may be made to see affective psychosis and non-affective psychosis as distinct, they really represent opposite ends of a spectrum, and this is reflected in considerable overlap in the candidate genes associated with the two conditions (Craddock and Owen, 2005; Craddock *et al.*, 2005; 2006).

Mood disturbances of some kind are almost invariable in cases of schizophrenia. Thus, up to 40% of people with schizophrenia also have clinical levels of depression (Birchwood, 2003; Sands and Harrow, 1999), 30% meet criteria for post-traumatic stress disorder (Mueser *et al.*, 1998), 20% have panic disorder (Turnbull and Bebbington, 2001) and up to 25%, obsessive compulsive disorder (Berman *et al.*, 1995). For a classification seeking to distinguish affective and non-affective forms of psychosis, this is an embarrassment. However, once we cease to worry about the overlap and think of emotional changes as potentially an integral part of the psychotic process, it becomes possible to see it as a doorway to explanation. This is easy for cognitive models of psychosis, which all involve an acknowledged role for affect (Birchwood, 2003; Garety *et al.*, 2001).

Aetiological processes

What then of the problems of explaining schizophrenia in biomedical terms? We define schizophrenia in relation to people's reports of their unusual mental experiences. It would make life much simpler if we had privileged access to some underlying condition or entity. However, all we have to go on is the disorder as defined, the phenomena, not the noumena. In other words, it is the strange beliefs, the hallucinations, and their contents, that we have to explain.

There has long been a prima facie assumption about aetiological theories in psychosis, a reductionist position placing genetic explanations at the beginning of the aetiological process. Virtually all genetic research in schizophrenia has been based on the assumption that genetic abnormalities lead to abnormalities in protein function, with consequent distortions of enzymatic activity, and that these in turn lead to corresponding deficits in neuronal function. These deficits then result in cognitive dysfunctions that form the substrate for the schizophrenic experiences that permit the diagnosis of the disorder. This is obviously a very useful working paradigm, but it must be treated with caution.

The high heritability of schizophrenia is easy to demonstrate from twin studies (Craddock *et al.*, 2005). However, recent research has served to emphasise that not only is schizophrenia a complex disorder to the clinical observer, it is also complex in genetic terms. Such disorders have relatively high population prevalence, are non-Mendelian and are imprecisely distinguished from the normal range. The search for genes linked to schizophrenia has been long, arduous and expensive (Norton *et al.*, 2006; Owen *et al.*, 2005). Candidates have been unearthed, but their association with schizophrenia remains tentative. The genes encoding dysbindin (DTNBP1) and neuroregulin (NRG1) are the strongest contenders, with evidence for other genes (*disrupted in schizophrenia* (DISC1), *D-aminoacid oxidase activator* (DAOA), *regulator of G-protein signalling 4* (RGS4) and *V-AKT murine thymoma viral oncogene homolog 1* (AKT1)) being at least suggestive (Norton *et al.*, 2006). Some have been associated with abnormalities of brain structure and enzyme function, which, albeit plausible, would seem to have a tenuous connection to the schizophrenic phenotype (Callicott *et al.*, 2005; Harrison and Weinberger, 2005; Meyer-Lindenberg *et al.*, 2005). Given the modern synthesis of evolutionary theory, genetics and developmental biology, focusing solely on encoding for enzymes is likely to prove simplistic, even though links with schizophrenia may be found. After all, only two percent or so of the DNA in human cells produce proteins that act as enzymes, while much more is involved in complex regulatory systems that switch the functions of protein-encoding genes on and off, something clearly of potential relevance to an acknowledged developmental disorder like schizophrenia. These issues have at last started to inform genetic research in schizophrenia (Glaser *et al.*, 2006; Law *et al.*, 2006; Lipska *et al.*, 2006).

Adjacent elements in the aetiological process seem likely to fall far short of a one-to-one relationship, with the implication that at every step on the way the specificity of relationships is progressively lost. The consequence is that the association of individual genes with schizophrenia must inevitably be attenuated, with small effect sizes (Norton *et al.*, 2006).

Moreover, the genes identified so far seem to be associated with neurocognitive deficits (Hariri *et al.*, 2003; Meyer-Lindenberg *et al.*, 2005). These are plausible antecedents of negative symptoms of schizophrenia, and there is appreciable empirical support for the association between them (Pinkham *et al.*, 2003). Thus genetic explanations so far lean towards an explanation of negative symptoms. However, the heritability of schizophrenia is the heritability of positive symptoms, since it is from these that the condition is identified. The potential association of the Val/Val allelic form of COMT with vulnerability to psychotic responses to cannabis might be one way round this difficulty (Caspi *et al.*, 2005). However, we fall far short of a comprehensive explanation in genetic terms for the positive symptoms responsible for the heritability of the condition in the first place.

There are further problems with the aetiological process. The implicit unidirectionality is an act of faith that almost certainly cannot be sustained. Thus the way in which heritability is calculated means that it actually includes gene–environment interaction. Moreover, gene–environment interaction covers environmental gene induction, and the inducing environment may be social as well as physical. Thus, natural variation in the competency of mouse mothers affects their offspring's responses to stress in later life (Meaney, 2001), apparently mediated by epigenetic changes involving histone regulation of DNA expression. This is then maintained, and affects the offspring's own parenting behaviour (Fish *et al.*, 2004; Weaver *et al.*, 2004). Thus the causal direction may sometimes run from the social to the physical, rather than the other way around. Furthermore, our knowledge about putative aetiological factors is based on induction. Thus, because some people with schizophrenia have, for example, a family history of the same condition, an inductive leap is made to the conclusion that *all* schizophrenia has a genetic basis. The frailty of the logic underpinning this inference is apparent. As the same caveat applies to social theories, aetiological modesty is imperative on all sides.

The final problem relates to the nature of schizophrenic symptoms themselves. Most of the experiences that form the basis of the identified symptoms of schizophrenia are *about* something: they carry within them representations of the social world (paranoid ideation is an obvious example of this). This is the characteristic of *intentionality* identified by Brentano (1874). Defining a medical condition in terms of experiences that have intentionality means that explanations in purely physical terms will always be incomplete.

This is the context in which models of psychosis involving social, emotional and cognitive elements have been developed. They do not deny an important role for the physical matrix of disorder, but they do add to the complexity and probably to the potential of explanation. They form one part of the overall model. There are several variants, and all are better described as social-cognitive-emotional models. They focus on the sorts of explanation that can be developed for considering the person with psychosis as an agent in a social and societal context. They also seek to explain psychosis by trying to explain single symptoms or coherent groups of symptoms.

Analysing single symptoms

The study of single psychotic symptoms, or single types of symptom, is assisted by a clear account of the symptoms themselves. Thus cognitive models encourage a return to the precision of the early psychopathologists. However, descriptions are amplified by attempts to discern processes that may underlie the mental experiences corresponding to the symptoms. This activity should be distinguished from actual explanation – it is more akin to exegesis, and increases the potential targets for explanation. An example of exegesis is provided by Frith in his persuasive account of passivity experiences as a combination of 'forward memory' and an exaggerated sense of agency ('if it is not me, it must be someone else') (Frith, 2005).

Phenomenological analyses may also clarify linkages between symptoms conventionally regarded as separate. For example, there are relationships between thought insertion, loud thoughts and thought broadcast. The essence of thought insertion is not the idea of external origin, but the loss of the sense of possession of the mental experience. This is shared by other passivity experiences, but also by auditory hallucinations. Loud thoughts are thoughts acknowledged by the person experiencing them, but they have the quality of loudness shared by our experience of sound waves. In this, they of course resemble auditory hallucinosis. Thought broadcast has been described imprecisely, but close attention to the self-reports of those who suffer from it reveals that the essential feature is the experience of thoughts that are externally projected. Such thoughts share this feature with some but not all forms of auditory hallucinosis. Thus these four types of symptoms exhibit variously the *loss of the sense of possession*, *loudness* and *external projection*, and the exact pattern of these three features determines what symptoms may be identified.

Projection and loudness merit further comment, as both can be seen as distortions of normal processes. It is probably of enormous evolutionary advantage to integrate the brain changes initiated by the immediate environment into an externally projected world. This capacity for projection is self-evidently inherent in human beings, and the external projection that characterises hallucination, thought broadcast and passivity experiences is thus also a failure of a normal mechanism. Loudness is the mental experience normally attached to the brain events corresponding to the impact of sound waves on the cochlea. As such, it flags up these events as relating to the external world. When the flag becomes attached to other mental experiences, they become anomalous (as in loud thoughts). Loudness and external projection may have a very similar neural embodiment, but their separation in particular psychotic symptoms suggests they are distinct.

A further example of this kind of analysis concerns the issue of meaning. This can be interpreted as an emotional component of mental experience. In psychiatric disorder, levels of meaning can be either increased or reduced, or both. The most obvious example of this reregulation occurs in depression and mania. People with depression lose a sense of meaning, just as those with mania acquire it. Perception carries an emotional charge that becomes apparent when it is lost. Loss of meaning underlies experiences such as dulled perception, depersonalisation and derealisation.

while in mania heightened perception affects the perceived intensity of colours and sounds and the beauty of music. However, meaning also attaches to non-perceptual mental experiences. In depression, this includes lost emotions: a painful sense of knowing and remembering the emotion but no longer being able to feel it. In general, reduction in the emotional component of mental experiences is negative if not always painful, while increases are more ambiguous. Thus, the increased signification attached to paranoid ideas is distressing while that attached to heightened perception and to some forms of ideas of reference may be pleasurable. Capgras' syndrome is a form of delusional depersonalisation, whereby the loss of the emotional component of person recognition results in delusional ideas concerning the replacement of known people by unknown impostors. In contrast, the Fregoli syndrome is associated with an increased signification of person perception, resulting in the belief that strangers are actually friends and relatives in disguise. It is also possible to conceive of mental experiences involving loss of the sense of possession as being down-regulations of the emotional significance of the experience.

There is, thus, a prima facie argument for suggesting that change in the emotional components of mental experience underlies many psychiatric symptoms including those involved in psychosis. This would again imply continuities between symptoms regarded as psychotic and those that are not. It remains possible, of course, that this proposition arises from over-interpretation and that there is no underlying commonality of the type described.

The distinctiveness of symptoms probably implies that there are also distinctions between the processes that generate them. Thus disorders like Fregoli and Capgras may include a specific malfunction of the part of the fusiform gyrus concerned with facial recognition (Pinkham *et al.*, 2005). Nevertheless, the possibility of a common contribution has been acknowledged by Kapur (2003) in his proposition that dopamine dysfunction in psychosis often increases *salience* but sometimes reduces it.

Cognitive models of psychosis

Over the last 10 years or so, several cognitive models of psychosis have been proposed (e.g., Bentall *et al.*, 2001; Birchwood, 2003; Broome *et al.*, 2005; Fowler, 2000; Freeman *et al.*, 2002; Garety *et al.*, 2001; Morrison, 2001). They seek to identify the origins of psychosis by explaining the causation of individual symptoms. To do this, they adduce interactions between social contexts, emotional tone and cognitive processing. They vary in the emphasis laid on these components and the extent to which the involved processes are regarded as unusual concatenations of normal internal and external circumstances.

Our own model emphasises the continuity of psychotic and non-psychotic experiences; a central role of appraisal; the role of low self-esteem and emotional changes; and findings relating to adverse social environments. While we do not specify biological explanations in the model, they are implicit. In other words, some of the components may be related to abnormal neural function. The model emphasises, *as one route to symptom development*, the significance of cognitive dysfunction leading to anomalous experiences, and the appraisal of these experiences as externally caused. Unlike Morrison (2001), we think this distinguishes psychosis from common mental disorders, such as anxiety and depression. Virtual reality experiments with normal subjects are of interest here. Some normal subjects develop persecutory thoughts even in neutral scenarios. Crucially, it seems that previous anomalous experiences of a schizotypal variety differentiate between people who are merely anxious in the situation and those who develop persecutory ideas (Freeman *et al.*, 2003, 2005a).

A considerable amount of recent work has tested hypotheses derived from these cognitive models. We ourselves start from the common assumption that people who develop a psychotic illness do so on the basis of a predisposition of biological or social origin that renders them vulnerable to stress. This vulnerability is expressed in emotional and cognitive changes that contribute to anomalies of conscious experience, of which the most salient example is auditory hallucinosis. Anomalous experiences seem likely to be embodied in information processing disturbances (Frith, 1992; Gray *et al.*, 1991; Hemsley, 1993, 2005). These authors have suggested that anomalous experiences are intrusions into conscious awareness arising from defects in the continuous integration of current experience with stored memories. However, the mere experience of anomalies does not lead to overt psychosis without an interpretation that lends them personal significance and attributes to them an external origin. Such interpretation is shaped by information processing biases, pre-existing schematic beliefs about the self and others, and emotional disturbance, all of which interact with (and sometimes originate from) the social contexts that individuals find themselves in. We will consider these elements in further detail.

Social influences on psychosis

Psychosocial factors are comprehended in a variety of ways. Research into the relationship between *life events* and various psychiatric conditions has been a major thrust in psychiatry over the past 40 years. Life events obviously range from the catastrophic to the relatively banal, and events of all types have been studied in relation to schizophrenia. Initial investigations involved recent events with significant social connotations (Bebbington *et al.*, 1996). More recent research has examined the ebb and flow of daily hassles (see Chapter 9).

Other research has involved quite complex aspects of the person's environment, for example, the immediate family environment (see Chapter 8) and social networks. Yet other studies focus on the wider context in which individuals are located. Examples are the overall experiences of people seeking asylum, migrating for other reasons to a new region or country (Cantor-Graae and Selten, 2005; McGrath, 2006), or forming part of an ethnic or cultural minority (Fearon *et al.*, 2006) (see Chapter 10). In the past 10 years or so there has been increasing interest in more distant social contexts. Some epidemiological studies have examined the impact of urban upbringing and changes of schooling (both are associated with later psychosis) (see Chapter 6). A number of research groups have examined the impact of traumatic events, in particular child sexual abuse (Bebbington *et al.*, 2004; Mueser *et al.*, 1998; Read *et al.*, 2005) (see Chapter 7). This has been accompanied by a convergence of ideas about post-traumatic stress disorder and psychotic experience (Fowler *et al.*, 2006). These new areas of research have raised questions about how early psychosocial experience might link with the later manifestation of psychosis.

Stressful events and psychosis

The study of life events occurring immediately before the onset or relapse of psychosis dates from the 1960s (Bebbington *et al.*, 1995). Even in nuclear schizophrenia, many cases experience stressful and personally significant events in the few weeks or months before an episode. The association of recent stressful life events with relapse into *positive* symptoms is well established (Bebbington *et al.*, 1995; Nuechterlein *et al.*, 1994). A role for events before *first* episodes would suggest an effect going beyond the mere triggering of subsequent episodes in people who had already manifested the disorder, presumably for other reasons. While the evidence for events in relation to first episodes is still thin, it has recently been bolstered by an indication of specificity: the strength of the association is increased when the event has attributes that can be meaningfully associated with the content of psychosis. Thus, events characterised by intrusiveness seem to be especially linked to psychosis, and perhaps to paranoid ideation in particular (Harris, 1987; Raune *et al.*, 2006).

Distant trauma and psychosis

Until recently it was assumed that the impact of events would dissipate fairly rapidly, and this is almost certainly true for most sorts of event, as they quite clearly cluster in the vicinity of onset (Day *et al.*, 1987). However, recent studies have also made clear that a history of trauma and victimisation is very common in people with psychosis. Although these may both precede and accompany episodes of psychotic disorder (Mueser *et al.*, 1998), many have occurred long before onset, raising the possibility that they may have produced a longstanding vulnerability that has been translated later into a psychotic episode. These findings have been incorporated into current psychosocial models of psychosis (Garety *et al.*, 2001; Kuipers *et al.*, 2006), which also postulate that stressful events may contribute to the initial emergence of psychosis. The obvious mechanism is that they change persistent psychological styles and attributes, but they may also increase biological sensitivity to stress. Bullying and sexual abuse are particularly associated with negative self and other schemas, and with positive symptoms such as persecutory delusions and hallucinations. Such experiences lead to a psychosis particularly characterised by hallucinations, although direct links between trauma and hallucinatory content seemed to be relatively rare (Hardy *et al.*, 2005).

Recent research into cognitive processes

Recent research has confirmed the importance of *reasoning* biases in psychosis. However, such reasoning biases are common: people often hold with conviction ideas without much basis in fact, and it is normal for them not to consider alternatives impartially. This is the so-called confirmatory bias. People with psychoses show all these features of normal thinking. It has been found that they also tend to use less evidence before making a decision: the *jumping to conclusions* (JTC) reasoning bias (Garety and Hemsley, 1994). This has particular relevance for delusional thinking. Interestingly, JTC persists after recovery from delusions (Peters and Garety, 2005). Moreover, it appears to be related to belief inflexibility and an inability to generate alternative explanations for experiences (Freeman *et al.*, 2004). The JTC reasoning bias is thus a good candidate for a true trait vulnerability for psychosis. Not surprisingly, reasoning biases appear to make a specific contribution to the level of conviction with which delusions are held (Garety *et al.*, 2005).

Attributional biases may also contribute to psychosis, although here the evidence is inconclusive (Bentall and Kinderman, 1999; Jolley *et al.*, 2006). *Externalising* biases may be particularly characteristic of people with persecutory delusions, whereby they attribute blame for negative events to external factors, predominantly to other people. This is markedly different from the self-blame of people with depression. Extreme negative evaluations of the self and others mediate the link between emotional processes and positive symptoms of psychosis (Fowler *et al.*, 2006; Smith *et al.*, 2006). Low self-esteem in people with psychosis is often associated with criticism from carers (Barrowclough *et al.*, 2003).

There is other evidence linking negative affect and positive symptoms, both from prospective studies and from research using time-sampling. Thus, Krabbendam and her colleagues (2005) demonstrated that depression encourages the later development of delusions in people with pre-existing anomalies of experience, while Myin-Germeys *et al.* (2001) found that fluctuations in positive symptoms of psychosis were associated with time-sampled changes in negative affect.

People with psychosis also have well established cognitive deficits in attention and working memory, which may also contribute to symptom formation (Joyce, 2005), although the precise mechanism remains unclear. Hallucinations or passivity experiences may be specifically related to self-monitoring, another cognitive process (Blakemore *et al.*, 2003; Frith, 1992; Johns *et al.*, 2001). In this context, Hemsley has provided evidence for a disruption to a sense of self (Hemsley, 1998, 2005). The ability to process immediate experience may be disrupted by a poor use of contextual information (Barch *et al.*, 2004).

Appraisal is central

Depressed mood in people with psychosis is related to attributions of power and control to the people persecuting them or responsible for their hallucinations (Birchwood, 2003; Green *et al.*, 2006). Negative appraisals of symptoms, of self and of others are of great clinical importance because they relate to suicidal ideation and high alcohol intake (Fialko *et al.*, 2006). The appraisal of danger by people with psychosis leads to safety behaviours, which are important in the maintenance of delusions (Freeman *et al.*, 2003, 2007; Morrison, 2001). People with psychosis also appraise the consequences of their illness, just as anyone with a physical illness does (Lobban *et al.*, 2004). Unsurprisingly, these appraisals are likely to be negative, and thus associated with distress (Watson *et al.*, 2006). Moreover, disagreements between carers and patients about appraisals of the illness seem to be associated with negative affect in both (Kuipers *et al.*, 2007).

Stress and cognition

Many people with psychosis have experienced significant psychosocial trauma in the past, and many are troubled by memories of it (Bebbington *et al.*, 2004; Janssen *et al.*, 2004; Johns *et al.*, 2004; Krabbendam *et al.*, 2004; Mueser *et al.*, 1998; Read *et al.*, 2005). While links are now reasonably well established between trauma and psychosis, we must explain how those links might work. The original conceptualisation of post-traumatic stress disorder was that it required no further explanation: every person exposed to catastrophic and life-threatening stress would respond with a set of symptoms that were largely affective, but included the specific and interlinked experiences of re-enaction and avoidance. It is now apparent that the relationship between life-threatening stress and the features of PTSD is not guaranteed (Rechtman, 2004). Thus PTSD itself requires additional explanation, and a relationship between catastrophic stress and the emergence of psychosis certainly does. Why is it that in processing such stress a minority of people (and only a minority) develop psychosis? Is there any kind of meaningful link between the nature of the events and the form and content of psychosis? Are there particular attributes of events that encourage psychotic reactions, and is this effect enhanced by the psychological or indeed neurobiological attributes of the person experiencing them?

Post-traumatic stress disorder is of special interest because the re-experiencing phenomenon shares with psychotic experience the quality of intrusiveness, and yet is different. Is it possible that the intrusive phenomena of PTSD lend themselves to transmutation into the alien intrusive experiences of psychosis? If so, how does this happen? A special variant of cognitive models of psychosis seeks to explain this: the so-called catastrophic interaction thesis (Fowler *et al.*, 2006).

Fowler *et al.* (2006) propose four separate pathways between severe stress and psychosis. The first involves a direct link between intrusive memories of traumatic stress and the content of hallucinations. The next postulates that links between trauma and persecutory delusions may sometimes be mediated by characteristic styles of evaluating self and others that underpin perceptions of value and danger in social contexts. In a third potential mechanism, trauma may engender ruminations and self-criticism centring on the particular identity of voices. The final route involves the interactions between emotional responses to trauma and information processing abnormalities, such as contextual processing and source memory. These interactions may distort and exaggerate the current experience of anxiety associated with memories of past trauma.

The detailed study of the relationship between trauma and psychosis is in its early days, but the investigation of the emotional and cognitive processes common to trauma responses and to psychosis in our view carries considerable promise.

Conclusion

Psychosis is a complex phenomenon that demands complex and multilevel explanations. At any point, an aetiological factor, though present, may fail to result in psychosis; indeed, failure is almost certainly the rule. Moreover, the connections may sometimes operate in a direction that is the reverse of that implied by reductionism. Our ignorance of the interactions between influences at different levels will only yield to prolonged research. We are unlikely to return to the simplistic formulations that drove research as recently as 15 years ago, and a start has certainly been made on 'new' psychosis research programmes. In this chapter, we have argued that important contributions have been made by linking cognition, emotion and the social world with the emergence and maintenance of psychotic experiences. These have been framed within specific models, which have clearly already been productive. Future research will investigate the relationships between cognition, emotion and neuropsychological abnormalities, which may themselves be associated with specific genetic effects.

REFERENCES

Barch, D., Mitropoulou, V., Harvey, P. D. *et al.* (2004). Context-processing deficits in schizotypal personality disorder. *Journal of Abnormal Psychology*, **113**, 556–68.

Barrowclough, C., Tarrier, N., Humphreys, L. *et al.* (2003). Self-esteem in schizophrenia: relationships between self-evaluation, family attitudes, and symptomatology. *Journal of Abnormal Psychology*, **112**, 92–9.

Bebbington, P. E. and Broome, M. (2004). Exploiting the interface between philosophy and psychiatry. *International Review of Psychiatry*, **16**, 179–83.

Bebbington, P. E., Bowen, J., Hirsch, S. R. and Kuipers, E. (1995). Schizophrenia and psychosocial stressors. In *Schizophrenia*, ed. S. R. Hirsch and D. Weinberger. Oxford: Blackwell Science, pp. 587–604.

Bebbington, P. E., Bhugra, D., Brugha, T. *et al.* (2004). Psychosis, victimisation and childhood disadvantage: evidence from the second British National Survey of Psychiatric Morbidity. *British Journal of Psychiatry*, **185**, 220–6.

Bentall, R. P. (2003). *Madness Explained: Psychosis and Human Nature*. London: Penguin.

Bentall, R. P. and Kinderman, P. (1999). Self-regulation, effect and psychosis: the role of social cognition in paranoia and mania. In *Handbook of Cognition and Emotion*, 2nd edn, ed. T. Dalgleish and M. Power. Chichester: Wiley, pp 353–81.

Bentall, R. P., Corcoran, R., Howard, R. *et al.* (2001). Persecutory delusions: a review and theoretical integration. *Clinical Psychology Review*, **21**, 1143–92.

Berman, I., Kalinowski, A., Berman, S. M. *et al.* (1995). Obsessive and compulsive symptoms in chronic schizophrenia. *Comprehensive Psychiatry*, **36**, 6–10.

Birchwood, M. (2003). Pathways to emotional dysfunction in first-episode psychosis. *British Journal of Psychiatry*, **182**, 373–5.

Blakemore, S. J., Oakley, D. A. and Frith, C. D. (2003). Delusions of alien control in the normal brain. *Neuropsychologia*, **41**, 1058–67.

Brentano, F. (1874). *Psychologie vom empirischen Standpunkt*. Leipzig: Duncker and Humblot.

Broome, M. R., Wooley, J. B., Tabraham, P. *et al.* (2005). What causes the onset of psychosis? *Schizophrenia Research*, **79**, 23–34.

Callicott, J. H., Straub, R. E., Pezawas, L. *et al.* (2005). Variation in DISC1 affects hippocampal structure and function and increases risk of schizophrenia. *Proceedings of the National Academy of Sciences of the USA*, **102**, 8627–32.

Cantor-Graae, E. and Selten, J. P. (2005). Schizophrenia and migration: a meta-analysis and review. *American Journal of Psychiatry*, **162**, 12–24.

Caspi, A., Moffitt, T. E., Cannon, M. *et al.* (2005). Moderation of the effect of adolescent-onset cannabis use on adult psychosis by a functional polymorphism in the catechol-O-methyltransferase gene: longitudinal evidence of a gene X environment inter-action. *Biological Psychiatry*, **57**, 1117–27.

Craddock, N. and Owen, M. J. (2005). The beginning of the end for the Kraepelinian dichotomy. *British Journal of Psychiatry*, **186**, 364–6.

Craddock, N., O'Donovan, M. C. and Owen, M. J. (2005). The genetics of schizophrenia and bipolar disorder: dissecting psychosis. *Journal of Medical Genetics*, **42**, 193–204.

Craddock, N., O'Donovan, M. C. and Owen, M. J. (2006). Genes for schizophrenia and bipolar disorder? Implications for psychiatric nosology. *Schizophrenia Bulletin*, **32**, 9–16.

Day, R., Neilsen, J. A., Korten, A. *et al.* (1987). Stressful life events preceding the acute onset of schizophrenia: a cross national study from the World Health Organization. *Culture, Medicine and Psychiatry*, **11**, 123–206.

Fearon, P., Kirkbride, J. B., Morgan, C. *et al.* (2006). Incidence of schizophrenia and other psychoses in ethnic minority groups: results from the MRC ÆSOP study. *Psychological Medicine*, **36**, 1541–50.

Fialko, L., Freeman, D., Bebbington, P. E. *et al.* (2006). Understanding suicidal ideation in psychosis: findings from the Psychological Prevention of Relapse in Psychosis (PRP) Trial. *Acta Psychiatrica Scandinavica*, **114**, 177–86.

Fish, E. W., Shahrokh, D., Bagot, R. *et al.* (2004). Epigenetic programming of stress responses through variations in maternal care. *Annals of the New York Academy of Sciences*, **1036**, 167–80.

Fowler, D. (2000). Cognitive behaviour therapy for psychosis: from understanding to treatment. *Psychiatric Rehabilitation Skills*, **4**, 199–215.

Fowler, D., Freeman, D., Steel, C. *et al.* (2006). The catastrophic interaction hypothesis: how do stress, trauma emotion and information processing abnormalities lead to psychosis? In *Trauma and Psychosis*, ed. W. Larkin and A. Morrison. London: Routledge, pp. 101–24.

Freeman, D., Garety, P., Kuipers, E. *et al.* (2002). A cognitive model of persecutory delusions. *British Journal of Clinical Psychology*, **41**, 331–47.

Freeman, D., Slater, M., Bebbington, P. E. *et al.* (2003). Can virtual reality be used to investigate persecutory ideation? *Journal of Nervous and Mental Disease*, **191**, 509–14.

Freeman, D., Garety, P. A., Fowler, D. *et al.* (2004). Why do people with delusions fail to choose more realistic explanations for their experiences? An empirical investigation. *Journal of Consulting and Clinical Psychology*, **72**, 671–80.

Freeman, D., Garety, P. A., Bebbington, P. *et al.* (2005a). The psychology of persecutory ideation II: a virtual reality experimental study. *Journal of Nervous and Mental Disease*, **193**, 309–15.

Freeman, D., Garety, P. A., Bebbington, P. E. *et al.* (2005b). Psychological investigation of the structure of paranoia in a non-clinical population. *British Journal of Psychiatry*, **186**, 427–35.

Freeman, D., Garety, P., Kuipers, E. *et al.* (2007). Acting on persecutory delusions: the impor-tance of safety-seeking. *Behaviour Research and Therapy*, **45**, 89–99.

Frith, C. D. (1992). *The Cognitive Neuropsychology of Schizophrenia*. Hove: Lawrence Erlbaum Associates.

Frith, C. (2005). The neural basis of hallucinations and delusions. *Comptes Rendus Biologies* **328**, 169–75.

Garety, P. A. and Hemsley, D. R. (1994). *Delusions: Investigations into the Psychology of Delusional Reasoning*. Oxford: Oxford University Press.

Garety, P. A., Kuipers, E. A., Fowler, D. *et al.* (2001). A cognitive model of the positive symptoms of psychosis. *Psychological Medicine*, **31**, 189–95.

Garety, P., Freeman, D., Jolley, S. *et al.* (2005). Reasoning, emotions and delusional conviction in psychosis. *Journal of Abnormal Psychology*, **114**, 373–84.

Glaser, B., Moskvina, V., Kirov, G. *et al.* (2006). Analysis of ProDH, COMT and ZHHHC8 risk variants does not support individual or interactive effects on schizophrenia susceptibility. *Schizophrenia Research*, **87**, 21–7.

Gray, J., Feldon, J. and Rawlins, J. (1991). The neuropsychology of schizophrenia. *Behavioral and Brain Sciences*, **14**, 1–84.

Green, C. E. L., Garety, P. A., Freeman, D. *et al.* (2006). Content and affect in persecutory delusions. *British Journal of Clinical Psychology*, **45**, 561–77.

Hanssen, M., Peeters, F., Krabbendam, L. *et al.* (2003). How psychotic are individuals with non-psychotic disorders? *Social Psychiatry and Psychiatric Epidemiology*, **38**, 149–54.

Hanssen, M., Krabbendam, L., de Graaf, R. *et al.* (2005). Role of distress in delusion formation. *British Journal of Psychiatry*, **48** (suppl.), s55–s58.

Hardy, A., Fowler, D., Freeman, D. *et al.* (2005). Trauma and hallucinatory experience in psychosis. *Journal of Nervous and Mental Disease*, **193**, 503–7.

Hariri, A. R., Goldberg, T. E., Mattay, V. S. *et al.* (2003). Brain-derived neurotrophic factor val[66]met polymorphism affects human memory-related hippocampal activity and predicts memory performance. *Journal of Neuroscience*, **23**, 6690–4.

Harris, T. (1987). Recent developments in the study of life events in relation to psychiatric and physical disorders. In *Psychiatric Epidemiology*, ed. B. Cooper. London: Croom-Helm, pp. 81–103.

Harrison, P. J. and Weinberger, D. R. (2005). Schizophrenia genes, gene expression, and neuro-pathology: on the matter of their convergence. *Molecular Psychiatry*, **10**, 40–68.

Hemsley, D. R. (1993). A simple (or simplistic?) cognitive model for schizophrenia. *Behaviour Research and Therapy*, **31**, 633–45.

Hemsley, D. R. (1998). The disruption of the 'sense of self' in schizophrenia: potential links with disturbances of information processing. *British Journal of Medical Psychology*, **71**, 115–24.

Hemsley, D. R. (2005). The schizophrenic experience: taken out of context? *Schizophrenia Bulletin*, **31**, 43–53.

Janssen, I., Krabbendam, L., Bak, M. *et al.* (2004). Childhood abuse as a risk factor for psychotic experiences. *Acta Psychiatrica Scandinavica*, **109**, 38–45.

Jaspers, K. (1913). *General Psychopathology*. Translated (1963) by J. Hoenig and M. W. Hamilton. Manchester, UK: Manchester University Press.

Johns, L. C., Rossell, S., Ahmad, F. *et al.* (2001). Verbal self-monitoring and auditory verbal hallucinations in patients with schizophrenia. *Psychological Medicine*, **31**, 705–15.

Johns, L. C., Cannon, M., Singleton, N. *et al.* (2004). The prevalence and correlates of self-reported psychotic symptoms in the British population. *British Journal of Psychiatry*, **185**, 298–305.

Jolley, S., Garety, P., Bebbington, P. *et al.* (2006). Attributional style in psychosis: the role of affect and belief type. *Behaviour Research and Therapy*, **44**, 1597–607.

Joyce, E. (2005). Origins of cognitive dysfunction in schizophrenia: clues from age at onset. *British Journal of Psychiatry*, **186**, 93–5.

Kapur, S. (2003). Psychosis as a state of aberrant salience: a framework linking biology, phenomenology, and pharmacology in schizophrenia. *American Journal of Psychiatry*, **160**, 13–23.

Krabbendam, L. and van Os, J. (2005). Affective processes in the onset and persistence of psychosis. *European Archives of Psychiatry and Clinical Neuroscience*, **255**, 185–9.

Krabbendam, L., Myin-Germeys, I., De Graaf, R. *et al.* (2004). Dimensions of depression, mania and psychosis in the general population. *Psychological Medicine*, **34**, 1177–86.

Krabbendam, L., Myin-Germeys, I., Hanssen, M. *et al.* (2005). Development of depressed mood predicts onset of psychotic disorder in individuals who report hallucinatory experiences. *British Journal of Clinical Psychology*, **44**, 113–25.

Kuipers, E., Bebbington, P., Dunn, G. *et al.* (2006). The influence of carer expressed emotion and affect on relapse in non-affective psychosis. *British Journal of Psychiatry*, **188**, 173–9.

Kuipers, E., Watson, P., Onwumere, J. *et al.* (2007). Discrepant illness perceptions, expressed emotion and affect, in people with psychosis and their carers. *Social Psychiatry and Psychiatric Epidemiology*, **35**, 242–7.

Law, A. J., Lipska, B. K., Weickert, C. S. *et al.* (2006). Neuregulin 1 transcripts are differentially expressed in schizophrenia and regulated by 5 SNPs associated with the disease. *Proceedings of the National Academy of Sciences of the USA*, **103**, 6747–52.

Linney, Y. M., Murray, R. M., Peters, E. R. *et al.* (2003). A quantitative genetic analysis of schizotypal personality traits. *Psychological Medicine*, **33**, 803–16.

Lipska, B. K., Peters, T., Hyde, T. M. *et al.* (2006). Expression of DISC1 binding partners is reduced in schizophrenia and associated with DISC1 SNPs. *Human Molecular Genetics*, **15**, 1245–58.

Lobban, F., Barrowclough, C. and Jones, S. (2004). The impact of beliefs about mental health problems and coping on outcome in schizophrenia. *Psychological Medicine*, **37**, 1165–74.

McGrath, J. J. (2006). Variations in the incidence of schizophrenia: data versus dogma. *Schizophrenia Bulletin*, **32**, 195–7.

Meaney, M. J. (2001). Maternal care, gene expression, and the transmission of individual differences in stress reactivity across generations. *Annual Review of Neuroscience*, **24**, 1161–92.

Melzer, D., Tom, B. D. M., Brugha, T. S. *et al.* (2002). Common mental disorder symptom counts in populations: are there distinct case groups above epidemiological cut-offs? *Psychological Medicine*, **32**, 1195–201.

Meyer-Lindenberg, A., Kohn, P. D., Kolachana, B. *et al.* (2005). Midbrain dopamine and prefrontal function in humans: interaction and modulation by COMT genotype. *Nature Neuroscience*, **8**, 594–6.

Morrison, A. P. (2001). The interpretation of intrusions in psychosis: an integrative cognitive approach to hallucinations and delusions. *Behavioural and Cognitive Psychotherapy*, **29**, 257–76.

Mueser, K. T., Goodman, L. B., Trumbetta, S. L. *et al.* (1998). Trauma and posttraumatic stress disorder in severe mental illness. *Journal of Consulting and Clinical Psychology*, **66**, 493–9.

Myin-Germeys, I., van Os, J., Schwartz, J. *et al.* (2001). Emotional reactivity to daily life stress in psychosis. *Archives of General Psychiatry*, **58**, 1137–44.

Norton, N., Williams, H. J. and Owen, M. J. (2006). An update on the genetics of schizophrenia. *Current Opinion in Psychiatry*, **19**, 158–64.

Nuechterlein, K. H., Dawson, M. E., Ventura, J. *et al.* (1994). The vulnerability/stress model of schizophrenic relapse – a longitudinal study. *Acta Psychiatrica Scandinavica*, **89** (suppl. 382), 58–64.

Owen, M. J., Craddock, N. and Donovan, M. C. (2005). Schizophrenia: genes at last? *Trends in Genetics*, **21**, 518–25.

Peters, E. and Garety, P. (2005). Cognitive functioning in delusions: a longitudinal analysis. *Behaviour Research and Therapy*, **44**, 481–514.

Pinkham, A. E., Penn, D. L., Perkins, D. O. *et al.* (2003). Implications of the neural basis of social cognition for the study of schizophrenia. *American Journal of Psychiatry*, **160**, 815–24.

Pinkham, A., Penn, D., Wangelin, B. *et al.* (2005). Facial emotion perception and fusiform gyrus volume in first episode schizophrenia. *Schizophrenia Research*, **79**, 341–3.

Plomin, R., Owen, M. J. and McGuffin, P. (1994). The genetic basis of complex human behaviors. *Science*, **264**, 1733–9.

Raune, D., Bebbington, P., Dunn, G. *et al.* (2006). Event attributes and the content of psychotic experiences in first-episode psychosis. *Psychological Medicine*, **36**, 221–30.

Read, J., van Os, J., Morrison, A. P. *et al.* (2005). Childhood trauma, psychosis and schizophrenia: a literature review with theoretical and clinical implications. *Acta Psychiatrica Scandinavica*, **112** (5), 330–50.

Rechtman, R. (2004). The rebirth of PTSD: the rise of a new paradigm in psychiatry. *Social Psychiatry and Psychiatric Epidemiology*, **39**, 913–15.

Sands, J. R. and Harrow, M. (1999). Depression during the longitudinal course of schizophrenia. *Schizophrenia Bulletin*, **25**, 157–71.

Smith, B., Fowler, D. G., Freeman, D. *et al.* (2006). Emotion and psychosis: links between depression, self-esteem, negative schematic beliefs and delusions and hallucinations. *Schizophrenia Research*, **86**, 181–8.

Sturt, E. (1981). Hierarchical patterns in the incidence of psychiatric symptoms. *Psychological Medicine*, **11**, 783–94.

Turnbull, G. and Bebbington, P. (2001). Anxiety and the schizophrenic process: clinical and epidemiological evidence. *Social Psychiatry and Psychiatric Epidemiology*, **36**, 235–43.

van Os, J., Verdoux, H., Maurice-Tison, S. *et al.* (1999). Self-reported psychosis-like symptoms and the continuum of psychosis. *Social Psychiatry and Psychiatric Epidemiology*, **34**, 459–63.

Watson, P. W. B., Garety, P. A., Weinman, J. *et al.* (2006). Emotional dysfunction in schizophrenia spectrum psychosis: the role of illness perceptions. *Psychological Medicine*, **36**, 761–70.

Weaver, I. C., Carvoni, N., Champagne, F. A. *et al.* (2004). Epigenetic programming by maternal behaviour. *Nature Neuroscience*, **7**, 847–54.

Wiles, N. J., Zammit, S., Bebbington, P. *et al.* (2006). Self-reported psychotic symptoms in the general population. *British Journal of Psychiatry*, **188**, 519–26.

Wing, J. (1978). *Reasoning about Madness*. Oxford: Oxford University Press.

15

Society and psychosis: future directions and implications

Craig Morgan, Kwame McKenzie and Paul Fearon

Psychotic disorders may be more common than previously thought. In a recent Finnish study, one of the most rigorous and comprehensive to date, estimates of lifetime prevalence were in excess of 3% for all psychotic disorders combined, irrespective of data source used (Perala *et al.*, 2007). This is a substantial public health problem. Schizophrenia and other psychoses are often lifelong conditions, characterised by distressing symptoms and considerable social disability and exclusion. The impact extends to family, not infrequently leading to a lifetime of care. As we have seen in Chapter 12, the negative responses of others compound suffering and feelings of isolation. The social costs are equally significant, in terms of lost productivity and costs of providing care, both formal and informal. In the UK, for example, recent estimates put the total societal costs of schizophrenia at £6.7 billion, much of these costs arising from informal care and private expenditures borne by families (Mangalore and Knapp, 2006). This is the background against which all research needs to be set. The imperative that drives attempts to understand the aetiology, course and outcome of psychosis better is the need to create more effective responses, be these at the levels of public policy, service delivery or clinical practice, to alleviate suffering and reduce burden.

For some, the question of what role social conditions and experiences have in the onset, course and outcome of psychosis remains controversial. This is particularly the case for aetiology. Many researchers and clinicians subscribe to a broadly biopsychosocial view of schizophrenia and other psychoses. However, even within this framework, the relative importance of psychosocial factors is frequently downplayed and the overwhelming majority of current research efforts are directed towards investigating broadly biological risk factors and markers for psychosis. With regard to outcomes and interventions, there is less controversy. It appears to be generally accepted that socioenvironmental factors impinge on outcome

Society and Psychosis, ed. Craig Morgan, Kwame McKenzie and Paul Fearon. Published by Cambridge University Press. © Cambridge University Press 2008.

and that interventions designed to modify aspects of the social environment (e.g., family interactions, employment) can lead to improvements in quality of life and symptoms (see Chapter 11). Despite this, clinical research remains dominated by studies of antipsychotic medications.

We started *Society and Psychosis* by asserting that psychiatry had rediscovered its roots. The chapters in this book demonstrate just how deep these roots are. Together they suggest that society and psychosis may be more intricately linked than the current balance of research and clinical priorities indicates. In this concluding chapter, our aims are to provide an overview and summary of the research presented in this book, to suggest directions and challenges for future research and to discuss the implications of this research.

A conceptual framework

In attempting to understand the links between society and psychosis, there is a need to develop conceptual tools that allow the complexities of the social world to be studied. In Chapter 4, March and colleagues provide a framework in which social factors are conceptualised as operating at many different levels (e.g., the individual, the family, the neighbourhood) (see also Chapter 6) and over time and space. The chapters focusing on aetiology have reviewed evidence relating to social factors at one or more of these levels. While these findings are presented separately, there is a need to draw them back into this overarching framework. This serves as an important reminder that processes operating at different levels and time points are connected and interact in the aetiology and course of psychosis. This is illustrated in the research presented by Myin-Germeys and van Os (Chapter 9), which suggests that early adversity may be linked to psychosis through ongoing daily stress in adult life. As noted in a number of the chapters, there is also research suggesting that individual risk of schizophrenia may be moderated by character-istics of the wider social environment (e.g., Boydell *et al.*, 2001).

The complexities are further emphasised in the distinction between processes and conditions. The variables that we utilise in analyses are often 'conditions' (e.g., being a migrant) that are the product of social processes (e.g., the transition from one cultural setting to another). Both conditions and processes are embodied and influence a person's health status; measuring and assessing the impact of social processes as well as conditions is a central challenge for future research.

Individuals may encounter processes and conditions that increase risk of psy-chosis throughout the life course. In many diseases there can be long latent periods between the occurrence of risk increasing exposures (e.g., early disadvantage) and onset of disease or disorder (e.g., heart disease) (see Brunner, 2000). These exposures may operate by increasing susceptibility to disorder in the event of exposure to subsequent risk factors later in the life course. This idea of an accumulation of risk over time consequent on exposure to adverse environments in childhood, adolescence and adulthood is a common framework for understanding the aetiology of a number of multifactorial diseases, such as heart disease and diabetes, in the wider social epidemiology literature (see Berkman and Kawachi, 2000).

There is a further dynamic. In evaluating what is currently known about specific social processes and conditions associated with psychosis, it is useful to make a distinction between risk indicators (i.e., factors that index risk but that do not in themselves confer risk) and risk factors (i.e., factors involved in risk processes) (Rutter, 2005). This is an important consideration. For example, Rutter (2005) notes how in the 1970s it became apparent that the association between antisocial behaviour and 'broken homes' was a function, not of family breakdown, but of prior family discord and conflict. The current evidence, as will be seen below, may well be stronger for social risk indicators than it is for social risk factors; this should both temper the claims that can be made and further emphasise the need for research that directly investigates potential risk-generating processes over time.

The framework for investigating the impact of society on psychosis, sketched here and discussed more fully in Chapter 4, provides a means of synthesising information and knowledge, and generating testable hypotheses for future research. The question nonetheless remains of whether the research evidence on specific social risk factors is sufficient to support the conclusion that such factors are causally connected to psychosis.

Do social factors cause psychosis?

In 1965, Austin Bradford Hill (1965) proposed a series of criteria against which causation could be judged (see Table 15.1). These have been widely used and

Table 15.1 Bradford Hill's criteria for assessing causation

Temporality
Strength
Consistency
Dose–response gradient
Specificity
Biological (psychological) plausibility
Coherence
Experiment
Analogy

applied in epidemiology and other social sciences. Not all of the criteria are equally relevant for all disorders. Van Reekum *et al.* (2001), for example, suggest that temporal ordering, strength, consistency and biological (or psychological) plausibility may be most relevant to neuropsychiatric disorders; specificity and dose–response relationships were, interestingly, considered less central to establishing causation. Further, once complex models are produced in which social factors interconnect at different levels and over time, these criteria do not necessarily provide the basis for conclusive judgement. Several factors of relatively small effect may combine over time to increase risk. Nonetheless, they do offer a framework against which to evaluate the evidence that specific factors are causally related to an outcome. These criteria, then, provide one means of assessing the current evidence for a causal role of social factors in psychosis. The specific issue of biological (or psychological) plausibility is one of increasing importance in this field and will be addressed separately below.

Urbanicity

Perhaps the strongest and most consistent evidence relates to urbanicity. Almost invariably, an increased risk for schizophrenia has been found for those who live in cities (the condition); the risk is present from birth and appears to be related to being brought up in a city (the process). Further, there is now relatively robust evidence that the risk for schizophrenia increases in a dose–response fashion with the number of years spent living in an urban centre. Urbanicity, then, appears to meet many of Bradford Hill's criteria – consistency, strength and temporal ordering of association, and evidence of a risk gradient. However, precisely what it is about living in a city that increases risk is unclear. As Boydell and McKenzie (see Chapter 6) note, it is perhaps most useful to consider urbanicity as a risk indicator, indexing risks that coalesce in densely populated environments. Further, it is not clear whether such risks are social; they may equally plausibly relate to the physical environment. That said, innovative ecological level research utilising concepts such as ethnic density and social capital is beginning to hint at specific social risk factors that may be particularly evident in urban settings (see Chapter 6). Disaggregating the urban environment, understanding its different facets and working out how these interact will be a major but fruitful task for research given that up to 30% of the population risk for schizophrenia may be accounted for by urbanicity (Krabbendam and van Os, 2005).

Migration and ethnicity

There is now a substantial body of research demonstrating increased rates of psychosis in migrant groups (see Chapter 10). These increased rates arise only in the host country, i.e., post-migration, and are present in primary migrant populations and in their children and subsequent generations. Further, Cantor-Graae and Selten's (2005) review suggests that there is a risk gradient for migrant groups, with the risk being greatest for those from countries where the majority population is black, and for those from 'developing' countries. So far, so good. Migration and ethnicity appear to meet some of the criteria for causation – consistency, strength and temporal ordering of association, and evidence of a risk gradient. However, once again, what it is about being a migrant or member of an ethnic minority group that increases risk is unclear.

The fields of migration and ethnicity have become linked. However, these 'conditions' may index distinct processes, and further information may be gleaned by comparisons between those who have migrated and those who have not but who have similar ethnicities, i.e., subsequent generations. Thus, it is necessary to draw a distinction between the process of migration and migrant or ethnic minority group status. In one sense, migrant and ethnic group statuses are risk indicators in that they are social realities that index a series of social processes. In terms of identifying the risk generating processes, research is beginning to provide important clues in relation to ethnicity. For example, recent studies have implicated discrimination, early adversity and population-level risks, including ethnic density (see Chapter 10). However, much less work is currently being done about the risk processes linked to migration.

Adversity across the life course

Consideration of factors operating in early childhood and family life as potential contributory causes of psychosis is fraught with problems, not least because it conjures memories of regrettable theories in which mothers were blamed for causing schizophrenia. However, it is unfortunately true that many children are exposed to various forms of adversity and trauma, ranging from parental neglect and hostility to sexual and physical abuse (within and outside of the family). Such early experiences have been linked with a wide range of negative childhood and adult outcomes, including depression, anxiety, eating disorders and personality disorders (see Chapter 7).

In relation to psychosis, there is a limited amount of robust research, and this means that any conclusions have to be tentative. Nonetheless, the evidence is suggestive of a link between early negative experiences and the risk of psychosis. Certainly, in terms of strength and consistency of association, the evidence relating to childhood trauma and family interactions is not yet as striking as that for urbanicity and migration. However, the balance is increasingly in favour of an association between these exposures and psychosis, and some of the more robust studies have reported findings suggestive of a dose–response relationship, such that the risk of experiencing psychosis or psychotic-like symptoms increases in line with levels of exposure to early adversity (see Chapter 7). Further, there are plausible biological and psychological mechanisms (see below).

The separation between childhood and adult adversity, as the chapter by Myin-Germeys and van Os (Chapter 9) makes clear, is artificial; their data suggest that experiences of adversity over the life course increase susceptibility to the negative effects of subsequent adversity in the genesis, and exacerbation of, psychotic symptoms. The research they report on daily hassles provides a good example of how innovative designs and methods can help disentangle the relative effects of genes, biology and life experiences over time. It both supports a role for adult and childhood adversity, and suggests that risk accumulates over time, findings that echo those from broader studies of physical health in social epidemiology noted above. The implication is that distal risk factors may exert their effect by increasing vulnerability to the damaging effects of proximal exposures. These findings, nonetheless, require careful replication, and the question of whether significant discrete life events, as opposed to ongoing difficulties and daily stresses, increases risk of psychosis remains unresolved. There have been numerous studies, but difficulties separating cause and effect have limited the inferences that can be made from these (see Chapter 9).

Specificity

One issue that has not yet been directly addressed is that of specificity. Many of the social conditions and processes that have been linked with psychosis here are also associated with a range of other illnesses, both mental and physical. There are a number of ways of viewing this. It may be that social factors are indeed non-specific, and that what they do is create a generalised vulnerability to disorder, the precise form depending on interactions with other factors, including genes. However, it may also be that the variables studied to date have been too crude to identify any specific effects. For example, in relation to depression, through a series of studies, Brown and Harris (Harris, 2001) were able to identify specific types of significant life event that increased risk of depression, i.e., those involving loss, humiliation and entrapment. Tirril Harris (1987) has since gone on to suggest that life events involving threat and intrusiveness may be more important for psychosis, a proposition that has gained some support in Bebbington *et al.*'s (2004) study of psychosis and victimisation experiences.

Causal connections?

When set along Bradford Hill's criteria, the most cautious interpretation is that the data reviewed in the second part of this book, taken together, are strongly suggestive, but not conclusive. For each of the broad areas, there are fairly consistent and relatively strong associations, with some studies suggesting that risk increases in a dose–response fashion with level of exposure. Improvements in study design and available data have allowed for the temporal sequencing of risk and onset to be more clearly established and the findings do suggest that the risk factors precede onset. In short, many of the limitations that characterised early research have been addressed, and the evidence continues to implicate social processes. What is giving particular impetus to this research, and increasing the credibility of the proposition that social experience matters, is that there are now a number of potential mechanisms, with empirical support, that may link forms of social adversity and the development of psychosis.

Mechanisms

Many diseases are socially patterned, with those in the lowest socioeconomic groups being most at risk (see Berkman and Kawachi, 2000). These include heart disease, stroke, diabetes, various forms of cancer and many infectious diseases. There have been debates, parallel to those in psychiatry, about the nature of these associations, and whether social conditions and experiences are aetiologically relevant. There are now a number of plausible mechanisms through which social and environmental processes could impact on, and contribute to shaping, developing biology in such ways as to increase susceptibility to, and risk for, a range of illnesses (for a discussion see Brunner, 2000).

One of the products of the recent rapid advances in neuroscience and genetics is a developing understanding of how social processes influence brain development and interact with genotype to produce later outcomes. These are of direct relevance to mental disorder, including psychosis, and examples are given in a number of the chapters in this book. For example, Fisher and Craig (see Chapter 7) document some of the recent research that suggests stress during childhood can lead to changes in glucocorticoid levels and HPA axis function (see p. 101), in turn leading to a heightened sensitivity to stress. Further, there is evidence of elevated dopamine metabolism in abused girls compared with healthy controls, a finding that is particularly noteworthy given the recent resurgence of interest in the role of dopamine in the genesis of psychotic experiences (see p. 101). There is also evidence that early adversity is associated with alterations in brain structure and function in areas that have been implicated in schizophrenia (e.g., hippocampus, corpus callosum and amygdala) (see p. 102). Perhaps the most significant recent advance is the realisation that genes and environment frequently interact to shape adult outcomes; indeed, this may be the rule. This is a major theme in many of the chapters in this book, and relevant conceptual and methodological issues are discussed fully by Barnett and Jones (Chapter 5).

These developments have allowed us to move beyond vague notions of stress-diathesis, to models in which precise mediating biological and psychologica!

variables are specified. A number of the chapters in this book present models that attempt to link social processes and conditions across the life course and psychosis through such biological and psychological mechanisms. Bebbington and colleagues (Chapter 14), in addition, draw on developing cognitive models of psychosis, and in doing so perhaps offer the most complete framework (note similarities with the model proposed by Fisher and Craig, Chapter 7).

As with all models, they are heuristic. The ones noted here link individual-level experience, biological and psychological mechanisms and psychosis. They provide tentative frameworks and hypotheses that suggest areas for future research; it is the task of this future research to accept, reject and modify aspects of these. On a more critical note, it could be argued that so far the mechanisms postulated have failed to take sufficient account of the higher levels of social organisation set out as important in Chapters 4 and 6. This points to a major conceptual and methodological challenge. Nonetheless, the tentative models outlined in this book indicate genuinely integrated theories of psychosis aetiology, in which the epidemiological evidence that psychosis is associated with forms of social adversity is linked through known biological and psychological mechanisms to the development of symptoms.

Methodological considerations

The methodological issues and challenges inherent in studying society and psychosis have been discussed at length in a number of the chapters in this book. Here, we highlight two interconnected issues, which we consider central to the development of research in this area.

Conceptualising and measuring social processes

One of the reasons why there have been such recent rapid advances in neuroscience and genetics is that the technology available for studying the brain and the genome have developed at a staggering pace. Unfortunately, in epidemiological research the primary units of analysis are frequently crude dichotomies – urban versus rural, migrant versus non-migrant, abused versus non-abused. With regard to urbanicity and migration, one consequence is that the precise meaning of observed associations is unclear, and the social experiences that these variables may index remain unknown (see above). This provides fertile ground for unwarranted speculation. One of the reasons why the literature on child abuse remains so controversial and contested is that the measures of abuse have usually been extremely limited, with little or no account taken of the timing, duration and severity of abuse. There are exceptions, such as the use of the Experience Sampling Method (see Chapter 9) and the detailed assessments of family communication patterns used in the studies reviewed by Tienari and Wahlberg (Chapter 8), and these help to point a way forward.

As indicated above, we need to develop appropriate conceptual maps and measurement tools that allow us to study complex social processes and the contexts in which they occur, if we are to understand fully the nature of the crude associations between, say, ethnicity and psychosis. In this, however, there is no need to start from scratch. These are the very issues that social scientists have been grappling with for at least the past century. There are already available a range of well developed theoretical frameworks and methodological tools for investigating a wide variety of social contexts and experiences (see Chapter 3), including social fragmentation, social capital, social networks, discrimination, childhood trauma and abuse, and life events. Of course, the resources, number of subjects and complexity of analyses required to conduct such research are considerable, particularly given the added need to include data that cut across different levels of analysis (e.g., individual and neighbourhood) or domains (e.g., social, genetic, biochemical). However, this has to be the next step. It is questionable how much value there is in more studies showing associations between migration, or population density, or trauma (broadly defined) and risk of psychosis unless these are accompanied by more concerted attempts to collect data relevant to hypotheses about the risk factors and mechanisms at work.

Distinguishing cause and effect

There is an intrinsic difficulty in studying social factors and psychosis. The development of a psychotic mental illness is frequently preceded or accompanied by a decline in social functioning, which often includes loss of employment, disintegration of, or failure to establish, meaningful social networks and downward social mobility. It is consequently often unclear whether the social experience of interest is a cause or consequence of the developing psychosis. It may be, moreover, that these processes are not separate. It is possible, for example, that early behavioural manifestations of developing psychosis increase the risk of social isolation, which in turn further increases the risk that a full psychotic disorder will develop. Social isolation, in this sense, may be both consequence and cause. By too successfully parsing out all but that which precedes onset, or prodrome, the influence of social experience may be underestimated. It nevertheless remains the case that associations will be most persuasive of causation if they can be shown to precede onset and to be independent of early manifestations of the illness. The work of George Brown and Tirril Harris (Harris, 2001) in developing a sophisticated and detailed methodology for the study of life events and depression is instructive here (see Chapter 3). Their development of a measure that could identify life events that were independent of the illness offers one template for psychosis research.

There is an added complexity. Individuals are not simply passive in the face of unyielding environments. Individuals also make and choose, within constraints, their environments. For example, it cannot simply be assumed that associations between problematic child–parent interactions and disorder reflect socialisation practices; as Rutter (2005) points out, 'it might derive from the effects of a difficult child on family function' (p. 4). Environments, as well as disorder, may be heritable. Kendler and Baker (2007) recently conducted a systematic review of 55 studies that have examined the heritability of measures of environments relevant to psychiatry. Weighted heritability estimates for environments, including stressful life events and social support, ranged from 7% to 39%. The authors concluded that genetic influences on measures of the environment are pervasive in extent and modest to moderate in impact. This does not, however, necessarily mean that the environments evoked by individuals do not then confer additional risk.

Outcomes and interventions

There is much less controversy concerning the relationship between society and the course and outcome of psychosis. Evidence has accumulated over a number of years showing that recovery and risk of relapse are influenced by life events, family interactions, social support and employment, to mention a small number of relevant factors (see Chapter 11).

The chapters in this book that focus on society and outcomes reflect three specific areas of important ongoing concern and interest. The first, that by Richard Warner (Chapter 11), is important because what it shows is that intervening to modify social circumstances can affect recovery; it also points to the potential for preventive interventions, if social circumstances are relevant to onset (see below). It would be misleading to suggest that the social worlds of sufferers are ignored by mental health services. In many countries, not least the UK and USA, where multidisciplinary teams are the norm, there are myriad efforts to attend to the psychosocial needs of those with psychosis, through the provision of occupational therapy, social work interventions, day centres and the kinds of programmes outlined by Warner. However, it is also the case that provision of such services is often patchy and poorly coordinated, and some interventions for which there is good evidence are only rarely, if at all, offered (e.g., family therapy to reduce expressed emotion). Further, when set alongside the tasks of diagnosis, provision and monitoring of medication and use of in-patient care, social care services for those with psychosis are dwarfed. To make this point is not to deny the value of medication and in-patient care. Both are essential. However, the evidence presented in Chapter 11 demonstrates the need for social interventions to be much more prominent and integrated into mainstream service provision. In this, we include developing cognitive-behavioural therapies for psychosis (Kuipers *et al.*, 2006).

The principle that underpins the various social interventions outlined by Warner is the need for those with psychosis to be reintegrated into wider social life; that recovery is, to a significant extent, social participation. To use the terminology increasingly in use in the UK and Europe, those with psychosis are often among the most socially excluded in society. Mental health services can have a significant role in promoting social reintegration and inclusion. However, as Thornicroft and colleagues show (see Chapter 12), there are significant barriers to achieving this that arise from the stigma that attaches to psychosis or madness in most, if not all, cultures. The consequences of this stigma filter into all aspects of society, underpinning discrimination in employment, in housing, in access to leisure, and within families and informal social networks. Countering the debilitating stigma that attaches to psychosis is arguably the most important task we face in supporting those who suffer to lead socially valued lives. As Warner's work, among others, shows, this is commonly a realistic goal; in a very real sense, society creates, or at least contributes to sustaining, the disability experienced by many people with psychotic mental disorders. The magnitude of the task, and the research required to support it, are set out in Chapter 12.

The proposition that social reintegration promotes recovery from psychosis has been the most common explanation of the repeated finding from the WHO studies that outcomes are better in the developing world (see Chapter 13). In essence, the argument is that schizophrenia is less stigmatised in the developing world, and sufferers are more readily reintegrated back into meaningful social roles, thereby promoting recovery. Kim Hopper's chapter (Chapter 13) provides an important corrective to this kind of snap conclusion, a conclusion that has transformed into axiom. The reality, it seems, is likely to be much more complex. First, there is limited evidence to support the above conclusion. Second, the supposition that mental health service provision in developing countries does not contribute to promoting recovery is likely to be an oversimplification. Third, the social processes contributing to variations in outcome may not work in the ways assumed, as the striking example of marriage rates in India suggests (see p. 205). As with aetiology, the social world is likely to have a complex relationship with outcomes, and other factors including genes, biochemistry, psychology and treatment will all contribute. What perhaps comes across most strongly from Hopper's chapter is that we know surprisingly little about the everyday experience of living with psychosis. There are very few full scale ethnographies. Those that have been conducted warn against oversimplifying and reifying complex social processes.

Implications

There are many potential implications and suggestions for further research within each chapter, and throughout the previous pages. Can we tease out a small number of important implications?

Implications (1) Prevention

The implications of there being social roots to psychosis in early and adult social experiences, and in the organisation of society, are profound, and important questions about how to utilise this knowledge are raised. We should not, of course, get ahead of ourselves. As the cautious summary above indicates, our knowledge of the social conditions that increase risk for psychosis, and the mechanisms through which they operate, is still limited. The resulting dilemma is neatly summarised by Cooper (1992, p. 597): 'Here the investigator is confronted by a central dilemma of social psychiatry, a discipline whose search for causal factors of mental illness demands an increased complexity in theory and methods that will take time to develop, yet which in its practical and service aspects must deal with public health problems of great and growing urgency.' Cooper (1992) goes on to argue that: 'This dilemma may be partially resolved by adopting preventive goals ... since the history of public health epidemiology ... has repeatedly demonstrated that effective preventive measures can precede the full causal elucidation of disease.' (p. 597.) What might these preventive measures be? In a broad, and overly general, sense, knowledge that exposure to adverse social conditions and experiences increases risk of severe mental illness (if it holds up) gives added impetus to public policy efforts to reduce inequality, sponsor neighbourhood regeneration and promote social inclusion for those groups cast adrift by mainstream society. Psychiatrists and other mental health professionals should not shy away from these issues. However, is it possible to be more concrete?

Two tentative propositions can be made. First, if the roots of adult disorder are sown in early childhood, this points to a need for improved understanding of the impact of social processes at this stage in life and improved services and social policy to protect children from harm. For those who have suffered, there is a need to understand how this changes their life trajectory, what other developmental and social processes are disturbed, and what can be done to rectify damage and reduce the impact. More work on understanding the possibilities of primary and secondary prevention in childhood would seem to be an important area for further development. Second, there is a need to consider whether the knowledge we have gained is of particular relevance to those who are at increased risk of developing psychosis. For example, the research reviewed in this book suggests that social circumstances and stresses may be particularly important in those who have a relative with a psychotic disorder (e.g., Chapter 9). If we are to develop preventive strategies, it may be that such groups could be targeted, though this has to be set alongside the potential stigmatising consequences.

Implications (2) Intervention

Irrespective of whether social factors are causally related to psychosis, many of those who present to services have significant social needs. The available research suggests that the continuation of social problems, in the form of unemployment, poor housing, limited social networks and difficult family circumstances, increases the risk of a poor outcome. When sufferers themselves are asked, it is often these life domains that they consider most important and with which they want help (Morgan, 2004). All of the interventions detailed in Chapter 11 are indicated. In short, the social care needs of those with psychosis need to be given even more prominence in the packages of care delivered by mental health services. It may be, moreover, that providing such interventions early in the course of the illness, in effect to protect and rebuild existing social resources, will have maximal impact. This, of course, remains to be tested, but the proposition ties in with the idea that there is a critical period early in the course of psychosis when long-term outcomes are most malleable (Birchwood *et al.*, 1997).

Conclusion

In an editorial pondering the place of social psychiatry in the age of the human genome, Leon Eisenberg (2004) asked the question: 'Is this the time to hold a memorial mass to bury social psychiatry, an outmoded corpus of work, charming in its day but overtaken by the relentless pace of scientific advance?' (p. 101.) The question was, of course, rhetorical. Following a short review documenting insightful examples of the many ways in which the social, genetic and biological interact in the genesis of disease, he concluded: 'Thus, I am a celebrant: social psychiatry is not only alive and well, but it has a bright future precisely because of genomics.' (p. 102.) This latter point is one that has run throughout this book. Advances in genetics and neuroscience have revealed just how important interactions with environments are in development, and this has contributed to a resurgence of interest in social factors and psychosis. However, this also represents the major challenge for future research, how to investigate and model these interactions to test hypotheses and build viable models of the aetiology of psychosis. The primary purpose of this book has been to bring together a series of contributions that can lay some of the groundwork for investigating the social side of these complex equations. What they suggest is that society and psychosis are intricately linked, both in cause and consequence. The implications for how we respond to those who develop these devastating disorders may be far reaching.

REFERENCES

Bebbington, P. E., Bhugra, D., Brugha, T. *et al.* (2004). Psychosis, victimisation and childhood disadvantage. *British Journal of Psychiatry*, **185**, 220–6.

Berkman, L. F. and Kawachi, I. (2000). *Social Epidemiology*. Oxford: Oxford University Press.

Birchwood, M., McGorry, P. and Jackson, H. (1997). Early intervention in schizophrenia. *British Journal of Psychiatry*, **170**, 2–5.

Boydell, J., van Os, J., McKenzie, K. *et al.* (2001). Incidence of schizophrenia in ethnic minorities in London: ecological study into interactions with environment. *British Medical Journal*, **323** (7325), 1336–8.

Bradford Hill, A. (1965). The environment and disease: association or causation? *Proceedings of the Royal Society of Medicine*, **58**, 293–300.

Brunner, E. J. (2000). Toward a new social biology. In *Social Epidemiology*, ed. L. F. Berkman and I. Kawachi. Oxford: Oxford University Press, pp. 306–31.

Cantor-Graae, E. and Selten, J. P. (2005). Schizophrenia and migration: a meta-analysis and review. *American Journal of Psychiatry*, **162** (1), 12–24.

Cooper, B. (1992). Sociology in the context of social psychiatry. *British Journal of Psychiatry*, **161**, 594–8.

Eisenberg, L. (2004). Social psychiatry and the human genome: contextualising heritability. *British Journal of Psychiatry*, **184**, 101–3.

Harris, T. (1987). Recent developments in the study of life events in relation to psychiatric and physical disorders. In *Psychiatric Epidemiology*, ed. B. Cooper. London: Croom Helm, pp. 81–103.

Harris, T. (2001). Recent developments in understanding the psychosocial aspects of depression. *British Medical Bulletin*, **57**, 17–32.

Kendler, K. S. and Baker, J. H. (2007). Genetic influences on measures of the environment: a systematic review. *Psychological Medicine*, **37**, 615–26.

Krabbendam, L. and van Os, J. (2005). Schizophrenia and urbanicity: a major environmental influence – conditional on genetic risk. *Schizophrenia Bulletin*, **31** (4), 795–9.

Kuipers, E., Garety, P., Fowler, D. *et al.* (2006). Cognitive, emotional, and social processes in psychosis: refining cognitive behavioural therapy for persistent positive symptoms. *Schizophrenia Bulletin*, **32** (suppl. 1), s24–s31.

Mangalore, R. and Knapp, M. (2006). *Cost of Schizophrenia in England*. PSSRU Discussion Paper 2376. Canterbury, UK: Personal Social Service Research Unit

Morgan, C. (2004). The role of social care. *Psychiatry*, **3** (9), 29–31.

Perala, J., Suvisaari, J., Saarni, S. I. *et al.* (2007). Lifetime prevalence of psychotic and bipolar I disorder in a general population. *Archives of General Psychiatry*, **64**, 19–28.

Rutter, M. (2005). How the environment affects mental health. *British Journal of Psychiatry*, **186**, 4–6.

van Reekum, R., Streiner, D. L. and Conn, D. K. (2001). Applying Bradford Hill's criteria for causation to neuropsychiatry: challenges and opportunities. *Journal of Neuropsychiatry and Clinical Neuroscience*, **13**, 318–25.

Index

Printed in the United States
by Baker & Taylor Publisher Services